Metabolic Diseases of Dairy Cattle

Editor

THOMAS H. HERDT

VETERINARY CLINICS OF NORTH AMERICA: FOOD ANIMAL PRACTICE

www.vetfood.theclinics.com

Consulting Editor

ROBERT A. SMITH

July 2013 • Volume 29 • Number 2

ELSEVIER

1600 John F. Kennedy Boulevard • Suite 1800 • Philadelphia, Pennsylvania, 19103-2899

http://www.vetfood.theclinics.com

VETERINARY CLINICS OF NORTH AMERICA: FOOD ANIMAL PRACTICE Volume 29, Number 2
July 2013 ISSN 0749-0720, ISBN-13: 978-1-4557-7616-0

Editor: John Vassallo; j.vassallo@elsevier.com

Veterinary Clinics of North America: Food Animal Practice (ISSN 0749-0720) is published in March, July, and November by Elsevier Inc., 360 Park Avenue South, New York, NY 10010-1710. Subscription prices are $224.00 per year (domestic individuals), $308.00 per year (domestic institutions), $104.00 per year (domestic students/residents), $253.00 per year (Canadian individuals), $402.00 per year (Canadian institutions), $319.00 per year (international individuals), $402.00 per year (international institutions), and $159.00 per year (international and Canadian students/residents). To receive student/resident rate, orders must be accompained by name of affiliated institution, date of term, and the signature of program/residency coordinator on institution letterhead. *Clinics* subscription prices. All prices are subject to change without notice. **POSTMASTER:** Send address changes to *Veterinary Clinics of North America: Food Animal Practice*, Elsevier Health Sciences Division, Subscription Customer Service, 3251 Riverport Lane, Maryland Heights, MO 63043. Customer Service (orders, claims, online, change of address): Elsevier Health Sciences Division, Subscription Customer Service, 3251 Riverport Lane, Maryland Heights, MO 63043. Tel: 1-800-654-2452 (U.S. and Canada); 314-447-8871 (ouside U.S. and Canada). Fax: 314-447-8029. E-mail: journalscustomerservice-usa@elsevier.com (for print support); journalsonlinesupport-usa@elsevier.com (for online support).

Reprints. For copies of 100 or more, of articles in this publication, please contact the Commercial Reprints Department, Elsevier Inc., 360 Park Avenue South, New York, NY 10010-1710. Tel.: 212-633-3812; Fax: 212-462-1935; E-mail: reprints@elsevier.com.

Veterinary Clinics of North America: Food Animal Practice is covered in *Current Contents/Agriculture, Biology and Environmental Sciences, MEDLINE/PubMed (Index Medicus), and Excerpta Medica.*

Printed and bound by CPI Group (UK) Ltd, Croydon, CR0 4YY

Transferred to digital print 2012

Contributors

CONSULTING EDITOR

ROBERT A. SMITH, DVM, MS
Diplomate, American Board of Veterinary Practitioners; Veterinary Research and Consulting Services, LLC, Greeley, Colorado

EDITOR

THOMAS H. HERDT, DVM, MS
Diplomate, American College of Veterinary Nutrition; Diplomate, American College of Veterinary Internal Medicine; Professor, Department of Large Animal Clinical Sciences, College of Veterinary Medicine, Michigan State University, East Lansing, Michigan

AUTHORS

MICHAEL S. ALLEN, PhD
University Distinguished Professor, Department of Animal Science, Michigan State University, East Lansing, Michigan

DONAGH P. BERRY, PhD
Principal Research Officer, Animal Genetics, Teagasc, Moorepark Dairy Production Research Centre, Fermoy, County Cork, Ireland

GIUSEPPE BERTONI
Faculty of Agriculture; Former Head, Institute of Zootechnic, Professor, Università Cattolica del Sacro Cuore, Piacenza, Italy

JENNE D. DE KOSTER, DVM
PhD Student, Department of Reproduction, Obstetrics and Herd Health, Faculty of Veterinary Medicine, Ghent University, Merelbeke, Belgium

PETER J. DEGARIS, BVSc (Hons), PhD
Tarwin Veterinary Group, Leongatha, Victoria, Australia

TODD F. DUFFIELD, DVM, DVSc
Professor, Department of Population Medicine, Ontario Veterinary College, University of Guelph, Guelph, Ontario, Canada

NIC C. FRIGGENS, PhD
Head of INRA, AgroParisTech Research Unit 791, Modélisation Systémique Appliquée aux Ruminants, Paris, France

JESSICA L. GORDON, BS, DVM
Department of Population Medicine, Ontario Veterinary College, University of Guelph, Guelph, Ontario, Canada

JANE K. KAY, PhD
Team Leader, Dairy Cow Nutrition, DairyNZ, Hamilton, New Zealand

IAN J. LEAN, BVSc, DVSc, PhD, MANZCVS
SBScibus, Camden, New South Wales, Australia

STEPHEN J. LEBLANC, BSc, DVM, DVSc
Associate Professor, Department of Population Medicine, Ontario Veterinary College, University of Guelph, Guelph, Ontario, Canada

JUAN J. LOOR, PhD
Associate Professor, Animal Sciences and Nutritional Sciences, University of Illinois, Urbana, Illinois

JESSICA A. MCART, DVM, PhD
Assistant Professor, Department of Clinical Sciences, Colorado State University, Fort Collins, Colorado

DARYL V. NYDAM, DVM, PhD
Associate Professor, Department of Population Medicine and Diagnostic Sciences, Veterinary Medical Center, Cornell University, Ithaca, New York

GARRETT R. OETZEL, DVM, MS
Diplomate, American College of Veterinary Nutrition (Honorary); Associate Professor, Food Animal Production Medicine Section, Department of Medical Sciences, School of Veterinary Medicine, University of Wisconsin–Madison, Madison, Wisconsin

GEERT OPSOMER, DVM, PhD, Msc
Diplomate, European College of Animal Reproduction; Diplomate, European College of Bovine Health Management; Professor, Department of Reproduction, Obstetrics and Herd Health, Faculty of Veterinary Medicine, Ghent University, Merelbeke, Belgium

PAULA A. OSPINA, DVM, MPH, PhD
Senior Lecturer, Department of Animal Science, Cornell University, Ithaca, New York

THOMAS R. OVERTON, PhD
Associate Professor, Department of Animal Science, Cornell University, Ithaca, New York

PAOLA PIANTONI, Veterinaria, MS
Graduate Research Assistant, Department of Animal Science, Michigan State University, East Lansing, Michigan

WILLIAM RAPHAEL, BVSc, MS
Diplomate, American Board of Veterinary Practitioners (Dairy); Diplomate, American College of Veterinary Preventive Medicine; Department of Large Animal Clinical Sciences, College of Veterinary Medicine, Michigan State University, East Lansing, Michigan

JOHN R. ROCHE, PhD
Principal Scientist, Animal Science, DairyNZ, Hamilton, New Zealand

LORRAINE M. SORDILLO, MS, PhD
Department of Large Animal Clinical Sciences, College of Veterinary Medicine, Michigan State University, East Lansing, Michigan

TRACY STOKOL, BVSc, PhD
Diplomate; American College of Veterinary Pathologists, Associate Professor, Department of Population Medicine and Diagnostic Sciences, Cornell University, Ithaca, New York

ERMINIO TREVISI, PhD
Faculty of Agriculture, Institute of Zootechnic, Assistant Professor, Università Cattolica del Sacro Cuore, Piacenza, Italy

ROBERT VAN SAUN, DVM, MS, PhD
Diplomate, American College of Theriogenology; Diplomate, American College of Veterinary Nutrition; Professor, Department of Veterinary and Biomedical Sciences, Pennsylvania State University, University Park, Pennsylvania

Contents

Preface: Metabolic Diseases of Dairy Cattle xi

Thomas H. Herdt

Significance of Metabolic Stress, Lipid Mobilization, and Inflammation on Transition Cow Disorders 267

Lorraine M. Sordillo and William Raphael

The incidence and severity of disease in cows is greatest during the transition period, when immune functions are impaired. Intense lipid mobilization is associated with both metabolic and infectious diseases in the transition cow. Significant increases in plasma nonesterified fatty acids contribute to oxidative stress and uncontrolled inflammatory responses. A dysfunctional inflammatory response is the common link between metabolic and infectious diseases around the time of calving. Intervention strategies that can reduce lipid mobilization may improve inflammatory responses and reduce the economic losses associated with health disorders during the transition period.

Metabolic Control of Feed Intake: Implications for Metabolic Disease of Fresh Cows 279

Michael S. Allen and Paola Piantoni

The objective of this article is to discuss metabolic control of feed intake in the peripartum period and its implications for metabolic disease of fresh cows. Understanding how feed intake is controlled during the transition from gestation to lactation is critical to both reduce risk and successfully treat many metabolic diseases.

Insulin Resistance in Dairy Cows 299

Jenne D. De Koster and Geert Opsomer

Glucose is the molecule that drives milk production, and insulin plays a pivotal role in the glucose metabolism of dairy cows. The effect of insulin on the glucose metabolism is regulated by the secretion of insulin by the pancreas and the insulin sensitivity of the skeletal muscles, the adipose tissue, and the liver. Insulin resistance may develop as part of physiologic (pregnancy and lactation) and pathologic processes, which may manifest as decreased insulin sensitivity or decreased insulin responsiveness. A good knowledge of the normal physiology of insulin is needed to measure the in vivo insulin resistance of dairy cows.

Assessing and Managing Body Condition Score for the Prevention of Metabolic Disease in Dairy Cows 323

John R. Roche, Jane K. Kay, Nic C. Friggens, Juan J. Loor, and Donagh P. Berry

Body condition score (BCS) is an assessment of a cow's body fat (and muscle) reserves, with low values reflecting emaciation and high values equating to obesity. The intercalving profile of BCS is a mirror image of the milk lactation profile. The BCS at which a cow calves, her nadir

BCS, and the amount of BCS lost after calving are associated with milk production, reproduction, and health. Genetics, peripartum nutrition, and management are factors that likely interact with BCS to determine the risk of health disorders.

Energy and Protein Nutrition Management of Transition Dairy Cows **337**

Ian J. Lean, Robert Van Saun, and Peter J. DeGaris

The aims of this article are to briefly review some of the underlying physiology of changes that occur around calving, examine the potential to control the risk of disease in this period, increase milk production, and improve reproductive performance through better nutritional management. Practical guidelines for veterinarians and advisors are provided.

Mineral and Antioxidant Management of Transition Dairy Cows **367**

Ian J. Lean, Robert Van Saun, and Peter J. DeGaris

Transition management needs to be fully integrated to be effective. We discuss and demonstrate this concept in the context of a study that used these principles. The roles of calcium, magnesium, phosphorus and dietary anion cation difference in influencing the pathophysiology and incidence of hypocalcemia are highlighted. Recent understandings of the pivotal role of skeleton in metabolism are reviewed. Micronutrient mineral and vitamin needs are addressed in the context of exposure of periparturient cattle to oxidative stress and inflammatory disorders. This article provides a series of practical approaches to improving transition diets.

Using Nonesterified Fatty Acids and β-Hydroxybutyrate Concentrations During the Transition Period for Herd-Level Monitoring of Increased Risk of Disease and Decreased Reproductive and Milking Performance **387**

Paula A. Ospina, Jessica A. McArt, Thomas R. Overton, Tracy Stokol, and Daryl V. Nydam

Dairy cows visit a state of negative energy balance (NEB) as they transition from late gestation to early lactation. At the individual level, there are several metabolic adaptations to manage NEB, including mobilization of nonesterified fatty acids (NEFA) from body fat reserves and glucose sparing for lactogenesis. Based on current pen-level feeding and management practices, strategies to minimize excessive NEB in both the individual and herd should focus on herd-level testing and management. This article reviews strategies for testing and monitoring of excessive NEB at the herd level through individual testing of 2 energy markers: NEFA and β-hydroxybutyrate.

Use of the Liver Activity Index and Other Metabolic Variables in the Assessment of Metabolic Health in Dairy Herds **413**

Giuseppe Bertoni and Erminio Trevisi

The usefulness of the metabolic profile in dairy cows has been questioned because of poor standardization of procedures, high cost of analysis, and perceived inefficiency of the approach. Composite indices based on multiple variables, namely the Liver Activity Index and the Liver Functionality

Metabolic Diseases of Dairy Cattle

VETERINARY CLINICS OF NORTH AMERICA: FOOD ANIMAL PRACTICE

FORTHCOMING ISSUES

November 2013
Heifer Development in Beef Cattle
David J. Patterson, PhD, and
Michael Smith, PhD, *Editors*

March 2014
Bovine Orthopedics
David E. Anderson, DVM, MS, DACVS and
André Desrochers, DMV, MS, DACVS,
DECBHM, *Editors*

RECENT ISSUES

March 2013
Pain Management
Johann (Hans) Coetzee, BVSc,
Cert CHP, PhD, *Editor*

November 2012
Diagnostic Pathology
Vicky L. Cooper, DVM, MS, PhD, *Editor*

July 2012
Mastitis in Dairy Cows
Pamela L. Ruegg, DVM, MPVM, *Editor*

RELATED INTEREST

Veterinary Clinics of North America: Equine Practice
April 2013 (Vol. 29, No. 1)
Topics in Equine Anesthesia
Stuart C. Clark-Price, DVM, MS, *Editor*

Preface
Metabolic Diseases of Dairy Cattle

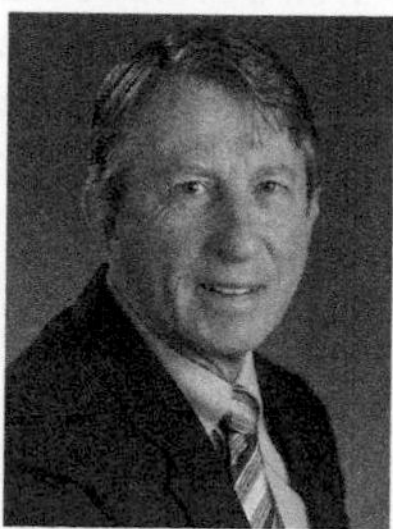

Thomas H. Herdt, DVM, MS
Editor

Metabolic disease continues to be a substantial challenge in the dairy industry, not only in North America but also in all other regions in which modern dairy cattle breeds are managed and fed for high milk yields. Undoubtedly, some of this continuing challenge is related to progressive improvement in dairy cow genetics and the ever-increasing average milk yields of modern dairy cattle. Improvements in production capacity challenge us to manage and feed cows to allow them to adapt to the tremendous metabolic demands of high milk production. More than this, however, I believe the continued and perhaps even enhanced interest in metabolic diseases of dairy cattle comes from our expanding understanding of the diverse ramifications of the metabolic events of early lactation. These ramifications go well beyond those associated with traditionally described metabolic diseases, such as milk fever and ketosis, and include the much broader realm of nearly all diseases common to early lactation cows. The intertwining associations among various metabolic stresses and their relationships to other diseases, particularly infectious and inflammatory diseases of early lactation, have now become a central focus of the interest in metabolic diseases of dairy cattle.

The issue leads off with articles addressing this complex association of metabolism with other health and nutritional challenges to the dairy cow. The article by Lorraine Sordillo and William Raphael illustrates the interrelationship of metabolism and inflammation and describes how metabolic events may lead to altered inflammatory responses and increased susceptibility to infectious diseases. The following article by Michael Allen and Paola Piantoni addresses new concepts in the potential relationship between metabolism and appetite regulation, particularly in early lactation cows. Ideas expressed in this article point to the potential of a "downward spiral" of metabolic events that may diminish feed intake at the exact time when feed intake should be increasing. The contributions by Jenne De Koster and Geert Opsomer, and by JR Roche and coworkers, discuss the long-term implications of body condition and body condition changes, their effects on insulin resistance, and subsequent effects

Vet Clin Food Anim 29 (2013) xi–xii
http://dx.doi.org/10.1016/j.cvfa.2013.05.001
0749-0720/13/$ – see front matter

on metabolic health. The articles by Ian Lean and colleagues, in addition to giving many practical recommendations for dry cow feeding and management, also present some new ideas and information describing potential mechanisms for an interrelationship and interaction between mineral and energy metabolism. I believe these articles all broaden the scope of what we've traditionally called "metabolic disease."

Other articles in this issue describe diagnostic tools for the herd-level evaluation of metabolic status and metabolic disease risk. Some of these are well developed and others are in development. The article by Paula Ospina and coworkers describes rigorous new approaches to the herd-level evaluation of serum nonesterified fatty acid and β-hydroxybutryic acid concentrations. These tests have been in wide application for some time and this article offers new insights, particularly into the herd-level interpretation of these values. The contribution from Giuseppe Bertoni and Erminio Trevisi points out the potential advantages in creating multivariate testing approaches to be applied at both the individual animal and the herd level. In this same vein of describing potentially new testing procedures to aid in the management of metabolic disease in dairy cows, Jenne Koester and Geert Opsomer describe diagnostic tests that may become practical in the field for the evaluation of insulin resistance in cows.

Finally, several articles in this issue, including some of those mentioned above, include sections describing very practical regimens for the management and prevention of metabolic disease in dairy cows. Included among these are those by Jessica Gordon and colleagues on ketosis therapy and Garrett Oetzel on the prophylactic use of oral calcium supplements.

I wish to express my admiration for and my appreciation to the contributing authors. They are a distinguished group of international scientists. This issue represents a worldwide contribution to continuing developments in the investigation, management, and prevention of metabolic diseases in dairy cattle.

Thomas H. Herdt, DVM, MS
Department of Large Animal
Clinical Sciences and Diagnostic
Center for Population and Animal Health
College of Veterinary Medicine
Michigan State University
East Lansing, MI 48824, USA

E-mail address:
Herdt@cvm.msu.edu

Significance of Metabolic Stress, Lipid Mobilization, and Inflammation on Transition Cow Disorders

Lorraine M. Sordillo, MS, PhD[a,*], William Raphael, BVSc, MS[b]

KEYWORDS

• Inflammation • Lipid mobilization • Oxidative stress • Transition period • Disease

KEY POINTS

- The incidence and severity of disease is greatest during the transition period. when immune functions are impaired.
- Intense lipid mobilization is associated with both metabolic and infectious diseases in the transition cow.
- Significant increases in plasma nonesterified fatty acids contribute to oxidative stress and uncontrolled inflammatory responses.
- A dysfunctional inflammatory response is the common link between metabolic and infectious diseases around the time of calving.
- Intervention strategies that can reduce lipid mobilization may improve inflammatory responses and reduce the economic losses associated with health disorders during the transition period.

Dairy cattle are susceptible to increased incidence of metabolic and infectious diseases during the physiologic transition from late pregnancy to early lactation. Dramatic changes in both metabolic activity and dysfunctional immune responses are closely associated with the development of many transition cow disorders.[1,2] Although dairy cows undergo several physiologic changes during the onset of lactation that may

Disclosure: the authors acknowledge research support through grants (2011-67015-30179 and 2012-67011-20019) from the Agriculture and Food Research Initiative Competitive Grants Programs of the USDA National Institute for Food and Agriculture and by an endowment from the Matilda R. Wilson Fund (Detroit, MI).

[a] Department of Large Animal Clinical Sciences, College of Veterinary Medicine, Michigan State University, 784 Wilson Road, G300 Veterinary Medical Center, East Lansing, MI 48824, USA; [b] Department of Large Animal Clinical Sciences, College of Veterinary Medicine, Michigan State University, 736 Wilson Road, D202 Veterinary Medical Center, East Lansing, MI 48824, USA
* Corresponding author.
E-mail address: sordillo@msu.edu

Vet Clin Food Anim 29 (2013) 267–278
http://dx.doi.org/10.1016/j.cvfa.2013.03.002 vetfood.theclinics.com
0749-0720/13/$ – see front matter

contribute to health problems, the mobilization of excessive body fat reserves and significant increases in plasma fatty acid concentration are important risk factors leading to enhanced disease.[3] The direct role that increased lipid mobilization has on liver function and the pathogenesis of certain metabolic diseases such as fatty liver and ketosis is well established. However, more recent evidence suggests that increased plasma fatty acid concentrations may indirectly affect both metabolic and infectious disease pathogenesis by compromising the function of cells involved in immune responses. Uncontrolled inflammatory reactions are especially important in the pathogenesis of several transition cow disorders. A better understanding of the interrelationship between metabolic stress, lipid mobilization, and immune dysfunction during the transition period facilitates the design of better control programs to prevent health disorders during this critical period in the production cycle of dairy cows. This article addresses the possible linkages between fat mobilization and dysfunctional inflammatory responses that may contribute to increased morbidity and mortality in transition dairy cows.

PHYSIOLOGIC ADAPTATIONS OF THE TRANSITION COW

The transition period for dairy cows is defined as approximately 3 weeks pre partum until 3 weeks post partum. Major physiologic, nutritional, metabolic, and immunologic changes occur within this time frame as the production cycle of the cow shifts from a gestational nonlactating state to the onset of copious milk synthesis and secretion. For example, cows must adjust metabolically to the dramatic increase in energy requirements that is needed to ensure optimal milk production in the ensuing lactation. Milk production requires large amounts of carbohydrates for lactose synthesis, and nearly all the available glucose in the body is diverted to the mammary gland for this purpose. Dairy cattle experience appetite suppression during the last week of gestation, and it can take up to a week after calving before dry matter intake (DMI) recovers.[4] The imbalance between energy consumed and the energy needed for production demands is termed negative energy balance (NEB). During times of NEB, sufficient energy must be mobilized from tissue stores to support energy-dependent needs of the body, and adipose tissues are a major fuel source for cows during the transition period. However, a balanced metabolic response during the onset of lactation is needed to regulate the appropriate amount of lipid mobilization. Initially, a decrease in blood glucose level occurs in response to both high demands of lactation and diminished DMI. The reduction in blood glucose results in lower insulin levels, which trigger the fat mobilization process through lipolysis. During lipolysis, nonesterified fatty acids (NEFAs) are cleaved from triglyceride molecules within adipocytes through the action of various hormone-sensitive lipases. NEFA is then transported into the blood by albumin, where it can be used as an energy source and also initiate negative feedback loops to regulate the amount of lipolysis (**Fig. 1**). The overall cumulative effect should result in relatively constant blood glucose concentrations needed for milk synthesis and secretion without excessive NEFA accumulation in the blood.[5]

Metabolic Stress

Cows successfully adapt to NEB when adipose mobilization is adequately regulated and the release of NEFA is limited to concentrations that can be fully metabolized for energy needs. Although lipid mobilization provides the energy needed to promote milk production, excessive release of lipids from adipose tissues and accumulation of high concentrations of free fatty acids in the blood are positively correlated to several metabolic problems in the transition cow.[6] The development of ketosis and fatty liver, severity. The major sources of these proinflammatory cytokines are macrophages and endothelial cells. Previous studies showed that these cells are more responsive to bacterial endotoxins during early lactation, which may contribute to exacerbated inflammation responses during coliform mastitis.[13,14] As a consequence, the delicate balance between a sufficient inflammatory response needed for optimal pathogen clearance and the prompt return to immune homeostasis is often lost during the transition period. Therefore, factors that contribute to either hyporesponsive or hyperresponsive inflammatory responses likely contribute to the pathophysiology of any inflammatory-based disease.

LINK BETWEEN METABOLIC AND INFLAMMATORY RESPONSES

In human medicine, there is ample evidence to suggest that obesity and the associated increase in plasma NEFA concentrations lead to a chronic inflammatory condition.[15,16] Systemic inflammation during obesity is characterized by the abnormal production of proinflammatory cytokines (ie, TNF-α and IL-6) and bioactive lipid mediators, which orchestrate the magnitude and duration of the inflammatory response. Adipocytes and macrophages that reside in adipose tissues are the cellular sources for these proinflammatory mediators and the resulting chronic inflammatory condition is believed to sensitize the body to both infectious and metabolic diseases in obese people.[15] Increased TNF-α concentrations also can block downstream signaling of insulin-mediated events. In humans, TNF-α is believed to be the link between obesity-induced insulin resistance and increased lipid mobilization.[16] The possibility that an overly aggressive or chronic inflammatory response during NEB can increase the incidence of transition cow disorders has been the subject of intense research interest.

Numerous studies suggest that certain aspects of energy metabolism, especially lipid mobilization, can negatively affect a balanced inflammatory response in transition dairy cattle. Dysfunction or unregulated inflammatory responses are believed to be the common link between the increased incidence of both metabolic and infectious diseases during the transition period. This assumption is based on the observations that metabolic and infectious diseases tend to occur in complexes with each other rather than as isolated events in cows during early lactation.[17] Moreover, increased incidence of any single transition cow disorder increases the chance that they succumb to other health issues. For example, epidemiologic studies indicated an association between the development of retained placenta and the incidence of mastitis.[18] In addition, cows suffering from ketosis were twice as likely to develop mastitis than healthy cows.[19] Although a direct causal link has not been established in cattle, there is ample evidence to suggest that increased health disorders during the transition period are symptomatic of a dysfunctional immune system.

Impact of Metabolic Stress on Inflammation

The relationships between metabolic factors and compromised immunity during the transition period have been investigated extensively.[2,20] Intense lipid mobilization during the transition period has long been recognized as a major contributing factor leading to immune dysfunction. The direct impact that metabolic stress has on immune functions around the time of calving was clearly shown using a mastectomy cow model.[21] In this study, pregnant dairy cows were mastectomized to assess the impact of milk production and NEB on immunity, but presumably maintaining the endocrine changes associated with late pregnancy and parturition. The mastectomy cows did not experience the dramatic shift in NEB, as indicated by only moderate increases in NEFA when compared with the intact cows. The functions of lymphocytes and neutrophils were significantly better in the mastectomy cows when compared with the intact cows during the transition period. The major conclusion from this study was that increased lipid mobilization caused by the metabolic demands of lactation can directly diminish the antimicrobial functional capabilities of immune cells during early lactation.[21] Another study[22] showed that certain metabolites associated with NEB also can negatively affect neutrophils and other immune cell functions. Ketotic cows are believed to be more susceptible to mastitis and other infectious conditions because of the adverse effects that BHB concentrations have on leukocyte antimicrobial mechanisms.[22,23] Plasma BHB concentrations are also significantly higher and neutrophil antimicrobial function lower during clinical cases of metritis.[20] Another important metabolic adaptation that may affect immunity is the change in glucose availability during the transition period as a consequence of NEB. Macrophages and neutrophils require considerable energy to support their antimicrobial functions, and glucose serves as a primary fuel source.[24] Therefore, the dramatic decrease in blood glucose concentrations during intense lipid mobilization and ketosis may also affect host defenses around the time of calving by limiting the fuels needed by immune cell populations.[22] The concept that an activated inflammatory reaction may compete with other production-related processes (ie, milk synthesis) for limited nutrients may account for the decreased productive efficiency of dairy cows during morbidity.

Fatty Acids Alter Inflammation

The possibility that the progressive increase in blood NEFA concentrations can directly affect inflammatory responses is supported by several recent investigations.[1] An increase in lipid mobilization in transition cows changes both the concentration and composition of plasma NEFA. The saturated fatty acids, palmitate and stearate, and the monosaturated oleic acid are the predominant fats found in plasma NEFA around the time of calving. Conversely, there is a decrease in some of the polyunsaturated fatty acid (PUFA) such as eicosapentaenoic acid (EPA) and docosahexaenoic acid (DHA). These changes are important to immunity because the fatty acid content of immune cells reflects the compositional changes seen in plasma NEFA during the transition period.[1] The fatty acid composition of immune cells can alter their functions in several ways. Once internalized by leukocytes and endothelial cells, fatty acids can play a significant role in intracellular signaling pathways, which can regulate the magnitude and duration of inflammation. In humans, for example, certain saturated and PUFAs can bind a family of nuclear receptors called peroxisome proliferator-activated receptors (PPARs). Both α-linolenic acid and DHA are ligands for PPAR and can downregulate inflammatory reaction in many cell types, including mononuclear leukocytes and endothelial cells.[15] In contrast, palmitate and stearate can enhance proinflammatory signaling pathways through the activation of nuclear factor κB (NFκB).[15] Although the direct effects that lipid mobilization may have on these signaling pathways have not been examined specifically in the dairy cow, changes in the composition of bovine NEFA around calving are consistent with the composition of human NEFA, which elicits a proinflammatory response.[15]

Another way that changes in NEFA composition could influence immunity is through the production of a class of lipid mediators called eicosanoids, which orchestrate many aspects of the inflammatory response. Macrophages and endothelial cells are major cellular sources of these lipid mediators, and some general categories of eicosanoids include prostaglandins, thromboxanes, leukotrienes, lipoxins, resolvins, and protectins. Eicosanoids are derived from either omega-6 and omega-3 PUFAs found in cell membrane phospholipids. The major omega-6 fatty acids used for eicosanoid biosynthesis include arachidonic and linoleic acids, whereas EPAs and DHAs are included in the omega-3 PUFA category. These fatty acids serve as substrates that become oxidized through either cycolooxygenase or lipoxygenase enzymatic pathways. In general, the omega-6–generated eicosanoids tend to enhance inflammatory responses and the omega-3–derived eicosanoids tend to promote the resolution of inflammation.[25] Thus, shifts in the phospholipid content of immune cells as a consequence of intense lipid mobilization can affect inflammatory responses by modifying the profile of eicosanoids produced.

Recent studies have begun to investigate how changes in NEFA concentration and composition may directly alter bovine inflammatory responses during times of intense lipid mobilization. Exposure to NEFA mixtures that mimic the composition and concentration found in cows during the transition period increased proinflammatory cytokine and eicosanoid expression by vascular endothelial cells.[26] Similar finding were reported in which high NEFA concentrations diminished the functional capabilities of mononuclear cells and antibacterial mechanisms of neutrophils.[27] However, increasing the omega-3 fatty acid content of endothelial cells could mitigate the proinflammatory responses to high NEFA concentrations.[28] The reduced inflammatory response could be a result of shifts in the eicosanoid profiles after omega-3 supplementation, in which more proresolving eicosanoids were produced, including resolvins, protectins, and lipoxins.[28]

Collectively, both epidemiologic observations and in vitro studies support the concept that the metabolic consequences of increased lipid mobilization around the time of calving are predictive for the subsequent development of health disorders, in which compromised immunity plays a significant role in pathogenesis.[6] Furthermore, changes in NEFA plasma concentrations and composition, as a consequence of intense lipid mobilization, can directly alter the magnitude and duration of the inflammatory response of certain immune cells through several mechanisms, including alterations in the balance of proinflammatory and proresolving eicosanoids biosynthesis.[2] However, inflammation can also be controlled through efficient disease prevention programs, which not only limit exposure to pathogens but also optimize vaccination protocols.

Oxidative Stress and Inflammation

Metabolically stressed cows also are known to produce excessive amounts of reactive oxygen species (ROS), which can damage cells involved in the inflammatory response. ROS is a general term used to describe several reactive molecules and free radicals derived from molecular oxygen (**Table 1**). Molecular oxygen is required as an electron donor for efficient energy production, and ROS are formed as a normal end product of cellular metabolism.[29] Most ROS are derived in metabolically active cells during aerobic energy metabolism through the mitochondrial electron transport chain. Other sources of ROS include various oxidizing enzyme pathways, especially nicotinamide adenine dinucleotide phosphate (NADPH) oxidase. Some examples of

Table 1
Examples of ROS

Free Radicals	Nonradicals
Superoxide anion ($O_2^{-\bullet}$)	Hydrogen peroxide (H_2O_2)
Hydroxyl radical ($OH^{\bullet}$)	Hypochlorous acid ($HOCl^{-}$)
Hydroperoxyl ($HO_2^{\bullet}$)	Single oxygen ($^1O_2$)

ROS produced during energy generation or as a result of increased NADPH oxidase activity include superoxide anion, hydroxyl radical, and hydrogen peroxide. Low to moderate concentrations of ROS are required for the regulation of normal cellular processes, including those that regulate the immune response. For example, ROS can activate NFκB signaling pathways in various immune cell populations and increase the expression of cytokines and vascular adhesion molecules needed to orchestrate inflammatory responses. Some ROS, such as nitric oxide, also play an important role in regulating vascular tone needed to increase blood flow to localized areas of infection. Larger amounts of ROS are produced by neutrophils and macrophages through NADPH oxidase activity. The ROS produced by these immune cells are essential for the destruction of invading pathogens after bacterial phagocytosis. Collectively, ROS are essential for optimizing immune defenses, especially during the early stages of disease.

Although ROS have numerous beneficial effects on immune and inflammatory responses, damage to host cells can occur if build-up of these highly reactive molecules becomes excessive. Several endogenous antioxidant defense mechanisms are present to tightly regulate ROS accumulation and are capable of slowing or preventing the oxidation of other molecules. Antioxidant defenses are diverse, can be either synthesized in the body or derived from the diet, are localized transiently throughout tissues and different cell types, and can be characterized as either radical scavengers or detoxifying enzyme systems.[11] Certain vitamins and trace minerals are important dietary sources of antioxidant defenses. **Table 2** summarizes some antioxidant defenses that are needed to protect host tissues from excessive ROS. A combination of both radical scavengers and detoxifying enzymes systems is required to maintain an ROS homeostasis. Although small fluctuations in the steady-state concentrations of ROS are necessary for optimal immune and inflammatory responses, dramatic imbalances can result in tissue damage and loss of normal cell function.

Oxidative stress is a term used to describe various deleterious processes resulting from an imbalance between excessive formation of ROS or reduced antioxidant defenses. Disturbances in the balance between ROS production and antioxidant defenses can result in substantial damage to nearby tissues by oxidizing cellular lipids, proteins, and DNA. Membrane phospholipids, for example, are especially susceptible to peroxidation and the subsequent formation of lipid radicals. If allowed to accumulate, these lipid peroxy radicals can act on adjacent fatty acids in the cellular plasma membranes and induce even more radical formation through positive feedback loops. As a result, excess ROS accumulates and can lead to a loss of normal membrane function and even cell death if the condition persists.[11] Increased metabolic demands associated with the onset of lactations increased oxidative stress in the transition cow. There is ample evidence to suggest that oxidative stress can contribute to dysfunctional inflammatory responses in metabolically stressed cows.[2,10,30]

Table 2
Examples of antioxidant defenses

Radical Scavengers	Detoxifying Enzymes Systems
Ascorbic acid (vitamin C)	Super oxide dismutase: copper, zinc, or manganese-containing enzyme that reduces superoxide anion
α-Tocopherol (vitamin E)	Catalase: catalyzes the reduction of hydrogen peroxide
β-Carotene (vitamin A)	Glutathione peroxidase: selenium-dependent enzyme that catalyzes the degradation of hydrogen peroxide and organic peroxides to less reactive water and alcohols

In humans, oxidative stress can lead to chronic inflammation and contribute to the pathogenesis of several inflammatory-based diseases including atherosclerosis, diabetes, and cancer.[11] Oxidative stress and inflammation are closely linked and act synergistically to perpetuate chronic inflammatory states that lead to these health disorders. Oxidative stress increases inflammation primarily through the activation of proinflammatory signaling pathways. For example, ROS can activate the redox-sensitive transcription factor, NFκB, which in turn increases the expression of proinflammatory cytokines, eicosanoids, and other lipid mediators. Exposure of macrophages and endothelial cells to TNF-α can increase mitochondrial ROS formation and escalate oxidative stress.[11] There also is a close association between oxidative stress and inflammation in transition dairy cattle.[30] The enhanced expression of TNF-α and other proinflammatory cytokines was linked with the severity of coliform mastitis during the transition period, when cows experience oxidative stress.[31,32] Macrophages obtained from early lactation cows were especially more sensitive to bacterial endotoxin stimulation and produced more TNF-α when compared with cells obtained from late-lactation cows.[14] More recent studies showed an inverse relationship between antioxidant activity and TNF-α production by mononuclear leukocytes obtained from cows experiencing oxidative stress.[33] Collectively, these studies support the contention that oxidative stress and inflammation can work in concert to aggravate the pathology of transition cow disorders.

The degree of inflammation and oxidative stress in transition cows can be enhanced further by several other factors, including environmental stress (eg, heat stress), disease challenge, obesity, and increased plasma NEFA concentrations. For example, increased lipid mobilization can increase the severity of oxidative stress and inflammation in several ways. Enhanced uptake of NEFA by the liver is accompanied by an increase in peroxisomal oxidation. Although peroxisomal oxidation increases the total oxidative capacity of hepatocytes, hydrogen peroxide is produced as an initial metabolite, which can escalate ROS accumulation during time of increased NEFA availability.[34] Increased plasma NEFA concentrations also can cause more oxidative stress by increasing lipid hydroperoxide formation. The transition to lactation, especially with obese cows, causes increased plasma markers of lipid peroxidation, which correlate with higher NEFA concentrations.[35,36] Several in vitro studies[26,37,38] also provide direct evidence that increases in NEFA concentration and individual lipid hydroperoxides resulting from oxidative stress can increase the proinflammatory phenotype and alter eicosanoid biosynthesis in bovine endothelial cells. Collectively, these data support the contention that oxidative stress and enhanced systemic inflammatory status in transition cows may be the common factors that contribute to metabolic and infectious disorders in transition cows.[2,30]

To elicit effective antioxidant responses and fuel immune cell activation, cows must use energy that could otherwise be used for production. As a result, increased oxidative stress and systemic inflammation can diminish the productive efficiency of dairy cows during the transition period indirectly by diverting available energy. Given the detrimental impact that oxidative stress has on immunity and associated health disorders, maintenance of oxidative balance should be a priority in managing the transition cow.

Impact of Inflammation on Metabolism

Metabolic stress can disrupt appropriate inflammatory responses, but there is sufficient evidence to suggest that inflammation can contribute to metabolic disorders as well.[34] During the pathogenesis of infectious diseases, such as coliform mastitis, there is a significant increase in proinflammatory cytokines, including TNF-α, IL-1β, and IL-6, which contribute to systemic inflammatory responses.[39] The increased concentrations of plasma TNF-α are especially associated with the severe clinical symptoms during acute inflammation. There is compelling evidence in both humans and cattle that TNF-α can promote the breakdown of fat stores and significantly increase blood NEFA concentrations not only by decreasing feed intake but also by directly stimulating lipolysis.[15,40] Therefore, pathogen-induced systemic inflammation can exacerbate the already significant increases in plasma NEFA that occur during the transition period. As a consequence, acute systemic inflammation can contribute to metabolic disorders by increasing lipid mobilization, impairing insulin sensitivity, promoting triglyceride accumulation in the liver, and reducing liver glucose production.[5,40]

SUMMARY AND INTERVENTION STRATEGIES

Historically, strategies to control metabolic and infectious diseases during the transition period have been treated as independent issues. However, more recent evidence suggests that changes in nutrient metabolism and changes in immunologic function are interdependent and it is the collective changes in these factors that affect the overall health of the transition cow. Therefore, strategies that help manage NEB, blood NEFA, and BHB concentrations around the time of calving can have a beneficial influence of immune and inflammatory responses. This goal can be achieved by optimizing diet ingredients, energy consumption, and rumen fermentation in the prepartum and postpartum period to minimize NEB during the transition period. Maintaining moderate BCS and not overfeeding during the prepartum period also helps to keep blood NEFA and BHB concentrations lower than detrimental threshold levels. Because inflammation and oxidative stress are intricately linked with most transition cow disorders, the control of these factors should be addressed as well. Inflammation can be controlled through efficient disease prevention programs that not only limit exposure to infectious pathogens but also optimize vaccination protocols. Providing adequate amounts of dietary antioxidant micronutrients, such as vitamin E and selenium, has proved to be an effective way of controlling oxidative stress and reducing some infectious diseases such as mastitis. Another approach to control oxidative stress and inflammation is to reduce other physiologic stressors associated with the management of transition cows. For example, housing conditions should be optimized to avoid overcrowding, improved stall design, cooling, and ventilation. Minimizing grouping changes around calving not only decreases social stress but also minimizes DMI depression by improving nutritional management. A better understanding of the complex interaction between metabolic stress and dysfunctional inflammatory responses will most likely lead to additional strategies that effectively reduce transition cow disorders and the large economic losses to the dairy industry.

REFERENCES

1. Contreras GA, O'Boyle NJ, Herdt TH, et al. Lipomobilization in periparturient dairy cows influences the composition of plasma nonesterified fatty acids and leukocyte phospholipid fatty acids. J Dairy Sci 2010;93(6):2508–16.
2. Sordillo LM, Contreras GA, Aitken SL. Metabolic factors affecting the inflammatory response of periparturient dairy cows. Anim Health Res Rev 2009;10(1):53–63.
3. Dechow CD, Rogers GW, Sander-Nielsen U, et al. Correlations among body condition scores from various sources, dairy form, and cow health from the United States and Denmark. J Dairy Sci 2004;87(10):3526–33.

4. Grummer RR, Mashek DG, Hayirli A. Dry matter intake and energy balance in the transition period. Vet Clin North Am Food Anim Pract 2004;20(3):447–70.
5. Herdt TH. Ruminant adaptation to negative energy balance. Influences on the etiology of ketosis and fatty liver. Vet Clin North Am Food Anim Pract 2000; 16(2):215–30, v.
6. Ospina PA, Nydam DV, Stokol T, et al. Evaluation of nonesterified fatty acids and beta-hydroxybutyrate in transition dairy cattle in the northeastern United States: critical thresholds for prediction of clinical diseases. J Dairy Sci 2010;93(2):546–54.
7. Kim IH, Suh GH. Effect of the amount of body condition loss from the dry to near calving periods on the subsequent body condition change, occurrence of postpartum diseases, metabolic parameters and reproductive performance in Holstein dairy cows. Theriogenology 2003;60(8):1445–56.
8. Wellen KE, Hotamisligil GS. Inflammation, stress, and diabetes. J Clin Invest 2005;115(5):1111–9.
9. Pires J, Souza A, Grummer R. Induction of hyperlipidemia by intravenous infusion of tallow emulsion causes insulin resistance in Holstein cows. J Dairy Sci 2007; 90(6):2735–44.
10. Contreras GA, Sordillo LM. Lipid mobilization and inflammatory responses during the transition period of dairy cows. Comp Immunol Microbiol Infect Dis 2011; 34(3):281–9.
11. Valko M, Leibfritz D, Moncol J, et al. Free radicals and antioxidants in normal physiological functions and human disease. Int J Biochem Cell Biol 2007;39(1): 44–84.
12. Aitken SL, Corl CM, Sordillo LM. Immunopathology of mastitis: insights into disease recognition and resolution. J Mammary Gland Biol Neoplasia 2011;16(4): 291–304.
13. Aitken SL, Corl CM, Sordillo LM. Pro-inflammatory and pro-apoptotic responses of TNF-alpha stimulated bovine mammary endothelial cells. Vet Immunol Immunopathol 2011;140(3–4):282–90.
14. Sordillo LM, Pighetti GM, Davis MR. Enhanced production of bovine tumor necrosis factor-alpha during the periparturient period. Vet Immunol Immunopathol 1995;49(3):263–70.
15. de Heredia FP, Gomez-Martinez S, Marcos A. Obesity, inflammation and the immune system. Proc Nutr Soc 2012;71(2):332–8.
16. Hotamisligil GS. Mechanisms of TNF-alpha-induced insulin resistance. Exp Clin Endocrinol Diabetes 1999;107(2):119–25.
17. Curtis CR, Erb HN, Sniffen CJ, et al. Association of parturient hypocalcemia with eight periparturient disorders in Holstein cows. J Am Vet Med Assoc 1983;183(5): 559–61.
18. Emanuelson U, Oltenacu PA, Grohn YT. Nonlinear mixed model analyses of five production disorders of dairy cattle. J Dairy Sci 1993;76(9):2765–72.
19. Oltenacu PA, Ekesbo I. Epidemiological study of clinical mastitis in dairy cattle. Vet Res 1994;25(2–3):208–12.
20. Hammon DS, Evjen IM, Dhiman TR, et al. Neutrophil function and energy status in Holstein cows with uterine health disorders. Vet Immunol Immunopathol 2006; 113(1–2):21–9.
21. Kimura K, Goff JP, Kehrli ME Jr. Effects of the presence of the mammary gland on expression of neutrophil adhesion molecules and myeloperoxidase activity in periparturient dairy cows. J Dairy Sci 1999;82(11):2385–92.
22. Suriyasathaporn W, Heuer C, Noordhuizen-Stassen EN, et al. Hyperketonemia and the impairment of udder defense: a review. Vet Res 2000;31(4):397–412.

23. Grinberg N, Elazar S, Rosenshine I, et al. Beta-hydroxybutyrate abrogates formation of bovine neutrophil extracellular traps and bactericidal activity against mammary pathogenic *Escherichia coli.* Infect Immun 2008;76(6):2802–7.
24. Calder PC, Dimitriadis G, Newsholme P. Glucose metabolism in lymphoid and inflammatory cells and tissues. Curr Opin Clin Nutr Metab Care 2007;10(4):531–40.
25. Serhan CN. Systems approach to inflammation resolution: identification of novel anti-inflammatory and pro-resolving mediators. J Thromb Haemost 2009; 7(Suppl 1):44–8.
26. Contreras GA, Raphael W, Mattmiller SA, et al. Nonesterified fatty acids modify inflammatory response and eicosanoid biosynthesis in bovine endothelial cells. J Dairy Sci 2012;95(9):5011–23.
27. Ster C, Loiselle MC, Lacasse P. Effect of postcalving serum nonesterified fatty acids concentration on the functionality of bovine immune cells. J Dairy Sci 2012;95(2):708–17.
28. Contreras GA, Mattmiller SA, Raphael W, et al. Enhanced n-3 phospholipid content reduces inflammatory responses in bovine endothelial cells. J Dairy Sci 2012;95(12):7137–50.
29. Halliwell B, Gutteridege JM. Free radicals in biology and medicine. 4th edition. Oxford University Press; 2007.
30. Sordillo LM, Aitken SL. Impact of oxidative stress on the health and immune function of dairy cattle. Vet Immunol Immunopathol 2009;128(1–3):104–9.
31. Shuster DE, Kehrli ME Jr, Stevens MG. Cytokine production during endotoxin-induced mastitis in lactating dairy cows. Am J Vet Res 1993;54(1):80–5.
32. Sordillo LM, Peel JE. Effect of interferon-gamma on the production of tumor necrosis factor during acute *Escherichia coli* mastitis. J Dairy Sci 1992;75(8): 2119–25.
33. O'Boyle N, Corl CM, Gandy JC, et al. Relationship of body condition score and oxidant stress to tumor necrosis factor expression in dairy cattle. Vet Immunol Immunopathol 2006;113(3–4):297–304.
34. Drackley JK. Biology of dairy cows during the transition period: the final frontier. J Dairy Sci 1999;82(11):2259–73.
35. Bernabucci U, Ronchi B, Lacetera N, et al. Influence of body condition score on relationships between metabolic status and oxidative stress in periparturient dairy cows. J Dairy Sci 2005;88(6):2017–26.
36. Sordillo LM, O'Boyle N, Gandy JC, et al. Shifts in thioredoxin reductase activity and oxidant status in mononuclear cells obtained from transition dairy cattle. J Dairy Sci 2007;90(3):1186–92.
37. Cao YZ, Reddy CC, Sordillo LM. Altered eicosanoid biosynthesis in selenium-deficient endothelial cells. Free Radic Biol Med 2000;28(3):381–9.
38. Sordillo LM, Streicher KL, Mullarky IK, et al. Selenium inhibits 15-hydroperoxyoctadecadienoic acid-induced intracellular adhesion molecule expression in aortic endothelial cells. Free Radic Biol Med 2008;44(1):34–43.
39. Hoeben D, Burvenich C, Trevisi E, et al. Role of endotoxin and TNF-α in the pathogenesis of experimentally induced coliform mastitis in periparturient cows. J Dairy Res 2000;67(04):503–14.
40. Kushibiki S, Hodate K, Shingu H, et al. Metabolic and lactational responses during recombinant bovine tumor necrosis factor-α treatment in lactating cows. J Dairy Sci 2003;86(3):819–27.

Metabolic Control of Feed Intake

Implications for Metabolic Disease of Fresh Cows

Michael S. Allen, PhD[a,*], Paola Piantoni, Veterinaria, MS[b]

KEYWORDS

- Hepatic lipidosis • Hepatic oxidation • Insulin resistance • Ketosis • Lipolysis
- Metabolic disease • Propionic acid • Ruminal starch fermentability

KEY POINTS

- Metabolic diseases are associated with depression of feed intake in the peripartum period.
- Control of feed intake during the peripartum period is likely dominated by signals from hepatic oxidation of fuels.
- Cows are in a lipolytic state in the peripartum period that is initiated several weeks prepartum as insulin concentration in blood and insulin sensitivity of adipose tissue decrease.
- The continuous supply of NEFA to the liver during the lipolytic state at this time likely suppresses feed intake as they are oxidized.
- Diet interacts with the extent of lipolysis to affect feed intake.
- A better understanding of the metabolic control of feed intake can help implement strategies to reduce risk of metabolic disease.

INTRODUCTION

Suppression of appetite in dairy cows during the postpartum (PP) period results in negative energy balance (NEB), which increases the risk of metabolic disorders. Cows in the PP period are in a lipolytic state from low plasma insulin concentration and decreased insulin sensitivity of tissues, which results in a gradual increase in plasma nonesterified fatty acid (NEFA) concentration in the days before parturition. The liver extracts NEFA from the blood, and these can be esterified and stored as triglycerides (TG) or oxidized to acetyl CoA. Acetyl CoA is oxidized completely to CO_2 or

Funding Sources: USDA NIFA, Cargill, Milk Specialties Global Animal Nutrition, Malaysian Palm Oil Board, Kemin Industries, Diamond V, Inc (M.S. Allen); None (P. Piantoni).
Conflict of Interest: None.
[a] Department of Animal Science, Michigan State University, 474 South Shaw Lane, Room 2265A, East Lansing, MI 48824, USA; [b] Department of Animal Science, Michigan State University, 474 South Shaw Lane, Room 2200, East Lansing, MI 48824, USA
* Corresponding author.
E-mail address: allenm@msu.edu

Vet Clin Food Anim 29 (2013) 279–297
http://dx.doi.org/10.1016/j.cvfa.2013.04.001
vetfood.theclinics.com
0749-0720/13/$ – see front matter

incompletely to ketones, which are then exported to the general circulation. Excessive storage of NEFA as TG compromises liver function while oxidation of NEFA might suppress feed intake. Satiety caused by hepatic oxidation of fuels might be a dominant mechanism controlling feed intake, especially in the peripartum period.[1] Minimizing the rate of lipolysis and the duration of the lipolytic state are key to reducing incidence of metabolic disease; especially because feed intake is likely controlled by hepatic oxidation of NEFA. Lipolysis can be controlled by preventing excessive body condition, minimizing stress in the peripartum period, and maximizing energy intake in the PP period. Optimal body condition at parturition and increased energy intake PP can be achieved with strategic diet formulation. The objective of this article is to discuss metabolic control of feed intake in the peripartum period and its implications for metabolic disease of fresh cows. Understanding how feed intake is controlled during the transition from gestation to lactation is critical to both reduce risk and successfully treat many metabolic diseases.

LIPOLYTIC STATE OF COWS IN THE PERIPARTUM PERIOD

The lipolytic state begins several weeks prepartum, with the decline in plasma insulin concentration and the decrease in insulin sensitivity of adipose tissue and muscle, and extends for up to several weeks PP. The decrease in insulin sensitivity of tissues is likely caused by the gradual increase in growth hormone,[2] proinflammatory cytokines, such as tumor necrosis factor α[3] from the placenta and adipose tissue, and increased plasma NEFA concentration.[4] Signals related to the concomitant gestation initiate lipolysis to provide NEFA as a fuel to the liver and extrahepatic tissues, sparing the glucose required for fetal development. Euglycemia is maintained until initiation of lactogenesis,[5,6] likely because glucose is spared by use of NEFA as a fuel. In addition, elevated NEFA concentration in blood is required to increase fat concentration of colostrum and milk in early lactation to meet the energy requirements of the calf. However, excessive fat mobilization can result in hepatic lipidosis, ketosis, and other metabolic disorders related to low feed intake and NEB. Importantly, oxidation of NEFA in the liver likely induces satiety, which might be the cause of the depression in feed intake.[1] Suppressed feed intake following parturition prevents restoration of euglycemia, extending the lipolytic state for days or weeks PP. The depression in feed intake that occurs during the peripartum period is likely caused by the lipolytic state that is established several weeks prepartum and increases greatly in the days before parturition.

Hepatic export of ketones is beneficial to some extent because complete oxidation of NEFA might depress feed intake further. Therefore, in the PP period, a limited increase in ketone body concentrations in blood (plasma [BHB] <1.2 mmol/L[7]) should be considered normal, because lipid mobilization and NEFA oxidation is the expected response to decreased insulin sensitivity and plasma insulin concentration around parturition. Nevertheless, concentrations of BHB in plasma lower than 1.2 mmol/L are indicators of a good transition from gestation to lactation. In contrast, elevated plasma ketone body concentrations indicate a lipolytic state that likely suppresses feed intake. In this case, peripartum cows would benefit from a diet composition different from what might be optimal days or weeks later,[1] when control of feed intake by hepatic oxidation subsides and signals from ruminal distention begin to dominate.

METABOLIC DISEASES RELATED TO DEPRESSED FEED INTAKE

The depression in dry matter intake (DMI) PP results in a period of NEB for most cows, increasing the risk of metabolic disorders.[8] The extent of lipid mobilization and, therefore, the depression in DMI, will determine if the cow will have normal plasma ketone body concentrations or will develop either subclinical or clinical ketosis. Incidence of ketosis is related to plasma concentrations of NEFA both prepartum[9] and PP[10] and to high body condition score (BCS) at parturition.[11] Although ketosis might be secondary to other disease(s) that can depress DMI and increase NEB, it can also be primary, with no apparent cause. In both cases, feed intake suppression from hepatic oxidation of NEFA is probably a contributing factor.

The decline in DMI in the peripartum period is greater for cows with higher BCS,[12] and this predisposes them to increased incidence of metabolic disorders, including ketosis and hepatic lipidosis. Cows with excessive body condition (BCS $\geq$3.5 on a 1 to 5 scale) during the transition period, likely have a greater rate and extent of lipolysis than cows with lower BCS because they have a larger mass of adipose tissue that can be mobilized and because the release of proinflammatory cytokines that contribute to insulin resistance[13] is increased when the mass of adipose tissue is greater. Prolonged lipolysis is likely associated with a longer period of depressed feed intake and, therefore, NEB.

Liver uptake of NEFA is proportional to their concentration in the blood.[14] Excessive hepatic TG concentration is a result of high blood NEFA concentration and compromises liver function, reducing gluconeogenesis[15] and, therefore, restoration of blood glucose and insulin concentrations, further extending the lipolytic state. Because ruminant liver has limited capacity to export TG as very low density lipoproteins (VLDL),[16] limiting lipolysis is the primary goal for a successful transition from gestation to lactation.

Other health disorders are associated with depressed feed intake around parturition. Depression in feed intake in the first several days PP greatly alters the balance between calcium absorbed and secreted in milk, increasing the risk of hypocalcemia. In addition, elevated blood NEFA concentration, and the resulting feed intake depression and increased ketones, will likely compromise the immune system response, increasing the risk of retained fetal membranes and metritis.[17–19] Furthermore, depressed feed intake results in lower rumen digesta mass and volume increasing the risk of displaced abomasum from lower rumen fill and subacute ruminal acidosis from reduced buffer capacity of ruminal digesta.[20]

CONTROL OF FEED INTAKE

A variety of factors interact to affect feed intake of dairy cows, including diet, management, environment, milk yield, and their physiological state (eg, insulin concentration and insulin sensitivity of tissues). Feeding behavior is controlled by brain feeding centers in the hypothalamus that receive peripheral signals from afferents in the liver and gut, as well as from metabolites and hormones. Feed intake is determined by the size and frequency of meals. Meal size is a function of eating rate and meal length, and the length of meals is determined by satiety. Meal frequency is affected by the time interval between meals, which is determined by hunger. Diet, social interactions, and stress affect feeding behavior and these are at least partially under management control (eg, cow comfort, strategic grouping, overcrowding, diet composition). Therefore, an understanding of how feeding behavior is controlled is vital to improve feed intake in dairy cows during the peripartum period.

Feed intake control mechanisms are complex and involve multiple signals, redundancies, and levels of integration. Signals include distention from rumen fill (physical regulation), gut peptides (endocrine regulation), and oxidation of fuels (metabolic regulation). These signals are additive,[21,22] and decisions to initiate and end meals are a result of integration of signals within brain feeding centers. The dominant signals controlling feeding behavior will likely vary temporally, within days, as well as through lactation.

Physical Regulation

Physical fill in the rumen has been studied extensively and previously reviewed.[23] The filling effect of diets is determined primarily by forage neutral-detergent fiber (NDF), forage fragility (susceptibility to particle size breakdown by digestion and chewing), and digestion characteristics affecting turnover rate of fiber, such as the potentially digestible fraction and its rates of digestion and passage.[24] Rumen distention is sensed by tension receptors located primarily in the reticulum and cranial sac of the rumen,[25] conveyed to brain feeding centers, and integrated with other signals to determine feeding behavior. Signals from ruminal distention from physical fill likely dominate control of feed intake during the periods of highest milk production. This is in contrast to periods earlier and later in lactation, as discussed later in this article.

Endocrine Regulation

Gut peptides that potentially contribute to the control of feed intake include ghrelin, cholecystokinin (CCK), and the incretin glucagon like peptide 1 (GLP-1), which also may stimulate insulin secretion.[26] Several of these have been studied in the ruminant animal[27,28] but most of the work has been done in nonruminants because of their potential use as satiety factors in the treatment of obesity in humans.[29,30] Ghrelin is known as the "hunger hormone" and is secreted by abomasal tissues. It is the only gut peptide known currently to stimulate feed intake, likely by increasing gastric emptying and passage rate from the rumen. Other gut peptides are secreted by the small intestine in response to various nutrients in the chyme. They may affect feed intake, gastric emptying, and favor digestion of nutrients through an increase in secretion of digestive enzymes or bile. A decrease in gastric emptying will likely result in longer retention times in the rumen and small intestine, favoring digestion and absorption of nutrients. Gut peptide signals (direct and indirect through effects on motility and distention as well as insulin and metabolism) are also integrated by brain feeding centers to determine feeding behavior.

Metabolic Regulation

Metabolites derived from the diet and mobilized from body reserves affect feed intake, which is likely related to their ability to be oxidized in the liver. This has been previously reviewed[1,31] and is discussed in relation to metabolic diseases in the sections that follow.

SIGNAL FROM HEPATIC OXIDATION OF FUELS

Research with laboratory species suggests that hepatic oxidation of fuels affects feeding behavior and that these signals are carried to brain feeding centers via hepatic vagal afferents; stimulation of oxidation inhibits feeding, whereas inhibition of fuel oxidation stimulates feeding. Various metabolic inhibitors have increased the discharge rate of hepatic vagal afferents and stimulated feeding, whereas hepatic vagotomy has blocked the stimulation of satiety by a variety of fuels in multiple species.[31] This research indicates that fuel oxidation in peripheral tissues is involved in the control of feeding and that the transmission of signals to brain feeding centers is via hepatic vagal afferents. We call this the Hepatic Oxidation Theory (HOT) of control of feed intake[1] and think it merits consideration for a better understanding of the prevention and treatment of metabolic diseases.

Energy Charge in the Liver

A series of experiments conducted by Friedman and colleagues[32] showed that feeding behavior was related to hepatic energy status rather than fuel oxidation and ATP production per *se*. Energy status is measured by adenylate energy charge ([ATP] + 0.5[ADP])/([ATP] + [ADP] + [AMP]) and is related to phosphorylation potential. It is determined by the balance between the rate of production of high-energy phosphate bonds from oxidation of fuels and their rate of utilization by energy-consuming reactions. An increase in hepatic energy status has been related to decreased firing rate of hepatic vagal afferents and satiety. Firing rate increases in the period between meals as hepatic oxidation subsides and energy charge is depleted, resulting in hunger and meal initiation (**Fig. 1**). Even though we know the hypophagic response to fuel oxidation is likely linked to an increase in hepatic energy status, the mechanisms by which oxidation of fuels in hepatocytes affect the firing rate of the hepatic vagus are yet to be discovered.[1]

Fuels Oxidized in the Liver

Fuels extracted from the blood and oxidized in ruminant liver include NEFA, glycerol, lactate, and amino acids (mobilized from body reserves, produced by metabolism of other fuels, and provided by the diet), as well as propionate and butyrate, produced by microbial fermentation in the gastrointestinal tract. All these fuels have the potential to induce satiety at different degrees. Acetate and glucose are not extracted from the blood by the liver because the activity of the enzymes required for their activation and subsequent metabolism are low in ruminant liver.[24] Consistent with HOT, their hypophagic effects in ruminants are much lower than fuels that are metabolized by ruminant liver.[33]

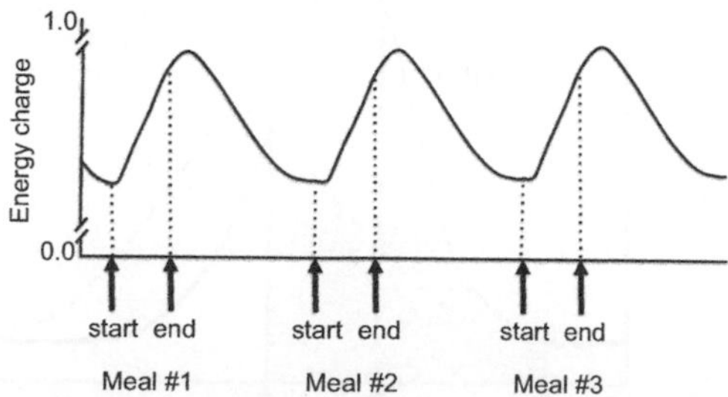

Fig. 1. Theoretical temporal relationship between hepatic energy charge and feeding behavior in the postpartum period. Energy charge ([ATP] + 0.5[ADP])/([ATP] + [ADP] + [AMP]) is related to phosphorylation potential. Energy charge increases over time within a meal as propionate and other glucogenic metabolites stimulate oxidation of acetyl CoA in the TCA cycle. Increased energy charge results in a decrease in the discharge rate of hepatic vagal afferents, causing satiety and end of the meal (*arrows*). Energy charge likely continues to increase as metabolites are absorbed following the end of meals, and, as absorption subsides, energy charge decreases. The discharge rate of hepatic vagal afferents gradually increases, causing hunger and initiation of meals (*arrows*). The pattern of change in energy charge within and following meals (represented the same here for simplicity) is likely determined by several factors, including extent of lipolysis, eating rate, and diet starch concentration and ruminal fermentability.

Effects of Propionate on Feed Intake

Hypophagic effects of propionate infusions (as propionic acid or sodium propionate) have been documented extensively for ruminants.[24] Propionate is more hypophagic than acetate or butyrate when infused into the portal vein of sheep,[34] and infusion of propionate into the mesenteric vein of steers reduced feed intake, whereas acetate infused at similar rates did not.[35] Although propionate might be expected to decrease feed intake compared with acetate when infused at the same rate because it has a higher energy concentration, propionate linearly decreased metabolizable energy intake in lactating cows when infused intraruminally as iso-osmotic mixtures compared with acetate.[36] The liver is likely involved in control of feed intake by propionate because hypophagic effects of portal infusions of propionate were eliminated by hepatic vagotomy.[37] These studies suggest that hypophagic effects of propionate cannot be explained simply by the additional energy supplied compared with acetate. It is unlikely that animals consume feed to meet their energy requirements per *se* but rather have fuel-specific mechanisms regulating satiety and hunger.

Propionate is produced primarily by ruminal fermentation of starch. Of fuels metabolized by the ruminant liver, propionate is likely a primary satiety signal because its flux to the liver increases greatly during meals.[38] Rate of propionate production and flux to the liver within meals (**Fig. 2**) is determined primarily by rate of eating, as well as the concentration and ruminal fermentability of dietary starch.[24] Propionate is efficiently extracted by the liver and can be oxidized by conversion to acetyl CoA when its rate of extraction exceeds its rate of use for glucose production and acetyl CoA concentration is low. When cows are in a lipolytic state and hepatic acetyl CoA concentration is elevated, propionate oxidation is inhibited and propionate will be used as a glucose precursor. However, propionate entry into the tricarboxylic acid (TCA) cycle can stimulate oxidation of the existing pool of acetyl CoA (**Fig. 3**),[1] generating ATP and increasing energy charge. Control of feed intake by propionate in the PP period as well as implications for diet formulation will be discussed in later sections.

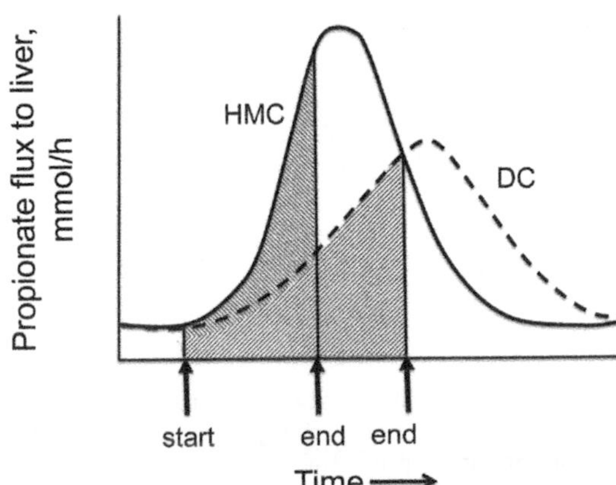

Fig. 2. Probable temporal relationship between ruminal fermentability of starch and propionate flux to the liver within meals. Ruminal starch fermentability of high-moisture corn (HMC, *solid line*) is greater compared with dry corn (DC, *dashed line*), resulting in increased propionate flux to the liver during meals assuming the same starch concentration in the diet. Propionic acid stimulates hepatic oxidation, increasing energy charge. A faster flux of propionate to the liver during meals elevates energy charge and decreases the firing rate of vagal afferents, causing satiety and ending meals sooner (*arrows*). A less fermentable starch source will likely allow a higher dietary starch concentration, increasing intake of total glucose precursors.

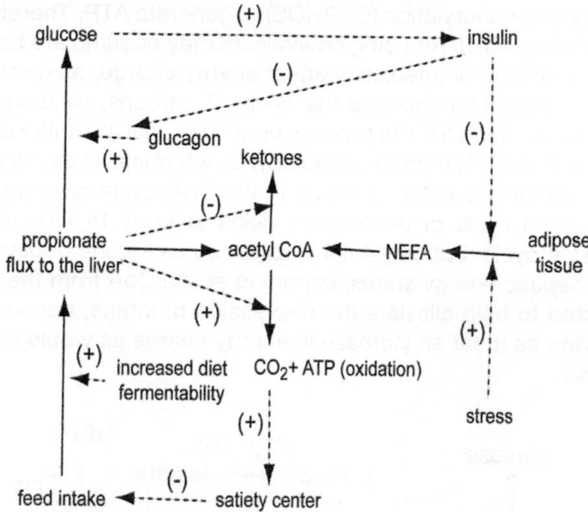

Fig. 3. Model by which feed intake might be controlled according to the hepatic oxidation theory. Solid lines show the flow of carbon, whereas dashed lines show stimulation/inhibition of flow. Propionate can be used by the liver for gluconeogenesis, using ATP, or oxidized in the TCA cycle through acetyl CoA, producing ATP. Acetyl CoA produced from β-oxidation of fatty acids and other ketogenic fuels is oxidized in the TCA cycle or exported as ketones. Decreased insulin concentration, increased insulin resistance, and stress increase lipolysis, thereby increasing the pool of acetyl CoA through β-oxidation of NEFA. Propionate uptake during meals stimulates oxidation of acetyl CoA to CO_2, generating ATP, increasing energy charge, and stimulating satiety. (*Adapted from* Allen MS, Bradford BJ, Oba M. The hepatic oxidation theory of the control of feed intake and its application to ruminants. J Anim Sci 2009;87:3317; with permission.)

CONTROL OF FEED INTAKE IN THE PP PERIOD

The "flood" of readily oxidizable NEFA to the liver is likely responsible for the depression of feed intake during the peripartum period consistent with the inverse temporal relationship between plasma NEFA concentration and DMI observed in many studies.[1] The following sections detail hepatic oxidation of fuels to provide a better understanding of how diet likely interacts with lipolytic state to affect energy intake.

Oxidation of NEFA in the Liver

Carnitine acyl transferase (CAT1) transports NEFA into mitochondria by binding them to carnitine. The balance between transport of NEFA into mitochondria and their esterification and storage as TG is affected by several factors, including availability of carnitine and concentration and activity of enzymes. Supplementation of carnitine to transition cows increased in vitro oxidation of palmitate[39] and depressed feed intake in the early PP period,[40] consistent with HOT.[1] Moreover, CAT1 is inhibited by malonyl CoA (an intermediate in fatty acid synthesis) and methylmalonyl CoA (an intermediate in propionate metabolism). Once inside the mitochondrion, reducing equivalents ($FADH_2$ and NADH) are generated by β-oxidation of NEFA. These reducing equivalents can then generate ATP, thus increasing the energy charge of the cell. It is important to recognize, however, that reducing equivalents must undergo oxidative phosphorylation (OXPHOS) to generate ATP. Therefore, there may be a lag phase during which reducing equivalents may accumulate before ATP generation, thus they may not immediately affect energy charge, as discussed later.

Each cycle of β-oxidation shortens the FA by 2 carbons, yielding 1 molecule of acetyl CoA, $FADH_2$, and NADH. The process continues until the entire chain is cleaved into acetyl CoA units (or until there is a propionyl CoA terminal in the case of odd-chain FA). Acetyl CoA, in turn, is either oxidized in the TCA cycle or exported as ketone bodies (**Fig. 4**). Each cycle of β-oxidation yields at least 14 ATP if acetyl CoA is oxidized in the TCA cycle, but only 4 if it is exported as ketone bodies. If feed intake is controlled by hepatic energy status, exporting acetyl CoA from the liver as ketone bodies is expected to help alleviate the depression of intake, because ketogenesis would not generate as great an increase in energy charge as would complete oxidation of acetyl CoA.

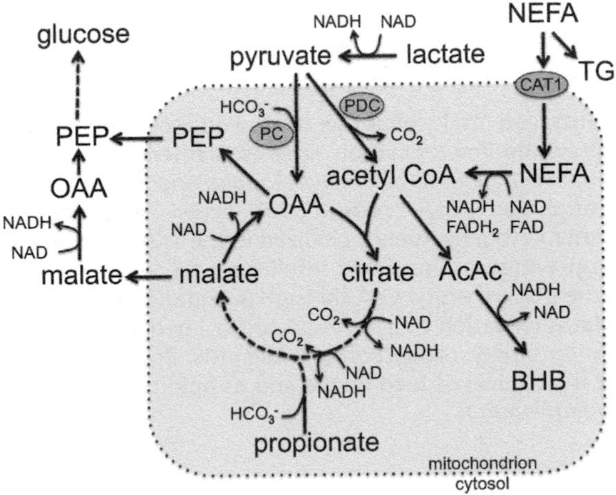

Fig. 4. Oxidation of fuels in hepatocytes of cows in the peripartum period. The lipolytic state during the peripartum period results in greater uptake of NEFA by the liver. NEFA are either transported via CAT1 into the mitochondria for β-oxidation or converted to TG. TG are stored in the cytosol for later oxidation or exported as very low-density lipoproteins. Oxidation of NEFA generates acetyl CoA, $FADH_2$, and NAD. The acetyl CoA produced can enter the TCA cycle in the citrate synthase reaction and be oxidized completely to CO_2 or exported as acetoacetate (AcAc) or beta-hydroxybutyric acid (BHB). Oxidation of acetyl CoA in the TCA cycle is dependent on availability of TCA intermediates. In the PP period, gluconeogenesis is stimulated because of the high glucose demand, increasing transport of malate and phosphoenolpyruvate (PEP) to the cytosol and depleting TCA intermediates. Increased concentration of acetyl CoA from β-oxidation conserves glucose precursors by stimulating pyruvate carboxylase (PC), enhancing pyruvate conversion to oxaloacetate (OAA), and decreasing activity of pyruvate dehydrogenase complex (PDC), decreasing pyruvate conversion to acetyl CoA. Flux of intermediates through the cycle is also affected by enzyme concentration and activity, which, in turn, is affected by redox state. Reducing equivalents are generated in mitochondria by β-oxidation ($FADH_2$ and NAD) and by the TCA cycle (NADH), and exported as BHB, shuttled to the cytosol (eg, malate), or used by OXPHOS to generate high-energy phosphate bonds. Because TCA intermediates are likely limiting in the PP period, there is increased export of acetyl CoA as ketones. Supply of TCA intermediates is primarily from lactate, amino acids, and propionate. Propionate uptake by the liver within meals stimulates TCA activity, which generates ATP, NADH, and CO_2. The production of CO_2 stimulates OXPHOS, which converts reducing equivalents to ATP, increasing energy charge.

Oxidation of Acetyl CoA

Acetyl CoA is the metabolic crossroad by which all fuels pass through to be oxidized to CO_2 and water in the TCA cycle. The 2-carbon acetyl moiety enters the TCA cycle in the citrate synthase reaction by combining with oxaloacetate (OAA) to form citrate (see **Fig. 4**). A fast rate of oxidation of acetyl CoA within the time frame of meals is expected to increase energy charge in the liver, thus inducing satiety rapidly, decreasing meal size, and possibly overall DMI. The rate of oxidation of acetyl CoA is likely affected by the availability of TCA cycle intermediates that provide OAA required for this reaction. Availability of TCA intermediates is likely low in the PP period because high glucose demand results in an upregulation of gluconeogenesis, which depletes the pool of TCA intermediates and decreases oxidation of acetyl CoA, as suggested by Krebs.[41]

Oxidation of acetyl CoA in the TCA cycle is not only affected by the concentration of TCA intermediates in mitochondria, but also by the flux of these intermediates through the cycle. The speed at which the available intermediates complete the cycle is affected by the concentrations and activity of the enzymes involved. These enzyme activities are affected by the mitochondrial redox state with activities diminishing with the accumulation of reducing equivalents, as reflected in decreasing NAD^+/NADH and FAD/$FADH_2$ ratios. Reducing equivalents are produced by β-oxidation of fatty acids (FA) and by oxidation of acetyl CoA in the TCA cycle, thus high rates of β-oxidation (as occurs when serum NEFA concentrations are high) are expected to feedback negatively on the rate of acetyl-CoA oxidation. As a result, elevated NADH concentration in the mitochondria will inhibit the flux of acetyl CoA through the TCA cycle, providing less OAA available for the citrate synthase reaction over time (see **Fig. 4**). Therefore, the capacity of the liver to oxidize acetyl CoA is determined by total TCA intermediates, which, in turn are affected by the balance between their rates of entry (anaplerosis) and exit (cataplerosis), and their flux through the cycle (determined by enzyme concentration and activity and the redox state).

Supply of TCA Intermediates

TCA cycle intermediates are continuously removed and replenished; anaplerosis primarily from propionate entry through succinyl CoA, and lactate entry through OAA via pyruvate. Glucogenic amino acids enter as various TCA intermediates. Lactate is supplied by diets containing silages and fermented feeds (small amounts), and by anaerobic metabolism of glucose by splanchnic tissues, erythrocytes, and muscle. Oxidation of amino acids depends on their supply relative to demand, as well as amino acid profile. Amino acids absorbed from the gastrointestinal tract and mobilized from muscle are used for protein synthesis, but excess supply of individual glucogenic amino acids increases their entry into the TCA cycle. Greater entry of amino acids into the TCA cycle occurs when supply of all amino acids exceeds the demand for protein synthesis and when protein synthesis is limited by individual amino acids. Propionate, produced primarily by ruminal fermentation of starch, is the fuel that will most likely supply TCA intermediates within the time frame of meals when starch is fed, because of the potential for rapid production in the rumen and extraction by the liver. Diets with highly fermentable starch can greatly increase flux of propionate to the liver (see **Fig. 2**), increasing energy charge within meals (**Fig. 5**).

TCA Activity and Control of OXPHOS

Why do cows normally consume their largest meal(s) of the day just after feeding[42] when plasma NEFA concentration is highest?[33] Why do cows in a lipolytic state

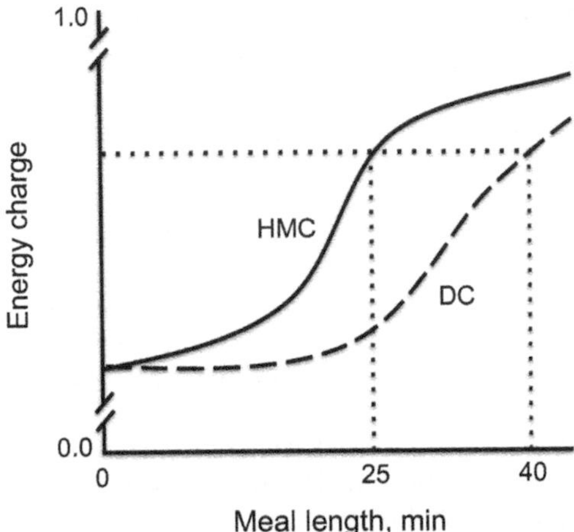

Fig. 5. Theoretical temporal relationship between ruminal fermentability of starch and hepatic energy charge within meals for cows in a lipolytic state. Energy charge ([ATP] + 0.5[ADP])/([ATP] + [ADP] + [AMP]) represents phosphorylation potential. Energy charge increases over time within a meal as propionic acid produced by ruminal fermentation of starch stimulates hepatic oxidation. Ruminal starch fermentability of high-moisture corn (HMC, *solid line*) is greater than dry corn (DC, *dashed line*), resulting in increased propionate flux to the liver during meals, assuming the same starch concentration in the diet. Propionic acid stimulates oxidation of acetyl CoA in the TCA cycle, increasing energy charge. As energy charge increases, the decreased firing rate of vagal afferents causes satiety, ending the meal (*dotted lines*). A less fermentable starch source will likely allow a higher dietary starch concentration, increasing intake of total glucose precursors.

(with copious reducing equivalents produced by β-oxidation) eat at all? Although this seems paradoxical, reducing equivalents produced by β-oxidation might not be used immediately by OXPHOS to produce ATP and increase energy charge in the liver. A key finding recently reported is that OXPHOS is controlled by bicarbonate from metabolically derived CO_2 within mitochondria.[43] The primary source of CO_2 is the TCA cycle (see **Fig. 4**), and no CO_2 is produced by β-oxidation. Rate of production of CO_2 likely corresponds to meals, when substrate entry into the TCA cycle is greatest, and declines following meals. The rapid increase in CO_2 during meals likely stimulates OXPHOS, greatly increasing energy charge by using reducing equivalents that might have accumulated since the previous meal. Consequently, the energy charge of the liver can increase very quickly depending on the flux of TCA intermediates to the liver within the time frame of meals. Following meals, acetyl CoA oxidation and CO_2 production decrease as TCA intermediates are likely depleted, decreasing OXPHOS activity, while high-energy phosphate bonds are used continuously by anabolic reactions in the liver. The conversion of reducing equivalents produced by β-oxidation to ATP will slow down, resulting in their accumulation between meals, a decrease in energy charge, and eventually hunger.

Interaction of Propionate and Lipolytic State

Rapid entry of TCA intermediates from propionate during meals might dramatically increase energy charge because of (1) increased oxidation in the TCA cycle of the existing pool of acetyl CoA in the liver, and (2) conversion of accumulated reducing equivalents to ATP by OXPHOS, which is stimulated by the CO_2 produced in the TCA cycle. Because propionate flux to the liver can increase greatly during meals, the rapid increase in energy charge might depress meal size and energy intake, counteracting its benefits as a glucose precursor.[24]

Little propionate carbon per *se* is oxidized in the PP period because of the elevated concentration of acetyl CoA; most of the propionate will enter the TCA cycle and then be routed to the gluconeogenic pathway. Acetyl CoA stimulates pyruvate carboxylase,[44] conserving glucose precursors in the TCA cycle, and inhibits pyruvate dehydrogenase complex,[45] preventing the conversion of pyruvate to acetyl CoA, which is the committed step in its oxidation. However, hypophagic effects of propionate may be enhanced because entry of propionate into the TCA cycle stimulates oxidation of the existing pool of acetyl CoA (see **Fig. 3**), which is abundant for most cows in the PP period.

Propionate was more hypophagic for cows in the PP period compared with cows in midlactation,[46] likely because propionate stimulated oxidation of the available pool of acetyl CoA supplied by β-oxidation of NEFA from mobilization of body lipid stores. Our recent research demonstrated that the hypophagic effects of propionate increased linearly with hepatic acetyl CoA concentration when propionate was infused intraruminally in cows in the PP period.[47] Therefore, although propionate is an important glucose precursor, enhanced propionate flux to the liver within meals might depress feed intake for cows in a lipolytic state and might be more hypophagic for cows with greater lipolysis.

KETOSIS TREATMENTS IN RELATION TO METABOLIC CONTROL OF FEED INTAKE

Hepatic oxidation of NEFA likely suppresses intake, predisposing cows to ketosis. Therefore, successful treatment of ketosis must focus on decreasing lipolysis to stimulate feed intake rather than reducing ketone body production alone. Common treatments for ketosis include oral administration of glucogenic precursors, including propylene glycol and calcium propionate (see article by Gordon and colleagues, elsewhere in this issue). Although both can theoretically increase plasma glucose and decrease plasma ketone body concentrations by stimulating oxidation of acetyl CoA in the liver, their efficacies vary. Results for both treatments are inconsistent in terms of plasma NEFA and ketone body concentrations: propylene glycol generally decreases plasma NEFA concentration and sometimes decreases concentration of ketone bodies, but calcium propionate is less effective.[48–50] Propylene glycol enters the TCA cycle as OAA (after conversion to lactate and pyruvate in the liver) and propionate enters the TCA cycle as succinyl CoA. Because both metabolites are intermediates of the TCA cycle, they can potentially inhibit feed intake through increased oxidation of acetyl CoA; however, propylene glycol might stimulate hepatic oxidation and depress feed intake to a lesser extent than propionate because its uptake by the liver and metabolism is slower.[51] Metabolism of lactate to pyruvate is not favored thermodynamically when cytosolic NADH (high concentration of reducing equivalents) is elevated and this may be the reason for a slower metabolism of propylene glycol, relative to propionate. Glycerol is another glucose precursor that has been used to treat ketosis but it has been cost-prohibitive until biodiesel production increased its supply recently.[52] Johnson[53] reported that oral administration of glycerol was more effective at increasing blood glucose compared with propylene glycol. Glycerol can enter the gluconeogenic pathway through dihydroxyacetone-phosphate without entering the TCA cycle, providing the potential advantage relative to propylene glycol or propionate of increasing glucose production with reduced risk of stimulating oxidation and suppressing feed intake.

Because the administration of these glucose precursors is oral, a portion of propylene glycol and glycerol will be metabolized in the rumen by ruminal bacteria. Glycerol is metabolized to propionic acid,[54] whereas propylene glycol is metabolized to propionic acid, as well as some propanol, and propanal;[51] however, administration in drenches or boluses overwhelms the metabolic capacity of ruminal bacteria. Therefore, a large proportion of these gluconeogenic precursors is expected to be absorbed intact. Adding small amounts of propylene glycol or glycerol in the diets is less likely to be effective at increasing plasma glucose concentration because ruminal microbes would partially metabolize them to propionate, decreasing their potential advantage by depressing feed intake.

Propionate decreases β-oxidation of NEFA in the liver by increasing their esterification to TG in the cytosol[55] or by inhibiting their transport into the mitochondria. This inhibition may occur because propionate is converted to methylmalonyl CoA, a molecule that can inhibit CAT1,[56] which is necessary for the transport of NEFA into the mitochondria. In addition, propionate decreases the activity of 3-hydroxy-3-methylglutaryl (HMG)-CoA synthase,[57] the rate-limiting enzyme in the conversion of acetyl CoA to ketone bodies, thus potentially decreasing the export of acetyl CoA from the liver as ketone bodies and increasing its availability for oxidation in the TCA cycle (see **Fig. 3**). Although a reduction in β-oxidation of NEFA might be expected to reduce energy charge, increased availability of acetyl CoA by reducing its export as ketone bodies would counteract the effect. In addition, increased fatty acid storage as TG might reduce hepatic function. Propylene glycol might also have opposite effects on oxidation of NEFA because it enters the TCA cycle through pyruvate, which increased β-oxidation of NEFA in liver cells in vitro.[58]

Monensin is an ionophore that selectively inhibits gram-positive bacteria, shifting ruminal populations of bacteria, generally increasing ruminal propionate production and affecting ruminant metabolism. A meta-analysis of treatment means from the literature indicated that monensin significantly reduced concentration of ketone bodies in lactating cows, including cows fewer than 30 days PP.[59] Monensin decreased feed intake slightly but effects of the ionophore on feed intake for cows in the PP period was not specified.[60] The reduction in ketone body concentration was attributed to a reduction in plasma NEFA concentration. Increasing propionate by inclusion of monensin in rations might be less hypophagic than by increasing ruminal starch fermentability, or direct addition of propionate or propionate precursors to the ration because the ionophore likely results in a more consistent supply of absorbed propionate over time.

Intravenous dextrose treatment has a direct effect on increasing plasma glucose concentration and insulin and, therefore, this treatment is more often used in extreme cases of ketosis. Insulin injections have also been reported in the treatment of ketosis, because insulin can inhibit lipolysis and ketogenesis. However, administration of exogenous insulin alone will exacerbate the existing hypoglycemia[61] and decrease gluconeogenesis so insulin should be administered in combination with other therapies. Indirect increases in insulin concentration by stimulation of gluconeogenesis (eg, by glucagon injection) would be preferable because hypoglycemia will be prevented.

Glucocorticoid injections might alleviate ketosis through effects on metabolism and production. However, their use is considered controversial by some scientists.[62] Intramuscular administration of glucocorticoids increases mobilization of amino acids from muscle, providing precursors for gluconeogenesis, reduces insulin sensitivity of tissues,[63] and can decrease milk yield. The reduction in insulin sensitivity of tissues and milk yield will assist in restoring euglycemia because glucose uptake by insulin-sensitive tissues and the mammary gland will be decreased. Increased supply of TCA cycle intermediates[64] might decrease synthesis and release of ketone bodies at the risk of anorexia from greater oxidation of acetyl CoA; however, greater production and lower use of glucose might increase plasma glucose concentration and insulin secretion, decreasing lipolysis and the supply of NEFA for oxidization in the liver.

Vitamin B complex and vitamin B_{12} alone are sometimes used in the treatment of ketosis. Several B vitamins act as cofactors of enzymes involved in the production of glucose from propionate. However, biotin and B_{12} are cofactors for enzymes involved in propionate entry into the TCA cycle, and treatment might result in a greater increase in energy charge within meals if the activities of the corresponding enzymes are limited by these cofactors. Therefore, although they might enhance glucose production, they might also decrease meal size and possibly feed intake.

Response to ketosis treatments varies greatly among cows. Cows with excessive body condition are at greater risk of ketosis in the days following parturition and are more recalcitrant to treatment. This is probably because they are more insulin resistant than cows with a lower BCS and, therefore, elevating plasma glucose for short periods (with dextrose administration) might not decrease plasma NEFA concentration enough to stimulate appetite. In addition, these cows are at greater risk of liver lipidosis, which will impair liver function. Moreover, FA stored as TG in the liver may be oxidized over time, continuing to suppress feed intake even when elevated glucose and insulin from treatment temporarily decrease adipose lipolysis. These cows will likely require an extended course of treatment to overcome ketosis. In contrast, other cows respond well to increased plasma glucose concentration from dextrose infusion or glucocorticoid injection. These latter cows tend to have a spontaneous increase in serum ketone body concentrations several weeks into lactation, and as they reach peak milk yield. In this case, fat is likely mobilized and plasma NEFA concentration increased because insulin is low from hypoglycemia or because of stress, but not because they are more insulin resistant as in cows with higher BCS. Like cows with insulin resistance, feed intake is likely depressed from increased oxidation of NEFA in the liver. However, increasing plasma glucose over the short term likely increases insulin enough to interrupt fat mobilization, resulting in increased feed intake and restored euglycemia, which will decrease plasma NEFA concentration and ketogenesis, alleviating anorexia.

STRATEGIES TO DECREASE METABOLIC DISORDERS

If feed intake during the PP period is controlled primarily by the hepatic oxidation of fuels, as much evidence suggests,[1,31] then the root cause of most fuel-related metabolic disorders is that feed intake is suppressed by the flood of NEFA to the liver during periods of excessive lipolysis. Therefore, minimizing the rate of lipolysis and the duration of the lipolytic state are key to reducing the incidence of metabolic diseases. Lipolysis can be reduced by (1) managing body condition, (2) minimizing stress, and (3) formulating diets to increase hepatic glucose production.

Managing Body Condition

Optimum BCS at parturition has been revised downward over the past couple of decades because cows with greater body condition have depressed feed intake, greater NEB, and greater risk of metabolic disease[65] (see also the article by Roche and colleagues, elsewhere in this issue). We currently recommend a BCS at parturition of 3.0 to 3.25 on a 1 to 5 scale at parturition. The best method to manage body condition of the herd without decreasing milk yield is to have an excellent reproductive program and to group cows by their physiological state.[66] Degree and extent of NEB can decrease fertility,[67] so methods to increase energy intake in early lactation will help improve reproductive performance and prevent extended lactations, which can lead to overconditioned cows. Grouping cows by their physiological state will also help increase lactation performance. Although low-fill, highly fermentable diets will allow greater energy intake and milk yield for cows in early to midlactation, they will likely result in depressed feed intake and increase risk of metabolic disorders if fed in the PP period. In addition, this diet will likely promote adiposity at the expense of milk yield as lactation proceeds. Insulin sensitivity of adipose tissue increases as plasma growth hormone concentration declines, and plasma insulin increases as glucose demand by the mammary gland is reduced as lactation progresses. When possible, recombinant bovine growth hormone might be used to increase energy partitioned to milk rather than body reserves. By mid to late lactation, once body condition has been restored, cows should be switched to a maintenance diet (see later in this article) to maintain BCS and milk yield, avoiding overconditioning.

Reduce Stress

Although the transition period is a stressful time by itself, stress can be reduced by considering factors under management control, including cow comfort, social interactions, housing, bunk space, grouping, feeding schedules, and the quality of human interactions. Poor management of the transition cow will not only decrease DMI directly, but indirectly by increasing lipolysis and plasma NEFA concentration. Stress hormones (catecholamines) are lipolytic, and their secretion exacerbates lipolysis from low insulin and insulin sensitivity that characterizes the transition period, resulting in higher plasma NEFA concentrations, a greater and prolonged depression in feed intake, and an extended period of NEB. Efforts to reduce stress in the transition period will likely be rewarded by enhanced feed intake and lower risk of metabolic diseases.

Diet Formulation and Grouping Strategy

As discussed previously, diets should be formulated to optimize energy intake and partitioning through lactation and this would require multiple diets for different groups of cows. The dominant factors controlling feed intake change with physiological state, which changes through lactation. Around parturition, feed intake is likely controlled primarily by hepatic oxidation of NEFA that interacts with the supply of propionate from the diet. Once lipolysis and the supply of NEFA to the liver decreases, feed intake increases until distention from rumen fill dominates control of feed intake. As lactation proceeds and milk yield declines, hepatic oxidation of fuels likely begins to dominate control of feed intake, probably due to a negative feedback on gluconeogenesis from elevated plasma glucose and insulin concentrations. In addition, energy partitioning is shifted from milk production to body reserves. Rations for cows with these 3 distinct physiological states are discussed as follows.

Fresh cow ration (first 2 weeks following parturition)

Cows in the PP period differ distinctly from cows later in lactation because they are in a lipolytic state caused by low plasma insulin concentration and reduced insulin sensitivity of tissues (for a further discussion of insulin resistance see the article by De Koster and Opsomer, elsewhere in this issue). These cows require glucose precursors and rations should contain higher starch concentrations to the extent possible. However, they also have lower rumen digesta mass, which increases risk of ruminal acidosis and displaced abomasum. Highly fermentable starch sources increase fermentation acid production, including propionic acid, which can stimulate oxidation of fuels in the liver, decreasing feed intake (see **Fig. 5**). Increased fermentation acid production can depress fiber digestibility if ruminal pH is reduced, depressing energy intake further. Therefore, highly fermentable starch sources should be limited during this period, which lasts up to 2 weeks for most cows but even longer for cows with excessive body condition at parturition or those stressed by disease or management. Highly fermentable starch sources (eg, wheat, barley, low-density steam-flaked corn, high-moisture corn), should be limited to allow greater starch concentrations (and glucose precursors) with less risk of acidosis or displaced abomasum, sometimes associated with less rumen fill. Dry ground corn is an excellent source of starch and allows a total starch concentration of 22% to 26% (DM basis). Because feed intake is less limited by ruminal distention during this period and greater rumen digesta mass is desirable, forage NDF concentration should be greater than 23%, using nonforage fiber sources to dilute starch concentration if necessary. Starch concentrations must be decreased when feeding highly fermentable starch sources (to prevent depressions in feed intake and ruminal pH), which would decrease energy intake. Because of large variation among cows in the duration of the lipolytic state, cows should be switched to a low-fill, highly fermentable diet when blood ketone body concentrations are low and control of feed intake begins to be dominated by rumen fill. Usually, such cows will have normal appetite (aggressive eating following feeding), stable and increasing milk production, and no signs of metabolic diseases.

Early to midlactation ration

Following the PP period, milk yield continues to rise steadily for several more weeks and control of feed intake is increasingly dominated by ruminal distention. Cows respond well to rations with lower forage NDF concentration (low fill) and highly fermentable starch. Starch concentration of rations should be in the range of 25% to 30% (DM basis), although the optimum concentration is dependent on starch fermentability, forage NDF concentration, and competition for bunk space. Higher starch, lower fill rations generally increase milk yield peaks and decrease loss of body condition in early lactation. Switching to this diet when cows are ready will help narrow the gap between glucose supply and glucose demand, decreasing risk of spontaneous ketosis around peak lactation. However, as lactation advances and cows replenish body condition lost in early lactation, they should be switched to a maintenance diet with lower starch concentration and ruminal fermentability to prevent excessive BCS.

Maintenance ration (>150 DIM and BCS of 3)

The maintenance ration is the key component of a ration formulation/grouping system to reduce variation in BCS at parturition. The goal of the maintenance ration is to maintain milk yield and body condition through the remainder of lactation. Cows should be offered the maintenance ration when they are replenishing body condition and have reached a BCS of 3. Cows at this stage are insulin sensitive; if they continue to receive a high-starch diet, BCS will continue to increase and they will be at increased risk of metabolic disease the following parturition. Cows gain condition when they are fed rations with greater starch concentrations than needed for their current milk production, which increases plasma glucose and insulin concentrations. In addition, lower-producing cows are more susceptible to altered biohydrogenation of unsaturated FA when fed a highly fermentable diet,[68] which can shift energy partitioned from milk to body condition.[66] Lowering starch concentration of the rations should limit body condition gain while maintaining and possibly improving feed intake and yields of milk and milk fat. The optimal concentration of starch will likely be in the range of

18% to 22% (DM basis). Starch sources that are highly fermentable (eg, high-moisture corn, bakery waste, aged corn silage) should be avoided. Dried ground corn is an excellent starch source because it has lower ruminal digestibility (50%–60%) but high total tract digestibility (>90%). The starch concentration of the maintenance ration should contain adequate, but not excessive forage NDF concentration to maintain DMI. It is important that the fiber source provided is highly digestible; nonforage fiber sources (eg, beet pulp, corn gluten feed, soyhulls) can be used to dilute starch to the target concentration. Monitoring BCS at dry-off is essential to adjust the starch concentration of the maintenance diet over time.

SUMMARY

Feed intake during the peripartum period is likely controlled by hepatic oxidation of fuels. At this time, cows are in a lipolytic state that is initiated several weeks prepartum, as insulin concentration in blood and insulin sensitivity of tissues decrease. Anorexia results from hepatic oxidation of the continuous flood of NEFA to the liver. Low plasma insulin concentration from the resulting imbalance of glucose production and use, combined with insulin resistance, stimulates further lipolysis and as lipolysis increases, the risk of metabolic disease and other health disorders also increases. Therefore, the lipolytic state is perpetuated during the PP period by hypophagia from the hepatic oxidation of NEFA. Cows with excessive body condition, and that are stressed, are at greater risk of metabolic disease from a greater suppression of feed intake. The diet interacts with the lipolytic state; rapid production of propionic acid within meals from highly fermentable dietary starch likely suppresses feed intake by stimulating hepatic oxidation. Strategic feeding can limit excessive body condition during late lactation and increase energy intake during the postpartum period, reducing the risk of metabolic disease.

REFERENCES

1. Allen MS, Bradford BJ, Oba M. Board invited review: the hepatic oxidation theory of the control of feed intake and its application to ruminants. J Anim Sci 2009;87(10):3317–34.
2. Bell AW, Bauman DE. Adaptations of glucose metabolism during pregnancy and lactation. J Mammary Gland Biol Neoplasia 1997;2(3):265–78.
3. Ohtsuka H, Koiwa M, Hatsugaya A, et al. Relationship between serum TNF activity and insulin resistance in dairy cows affected with naturally occurring fatty liver. J Vet Med Sci 2001;63(9):1021–5.
4. Pires JA, Souza AH, Grummer RR. Induction of hyperlipidemia by intravenous infusion of tallow emulsion causes insulin resistance in Holstein cows. J Dairy Sci 2007;90(6):2735–44.
5. Doepel L, Lapierre H, Kennelly JJ. Peripartum performance and metabolism of dairy cows in response to prepartum energy and protein intake. J Dairy Sci 2002;85(9):2315–34.
6. Gulay MS, Hayen MJ, Bachman KC, et al. Milk production and feed intake of Holstein cows given short (30-d) or normal (60-d) dry periods. J Dairy Sci 2003;86(6):2030–8.
7. McArt JA, Nydam DV, Oetzel GR. Epidemiology of subclinical ketosis in early lactation dairy cattle. J Dairy Sci 2012;95(9):5056–66.
8. Ingvartsen KL, Dewhurst RJ, Friggens NC. On the relationship between lactational performance and health: is it yield or metabolic imbalance that cause

production diseases in dairy cattle? A position paper. Livest Prod Sci 2003; 83(2–3):277–308.

9. Joshi NP, Herdt TH, Neuder L. Association of rump fat thickness and plasma NEFA concentration with postpartum metabolic diseases in Holstein cows. Prod Diseases Farm Anim 2006;9789(90–76952):46.
10. Ospina PA, Nydam DV, Stokol T, et al. Associations of elevated nonesterified fatty acids and b-hydroxybutyrate concentrations with early lactation reproductive performance and milk production in transition dairy cattle in the northeastern United States. J Dairy Sci 2010;93(4):1596–603.
11. Gillund P, Reksen O, Gröhn YT, et al. Body condition related to ketosis and reproductive performance in Norwegian dairy cows. J Dairy Sci 2001;84(6):1390–6.
12. Hayirli A, Grummer RR, Nordheim EV, et al. Animal and dietary factors affecting feed intake during the prefresh transition period in Holsteins. J Dairy Sci 2002; 85(12):3430–43.
13. Hotamisligil G, Shargill N, Spiegelman B. Adipose expression of tumor necrosis factor-alpha: direct role in obesity-linked insulin resistance. Science 1993; 259(5091):87–91.
14. Emery RS, Liesman JS, Herdt TH. Metabolism of long chain fatty acids by ruminant liver. J Nutr 1992;122(Suppl 3):832–7.
15. Murondoti A, Jorritsma R, Beynen AC, et al. Activities of the enzymes of hepatic gluconeogenesis in periparturient dairy cows with induced fatty liver. J Dairy Res 2004;71(2):129–34.
16. Grummer RR. Impact of changes in organic nutrient metabolism on feeding the transition dairy cow. J Anim Sci 1995;73:2820–33.
17. Sartorelli P, Paltrinieri S, Agnes F. Non-specific immunity and ketone bodies. I: in vitro studies on chemotaxis and phagocytosis in ovine neutrophils. Zentralbl Veterinarmed A 1999;46(10):613–9.
18. Sartorelli P, Paltrinieri S, Comazzi S. Non-specific immunity and ketone bodies. II: in vitro studies on adherence and superoxide anion production in ovine neutrophils. J Vet Med A Physiol Pathol Clin Med 2000;47(1):1–8.
19. Sordillo LM, Contreras GA, Aitken SL. Metabolic factors affecting the inflammatory response of periparturient dairy cows. Anim Health Res Rev 2009;10(1): 53–63.
20. Allen MS, Voelker JA, Oba M. Physically effective fiber and regulation of ruminal pH: more than just chewing. Prod Diseases Farm Anim 2006;978(90–76952): 270–8.
21. Mbanya JN, Anil MH, Forbes JM. The voluntary intake of hay and silage by lactating cows in response to ruminal infusion of acetate or propionate, or both, with or without distension of the rumen by a balloon. Br J Nutr 1993; 69(3):713–20.
22. Choi BR, Allen MS. Intake regulation by volatile fatty acids and physical fill. S Afr J Anim Sci 1999;29(ISRP):40–1.
23. Allen MS. Physical constraints on voluntary intake of forages by ruminants. J Anim Sci 1996;74(12):3063–75.
24. Allen MS. Effects of diet on short-term regulation of feed intake by lactating dairy cattle. J Dairy Sci 2000;83(7):1598–624.
25. Leek BF. Sensory receptors in the ruminant alimentary tract. In: Milligan LP, Grovum WL, Dobson A, editors. Control of digestion and metabolism in ruminants. Prentice-Hall, Englewood Cliffs, NJ 1986. pp. 3–17.
26. Strader AD, Woods SC. Gastrointestinal hormones and food intake. Gastroenterology 2005;128(1):175–91.

27. Della-Fera MA, Baile CA. CCK-octapeptide injected in CSF and changes in feed intake and rumen motility. Physiol Behav 1980;24(5):943–50.
28. Relling A, Reynolds C. Abomasal infusion of casein, starch and soybean oil differentially affect plasma concentrations of gut peptides and feed intake in lactating dairy cows. Domest Anim Endocrinol 2008;35(1):35–45.
29. Murphy KG, Bloom SR. Gut hormones in the control of appetite. Exp Physiol 2004;89(5):507–16.
30. Sam AH, Troke RC, Tan TM, et al. The role of the gut/brain axis in modulating food intake. Neuropharmacology 2012;63(1):46–56.
31. Allen MS, Bradford BJ. Control of food intake by metabolism of fuels: a comparison across species. Proc Nutr Soc 2012;71(3):401–9.
32. Friedman MI, Harris RB, Ji H, et al. Fatty acid oxidation affects food intake by altering hepatic energy status. Am J Physiol 1999;276(4 Pt 2):R1046–53.
33. Allen MS, Bradford BJ, Harvatine KJ. The cow as a model to study food intake regulation. Annu Rev Nutr 2005;25:523–47.
34. Anil MH, Forbes JM. Feeding in sheep during intraportal infusions of short-chain fatty acids and the effect of liver denervation. J Physiol (Lond) 1980;298:407–14.
35. Elliot JM, Symonds HW, Pike B. Effect on feed intake of infusing sodium propionate or sodium acetate into a mesenteric vein of cattle. J Dairy Sci 1985;68(5):1165–70.
36. Oba M, Allen MS. Intraruminal infusion of propionate alters feeding behavior and decreases energy intake of lactating dairy cows. J Nutr 2003;133(4):1094–9.
37. Anil MH, Forbes JM. The roles of hepatic nerves in the reduction of food intake as a consequence of intraportal sodium propionate administration in sheep. Q J Exp Physiol (Cambridge, England) 1988;73(4):539–46.
38. Benson J, Reynolds C, Aikman P. Effects of abomasal vegetable oil infusion on splanchnic nutrient metabolism in lactating dairy cows. J Dairy Sci 2002;85(7):1804–14.
39. Carlson DB, Litherland NB, Dann HM, et al. Metabolic effects of abomasal L-carnitine infusion and feed restriction in lactating Holstein cows. J Dairy Sci 2006;89(12):4819–34.
40. Carlson DB, McFadden JW, D'Angelo A, et al. Dietary L-carnitine affects periparturient nutrient metabolism and lactation in multiparous cows. J Dairy Sci 2007;90(7):3422–41.
41. Krebs HA. Bovine ketosis. Vet Rec 1966;78(6):187–92.
42. Dado RG, Allen MS. Variation in and relationships among feeding, chewing, and drinking variables for lactating dairy cows. J Dairy Sci 1994;77(1):132–44.
43. Acin-Perez R, Salazar E, Kamenetsky M, et al. Cyclic AMP produced inside mitochondria regulates oxidative phosphorylation. Cell Metab 2009;9(3):265–76.
44. Utter MF, Keech DB, Scrutton MC. A possible role for acetyl CoA in the control of gluconeogenesis. Adv Enzyme Regul 1964;2:49–68.
45. Patel MS, Korotchkina LG. Regulation of the pyruvate dehydrogenase complex. Biochem Soc Trans 2006;34(2):217.
46. Oba M, Allen MS. Dose-response effects of intraluminal infusion of propionate on feeding behavior of lactating cows in early or midlactation. J Dairy Sci 2003;86(9):2922–31.
47. Stocks SE, Allen MS. Hypophagic effects of propionate increase with elevated hepatic acetyl coenzyme A concentration for cows in the early postpartum period. J Dairy Sci 2012;95(6):3259–68.
48. Overton TR, Emmert LS, Clark JH. Effects of source of carbohydrate and protein and rumen-protected methionine on performance of cows. J Dairy Sci 1998;81(1):221–8.

49. Waldron MR, Kulick AE, Bell AW, et al. Acute experimental mastitis is not causal toward the development of energy-related metabolic disorders in early postpartum dairy cows. J Dairy Sci 2006;89(2):596–610.
50. Overton TR, Waldron M. Nutritional management of transition dairy cows: strategies to optimize metabolic health. J Dairy Sci 2004;87(Suppl E):E105–19.
51. Kristensen NB, Raun BML. Ruminal and intermediary metabolism of propylene glycol in lactating Holstein cows. J Dairy Sci 2007;90(10):4707–17.
52. Hippen AR, DeFrain JM, Linke PL. Glycerol and other energy sources for metabolism and production of transition dairy cows. Proc 19th Annual Florida Ruminant Nutrition Symposium. University of Florida, Gainesville. dairy.ifas.ufl.edu/rns/Hippen.pdf 2008.
53. Johnson RB. The treatment of ketosis with glycerol and propylene glycol. Cornell Vet 1954;44(1):6–21.
54. Krueger NA, Anderson RC, Tedeschi LO, et al. Evaluation of feeding glycerol on free-fatty acid production and fermentation kinetics of mixed ruminal microbes in vitro. Bioresour Technol 2010;101(21):8469–72.
55. Jesse BW, Emery RS, Thomas JW. Control of bovine hepatic fatty acid oxidation. J Dairy Sci 1986;69(9):2290–7.
56. Brindle NP, Zammit VA, Pogson CI. Regulation of carnitine palmitoyltransferase activity by malonyl-CoA in mitochondria from sheep liver, a tissue with a low capacity for fatty acid synthesis. Biochem J 1985;232(1):177–82.
57. Lowe DM, Tubbs PK. Succinylation and inactivation of 3-hydroxy-3-methylglutaryl-CoA synthase by succinyl-CoA and its possible relevance to the control of ketogenesis. Biochem J 1985;232(1):37–42.
58. Drackley JK, Beitz DC, Young JW. Regulation of in vitro palmitate oxidation in liver from dairy cows during early lactation. J Dairy Sci 1991;74(6):1884–92.
59. Duffield TF, Rabiee AR, Lean IJ. A meta-analysis of the impact of monensin in lactating dairy cattle. Part 1. Metabolic effects. J Dairy Sci 2008;91(4):1334–46.
60. Duffield TF, Rabiee AR, Lean IJ. A meta-analysis of the impact of monensin in lactating dairy cattle. Part 2. Production effects. J Dairy Sci 2008;91(4):1347–60.
61. Hayirli A, Bertics SJ, Grummer RR. Effects of slow-release insulin on production, liver triglyceride, and metabolic profiles of Holsteins in early lactation. J Dairy Sci 2002;85(9):2180–91.
62. Seifi HA, LeBlanc SJ, Vernooy E, et al. Effect of isoflupredone acetate with or without insulin on energy metabolism, reproduction, milk production, and health in dairy cows in early lactation. J Dairy Sci 2007;90(9):4181–91.
63. Kusenda M, Kaske M, Piechotta M, et al. Effects of dexamethasone-21-isonicotinate on peripheral insulin action in dairy cows 5 days after surgical correction of abomasal displacement. J Vet Intern Med 2012;27(1):200–6.
64. Baird GD, Heitzman RJ. Gluconeogenesis in the cow. The effects of a glucocorticoid on hepatic intermediary metabolism. Biochem J 1970;116(5):865–74.
65. Roche JR, Friggens NC, Kay JK, et al. Invited review: body condition score and its association with dairy cow productivity, health, and welfare. J Dairy Sci 2009;92(12):5769–801.
66. Allen MS. Adjusting concentration and ruminal digestibility of starch through lactation. In: Proc. four-state dairy and nutrition management conference. Madison (WI): Dept. Dairy Sci., Univ. Wisconsin; 2012. p. 24–30.
67. Butler WR, Smith RD. Interrelationships between energy balance and postpartum reproductive function in dairy cattle. J Dairy Sci 1989;72(3):767–83.
68. Bradford BJ, Allen MS. Milk fat responses to a change in diet fermentability vary by production level in dairy cattle. J Dairy Sci 2004;87(11):3800–7.

Insulin Resistance in Dairy Cows

Jenne D. De Koster, DVM, Geert Opsomer, DVM, PhD, Msc*

KEYWORDS

- Insulin resistance • Dairy cow • Glucose metabolism • Insulin sensitivity tests
- Pregnancy and lactation • Adipose tissue

KEY POINTS

- Insulin plays a pivotal role in the glucose metabolism of dairy cows.
- The glucose metabolism of ruminants is characterized by low peripheral glucose concentrations and a low insulin response of the peripheral tissues.
- The effect of insulin on the glucose metabolism is regulated by the secretion of insulin by the pancreas and the insulin sensitivity of the skeletal muscles, adipose tissue, and liver.
- A state of insulin resistance may develop as part of physiologic (pregnancy and lactation) and pathologic processes, which may manifest as decreased insulin sensitivity or decreased insulin responsiveness.

COWS ARE RUMINANTS AND POSSESS A VERY SPECIFIC GLUCOSE METABOLISM

The glucose metabolism is of major interest in all living mammals because certain vitally important cell types (erythrocytes, brain cells, and kidney cells) have to rely on glucose as the only energy substrate.[1] Therefore, maintenance of blood glucose levels within normal physiologic ranges is of utmost importance. In comparison with that of other mammals, the glucose metabolism of ruminants is characterized by low peripheral glucose concentrations[2–4] and a low insulin response of the peripheral tissues.[3,5–7] The glucose metabolism is regulated by the supply and removal of glucose and glucogenic precursors in the blood and is tightly controlled by different hormones. Within the ruminants, dairy cows occupy a special position regarding the glucose metabolism. The massive glucose drain toward the udder and the unique transition between pregnancy and lactation make the glucose metabolism of dairy cows an example of how intensive genetic selection can drive metabolism to extremes. A schematic overview of the glucose metabolism in dairy cows is given in **Fig. 1**.

Funding Sources: Ghent University (G. Opsomer); Special Research Fund, Ghent University, grant number 01D28410 (J.D. De Koster).
Conflict of Interest: None.
Department of Reproduction, Obstetrics and Herd Health, Faculty of Veterinary Medicine, Ghent University, Salisburylaan 133, Merelbeke 9820, Belgium
* Corresponding author.
E-mail address: geert.opsomer@ugent.be

Vet Clin Food Anim 29 (2013) 299–322
http://dx.doi.org/10.1016/j.cvfa.2013.04.002 vetfood.theclinics.com

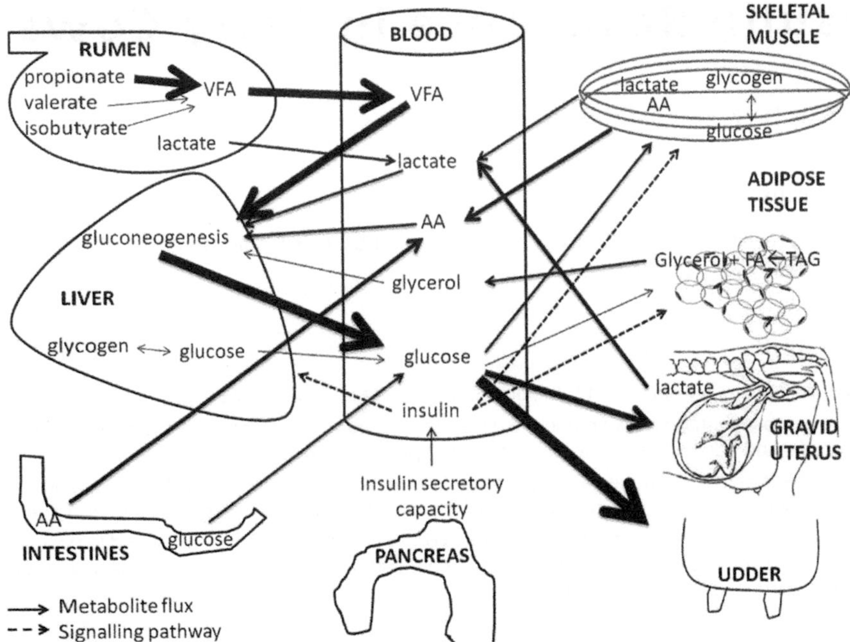

Fig. 1. Overview of the glucose metabolism in ruminants. Thickness of arrows indicates the importance of the metabolite or tissue in production or use. Volatile fatty acids (VFA) produced in the rumen are the most important precursors for hepatic gluconeogenesis. In addition, lactate (originating from the rumen, skeletal muscles, and gravid uterus), glycerol (from lipolysis of triglycerides [TAG] in the adipose tissue), and amino acids (AA) (from the intestines and skeletal muscles), all contribute to the total hepatic gluconeogenesis. Glucose absorbed from the intestines and glucose released from the liver (mostly gluconeogenesis, partly glycogenolysis) are the most important contributors to the blood glucose level. The lactating udder and the gravid uterus are quantitatively the most important glucose consumers. In late pregnancy and during early lactation, skeletal muscles and adipose tissues take up minimal amounts of glucose. The pancreas releases insulin into the bloodstream, which suppresses hepatic gluconeogenesis, glycogenolysis in liver and skeletal muscles, and adipose tissue lipolysis, whereas insulin stimulates glucose uptake in skeletal muscles and adipose tissues.

Glucose Supply

Propionate

Whereas monogastric species rely on intestinal glucose absorption as an exogenous supply of glucose, ruminants absorb only small amounts of glucose in the intestines.[1] Most of the circulating glucose in ruminants originates from hepatic and renal gluconeogenesis. Different endogenous and exogenous substrates are used for this gluconeogenesis. In the forestomachs, short-chain fatty acids are formed by microbial fermentation of carbohydrates in the feed. Among these short-chain fatty acids propionate, isobutyrate, and valerate are the main contributors to gluconeogenesis.[1] The relative contribution of glucogenic precursors changes during the different stages of lactation depending on feed intake, tissue mobilization, and energy balance. Quantitatively, propionate (60%–74%) is the most important glucogenic precursor, followed by lactate (16%–26%), alanine (3%–5%), valerate and isobutyrate (5%–6%), glycerol (0.5%–3%), and other amino acids (8%–11%).[1,8]

Lactate

Lactate can have an endogenous or exogenous origin. Rations based on high amounts of concentrates provoke a shift from a cellulolytic to an amylolytic flora in the rumen.[9] This amylolytic flora is responsible for the production of lactate in the rumen, which can be used by the liver for glucose production.[10] However, an overproduction of lactate may become detrimental to the health of the cow because of its low pH and concomitant higher risk of suffering from (sub)clinical ruminal acidosis. Another source of lactate is the anaerobe oxidation of glucose in the skeletal muscles and other peripheral tissues. During early lactation the expression of lactate dehydrogenase, the enzyme responsible for converting pyruvate into lactate, is upregulated, whereas the expression of the main enzymes of the citric acid cycle are downregulated in skeletal muscle. The latter indicates that the catabolism of glucose in skeletal muscle is diverted toward lactate production, indirectly supporting gluconeogenesis.[11] At the end of pregnancy, the uterus and placenta are important sources of lactate.[12] Therefore, the relative contribution of lactate in hepatic gluconeogenesis is maximal at the end of pregnancy and during early lactation.[8,13]

Glycerol

When adipose stores are mobilized, nonesterified fatty acids (NEFAs) and glycerol are released into the bloodstream. The fate of the NEFAs is well described in other reviews.[14,15] The released glycerol can be used in the gluconeogenic pathway. Its contribution to gluconeogenesis and, hence, in the overall glucose production depends on the size of the fat depots and the amount of fat mobilization, and is thus directly related to the negative energy balance.[8]

Amino acids

Circulating amino acids provide another determinant in gluconeogenic pathways. Especially during periods of high glucose requirements, more amino acids are converted into glucose. The extra amino acids originate from intestinal absorption (higher feed intake), decreased protein synthesis in skin and skeletal muscles, and increased protein breakdown in skeletal muscles.[8,16] The most important amino acids to contribute to glucose provision are alanine and glutamine.[8]

Glycogen

Glycogen stores in the liver and skeletal muscles provide a store of glucose in the body of the dairy cow. In periods of low glucose availability or high glucose requirements (end of pregnancy and early lactation), these stores can be mobilized. Only the glycogen stores in the liver can directly support the blood glucose level, because the liver is able to convert glucose-6-phospate into glucose. Skeletal muscles lack the enzyme, glucose-6-phosphatase, necessary for this conversion, therefore glycogen stores from skeletal muscle do not directly contribute to the blood glucose level.[17] Because of the limited size of the glycogen stores in the liver, this glucose reserve is regarded as a minor contributor to the overall blood glucose regulation at the end of pregnancy and at the beginning of lactation.[18–20] Glycogenolysis and glycolysis in skeletal muscle are upregulated at the initiation of lactation. In this period the oxidation of glucose in skeletal muscle is shifted in the direction of lactate. Because lactate can be converted to glucose by the liver, this shift in glucose metabolism within the skeletal muscle means that the muscular glycogen stores contribute indirectly to the blood glucose levels.[11]

Glucose Removal

Glucose uptake: a facilitated process

Glucose cannot pass the plasma membrane surrounding the cells.[21] Glucose uptake takes place by 2 different processes: facilitated diffusion and cotransport. Cotransport is mediated by sodium-dependent glucose transporters (SGLT), and is driven by a difference in sodium concentration between the intracellular and extracellular fluid. The sodium-dependent glucose transporters are located at the epithelial cells of the small intestine and the tubular cells of the kidney.[22] Most cells, however, take up glucose by facilitated diffusion via glucose transporter (GLUT) molecules. The uptake of glucose through these GLUTs is basically driven by the difference in glucose concentration between the extracellular and intracellular fluid.[7,22] There are 13 different isoforms of the GLUTs, all of them having a specific tissue distribution, expression profile, and specific properties regarding sensitivity to hormones. The GLUT1 molecule is expressed in all tissues throughout the body and is responsible for basal glucose uptake.[22] Of all the GLUT molecules, GLUT4 is the only one that is responsible for the insulin-stimulated glucose uptake in skeletal muscle, heart, and adipose tissue.[22] The quantitatively most important glucose-consuming tissues are the skeletal muscles, the udder, and the gravid uterus.

Glucose uptake in skeletal muscle and adipose tissue

In skeletal muscle and adipose tissue, glucose is transported into the cells by GLUT1 and GLUT4 molecules. GLUT1 accounts for the basal glucose supply while GLUT4 mediates the insulin-stimulated glucose uptake.[22,23] On insulin stimulation, intracellularly stored GLUT4s are translocated to and fused with the plasma membrane. The increased number of GLUT4s on the cell membrane is responsible for the insulin-induced blood glucose reduction.[21] The previously mentioned lower insulin response of skeletal muscle and adipose tissue in ruminants compared with monogastric animals is partly due to the lower number and lower insulin-induced translocation of GLUT4s in these tissues in ruminants.[7,23] Another typical feature in ruminants is that adipose tissue prefers to use acetate, a volatile fatty acid produced in the forestomachs, as a substrate for lipogenesis. Monogastrics use glucose for this purpose.[5,24] Therefore, the adipose tissues in ruminants account for only a small part of the total insulin-induced glucose disposal.

To preserve sufficient glucose for fetal growth and development, homeorhetic changes in glucose metabolism take place throughout the body during pregnancy and lactation. At the level of the skeletal muscle and adipose tissue, glucose consumption is reduced. According to Komatsu and colleagues,[25] GLUT4 mRNA expression was not altered in adipose tissue or skeletal muscle during lactation or the dry period. A recent study using Western blot analysis of skeletal muscle, however, revealed that GLUT4 content was reduced by 40% by the fourth week of lactation in comparison with the GLUT4 content during the dry period,[11] suggesting a posttranscriptional regulation of GLUT4 mRNA in the skeletal muscle to reduce muscular glucose uptake in early lactation.

In adipose tissue, expression and protein content of GLUT1 and GLUT4 are minimal during peak lactation, and increase at the end of lactation to remain elevated during the dry period.[25–27] This expression profile gives rise to a decreased basal and insulin-stimulated glucose uptake by the adipose tissue in early lactation, thereby sparing glucose for milk production. From these studies, it seems that homeorhetic changes at the level of the glucose metabolism of skeletal muscle and adipose tissue are regulated by different mechanisms.

Glucose uptake by the uterus, placenta, and fetus

The GLUT molecules responsible for glucose uptake in the ovine placenta are of the GLUT1 and GLUT3 isoform type.[6] Only during the last trimester of pregnancy do uterine, fetal, and placental glucose requirements substantially increase the total glucose requirement of the dam.[28] In sheep, this is associated with an increased number of GLUT3.[6]

In cattle, placental expression of GLUT1, GLUT3, GLUT4, and GLUT5 has been demonstrated.[29–31] The expression of GLUT4 mRNA in placental tissue during early pregnancy is a new finding in dairy cows and had been demonstrated previously in humans. However, no direct evidence exists that insulin stimulates the glucose uptake by placenta in humans or cattle.[31,32]

Glucose uptake by the mammary gland

Glucose consumption of the mammary gland in dairy cows is responsible for 50% to 85% of whole-body glucose consumption, and amplifies the glucose demand by 2.5-fold at the third week of lactation in comparison with the demand during the end of the dry period.[8,22,33] Seventy-two grams of glucose are needed to produce 1 kg of milk.[34] This glucose is transported into the epithelial cells of the alveoli and is converted into lactose, creating an osmotic pressure that ultimately determines the amount of milk produced. The uptake of glucose into the bovine mammary gland is regulated by GLUT1, GLUT8, GLUT12, SGLT1, and SGLT2,[22] GLUT1 being the most important. Its expression and protein content are almost undetectable during the dry period and increase severalfold at the initiation of lactation.[22,25] The insulin independence regarding the mammary glucose uptake is further demonstrated by the absence of GLUT4 in the mammary gland.[25]

Glucose uptake by the liver

In nonruminants, the liver is an appreciable glucose consumer.[35] Because of the sophisticated carbohydrate metabolism, the main function of the liver in ruminants is glucose production, with production rates increasing up to 3600 g per day during peak lactation.[13] The GLUT isoforms responsible for the transport of glucose out of (and into) the hepatocytes are of the GLUT2 and GLUT5 type.[35]

INSULIN RESISTANCE, INSULIN SECRETION, AND DIABETES MELLITUS: A NECESSARY DISTINCTION

Definition of Insulin Resistance

Insulin resistance is defined as a state whereby a normal concentration of insulin induces a decreased biological response in the insulin-sensitive tissues.[36] Insulin resistance can furthermore be subdivided based on 2 distinct features: insulin sensitivity and insulin responsiveness. The maximal effect of insulin determines the insulin responsiveness. The concentration of insulin to elicit a half-maximal response determines the insulin sensitivity.[36] Insulin resistance can hence be attributed to a decrease in insulin responsiveness (a downward shift of the insulin dose-response curve), a decrease in insulin sensitivity (a rightward shift of the insulin dose-response curve), or both (**Fig. 2**).[36,37] Insulin resistance can be specific for certain tissues and for certain biological processes within these tissues.[36,38]

Insulin Secretion and Diabetes Mellitus

A further necessary distinction needs to be made between insulin resistance and deficient insulin secretion. Insulin resistance is determined by the response of the insulin-sensitive tissues to a normal concentration of insulin. Insulin secretion is determined by the secretory capacity of the pancreas in response to a factor that stimulates insulin secretion. Deficient insulin secretion does not entail an altered state of insulin resistance. The best way to explain this is by observing the difference between type 1 and type 2 diabetes in human medicine. Type 1 diabetes is caused by a destruction of the β cells of the pancreas, resulting in an absolute insulin deficiency. Patients

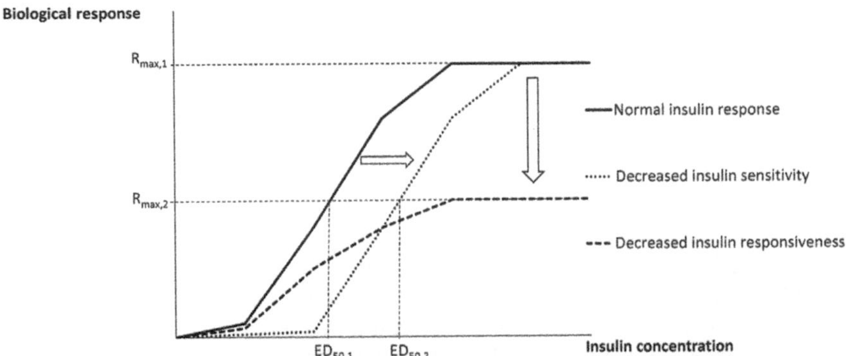

Fig. 2. The difference between insulin sensitivity and insulin responsiveness. The normal insulin response is characterized by a maximal biological effect ($R_{max,1}$) and an insulin concentration to elicit a half-maximal effect ($ED_{50,1}$). A decreased insulin sensitivity is visualized by a right shift of the normal curve and is characterized by a normal maximal biological effect ($R_{max,1}$) while an increased insulin concentration is needed to elicit half of the maximal effect ($ED_{50,2}$). A decreased insulin responsiveness is visualized by a downshift of the normal curve and is characterized by a decreased maximal biological effect ($R_{max,2}$) while a normal insulin concentration is needed to elicit a half-maximal effect ($ED_{50,1}$). (*Adapted from* Kahn CR. Insulin resistance, insulin insensitivity, and insulin unresponsiveness: a necessary distinction. Metabolism 1978;27(12 Suppl 2):1893–902; with permission.)

with type 1 diabetes have no insulin secretion but can have normal insulin sensitivity and responsiveness of their tissues.[39]

The most common form of type 2 diabetes is caused by a combination of insulin resistance and a relative deficiency of insulin secretion. In the early phase of the pathophysiology of type 2 diabetes mellitus, insulin resistance occurs but the pancreas compensates for this by increasing the secretion of insulin, giving rise to a secondary hyperinsulinemia. If the insulin resistance is not ameliorated, the pancreas may become exhausted, which may lead to β cells failing to compensate for the increased insulin resistance. Relative to the degree of insulin resistance, the pancreas cannot produce enough insulin (relative insulin deficiency) and levels of blood glucose rise, thus type 2 diabetes develops.[39–41] Insulin secretion in type 2 diabetes can be normal, but is insufficient to compensate for the higher degree of peripheral insulin resistance.

Diabetes mellitus has been described in young cattle and dairy cows.[42,43] The role of insulin resistance in the development of diabetes in cattle is unknown, but diabetes mellitus is considered to be a rare endocrine disease in dairy cows owing to its irreversible nature. By contrast, the insulin-secretory capacity of the pancreas seems to be influenced by NEFAs in dairy cows. Bossaert and colleagues[44] demonstrated a negative impact of chronically elevated NEFA levels on the insulin-secretory capacity of the pancreas. Similarly, lower insulin secretion following an intravenous glucose bolus has been demonstrated in ketonemic and starved cows.[45–47] Opsomer and colleagues[48] demonstrated blunted insulin secretion in cows suffering from cystic ovarian disease, suggesting a role of insulin in the pathogenesis of this ovarian disease in dairy cows.

EFFECT OF INSULIN RESISTANCE IN DIFFERENT TISSUES

Insulin elicits different effects on the carbohydrate, lipid, and protein metabolism of different insulin-sensitive tissues (**Table 1**).

Table 1
Overview of insulin effects on different metabolic pathways in the different insulin-sensitive tissues

Tissue	Metabolic Pathway	Insulin Effect	Authors,Ref. Year
Liver	Glycogenesis	Stimulation	Brockman & Laarveld,[5] 1986
	Ketogenesis	Suppression	Brockman & Laarveld,[5] 1986
	Triglyceride synthesis	Stimulation	Andersen et al,[49] 2002
	Gluconeogenesis	Suppression	Brockman & Laarveld,[5] 1986
	Glycogenolysis	Suppression	Brockman & Laarveld,[5] 1986
	Glycolysis	Stimulation	Hayirli,[4] 2006
	Protein synthesis	Stimulation	Sjaastad et al,[50] 2010
	Protein degradation	Suppression	Sjaastad et al,[50] 2010
Skeletal muscle	Glucose uptake	Stimulation	Brockman & Laarveld,[5] 1986
	Ketone body use	Stimulation	Brockman & Laarveld,[5] 1986
	Protein synthesis	Stimulation	Brockman & Laarveld,[5] 1986
	Protein degradation	Suppression	Brockman & Laarveld,[5] 1986
	Glycolysis	Stimulation	Hayirli,[4] 2006
	Glycogenolysis	Suppression	Hayirli,[4] 2006
	Glycogenesis	Stimulation	Hayirli,[4] 2006
Adipose tissue	Lipolysis	Suppression	Brockman & Laarveld,[5] 1986
	Lipogenesis	Stimulation	Brockman & Laarveld,[5] 1986
	Glucose uptake	Stimulation	Brockman & Laarveld,[5] 1986

Besides these effects on glucose, amino acid, and lipid metabolism, insulin has some additional functions on several tissues throughout the body. In general, insulin is known to stimulate cell proliferation and differentiation.[40] In the ovary, insulin stimulates steroidogenesis and the proliferation of granulosa cells, and hence influences follicular growth.[51,52] Lower peripheral insulin levels have been associated with the development of ovarian cysts in postpartum dairy cows.[53]

As previously mentioned, the development of insulin resistance may be specific for a certain metabolic pathway in a certain tissue. For dairy cows, the most important pathways that have an altered insulin response during the transition period are: glucose uptake by skeletal muscle and adipose tissue; lipogenesis and lipolysis in adipose tissue; gluconeogenesis in the liver; and protein metabolism of skeletal muscle. The role of insulin and insulin resistance in the adaptation of these metabolic pathways during the transition period are further explored here.

Insulin-Stimulated Glucose Uptake by Skeletal Muscle and Adipose Tissue

General aspects of insulin-stimulated glucose uptake

Insulin-stimulated glucose uptake is probably the most intensively studied metabolic pathway of insulin in dairy cows. Based on the effect of insulin on this pathway, conclusions are drawn for other metabolic pathways, which may give rise to incorrect or at least insufficiently substantiated conclusions. In humans, skeletal muscles account for 80% of the insulin-stimulated whole-body glucose uptake, whereas adipose tissues contribute to only 5%.[40] In dairy cows, where acetate is the major precursor of triglyceride synthesis, the skeletal muscles account for most of the insulin-stimulated whole-body glucose uptake.[23] Therefore, glucose uptake in adipose tissue is limited in dairy cows.[5] The fact that dairy cows are in a lactating and/or pregnant state means that a considerable amount of glucose is taken up by the pregnant uterus or the lactating udder. One should consider this carefully when comparing glucose-uptake experiments in cows at different stages of lactation or in cows with a different level of milk production.

Insulin resistance for glucose uptake by skeletal muscles and adipose tissues is a well-known feature in pregnant women, obese people, and people suffering from type 2 or gestational diabetes.[40,54–57] Some of these metabolic states in humans show remarkable similarities with insulin resistance in cattle.[58]

Insulin resistance as homeorhetic mechanism during pregnancy and lactation

Nowadays it is generally accepted that dairy cows are insulin resistant at the end of gestation and in early lactation. These homeorhetic adaptations are necessary to ensure a sufficient glucose supply for the gravid uterus and lactating mammary gland in support of the growing offspring, both prenatally and postnatally.[6] The adaptation toward an insulin-resistant state seems to be conserved in mammals among different species.

Different studies have been performed to assess insulin resistance in glucose metabolism during pregnancy and lactation in ruminants, and these are summarized in **Table 2**.

Overall, most of these studies confirm the state of increased insulin resistance in glucose metabolism during early lactation. The onset of this lactational insulin resistance may be traced to the end of pregnancy.

Table 2
Different studies assessing insulin resistance in ruminants during lactation and pregnancy

Authors,[Ref.] Year	Species	Test	Conclusion
Vernon et al,[59] 1990	Sheep	HEC test with measurement of arteriovenous glucose difference in the hindlimb	Decreased sensitivity and decreased responsiveness of insulin-stimulated glucose uptake in skeletal muscles of lactating animals vs nonlactating and nonpregnant animals
Vernon & Taylor,[60] 1988	Sheep	In vitro culture adipose tissue	Decreased responsiveness and decreased sensitivity of insulin-stimulated glucose uptake in adipose tissue of lactating sheep vs nonlactating and nonpregnant animals
Debras et al,[61] 1989	Goat	HEC test	Decreased responsiveness of whole-body insulin-stimulated glucose uptake in goats in early lactation vs late lactating and dry goats
Kerestes et al,[46] 2009	Dairy cow	IVITT	Lower insulin-stimulated blood glucose reduction in early lactating dairy cows vs dry and midlactating cows
Petterson et al,[62] 1993	Sheep	HEC test	Decreased insulin sensitivity of whole-body insulin-stimulated glucose uptake in late pregnant sheep vs nonpregnant and nonlactating sheep
Ji et al,[26] 2012	Dairy cow	In vitro culture adipose tissue	Reduced insulin signaling (IRS-1 tyrosine phosphorylation) in adipose tissue of early lactating vs dry dairy cows

Abbreviations: HEC, hyperinsulinemic euglycemic clamp; IVITT, intravenous insulin tolerance test; IRS-1, insulin receptor substrate 1.

Adipose tissue and its derivatives

The adipose tissue and its derivatives undoubtedly play a crucial role in the determination and modulation of insulin sensitivity in the glucose metabolism of dairy cows. A first indication in this regard was given by McCann and Reimers in 1985.[63] Using the intravenous insulin tolerance test (IVITT), they demonstrated a lower reduction of glucose in obese heifers when compared with lean heifers.

In the last decade, different researchers have focused on the role of NEFAs in the insulin sensitivity of dairy cattle. In experimental studies using nonpregnant and nonlactating dairy cows, an artificial elevation of circulating NEFAs following a fasting period or by the intravenous administration of a tallow infusion has been shown to cause an impaired insulin-stimulated glucose uptake by insulin-sensitive tissues.[47,64,65] On the other hand, reduction of the NEFA load by means of abomasal delivery of nicotinic acid improved the insulin-stimulated glucose uptake.[66]

Other studies provided evidence for the extrapolation of these experimental results in practice. Overfeeding dairy cows during the dry period provoked an excessive condition score at parturition.[67] In the dry period, these overfed cows showed higher peripheral levels of insulin in response to a glucose bolus, which may point to a higher insulin resistance of the peripheral tissues eliciting a secondary hyperinsulinemia at that time. In the subsequent lactation, these overfed cows showed prolonged elevated levels of NEFAs and a lower glucose clearance after an intravenous glucose tolerance test (IVGTT), indicating a higher degree of insulin resistance.[68] In dairy cows suffering from different degrees of fatty liver, NEFA levels were negatively correlated with the insulin-stimulated reduction in blood glucose after an insulin challenge.[69] In a study using cows suffering from different forms of ketonemia, the cows with chronically elevated concentrations of β-hydroxybutyrate (BHB) (more than 1 mmol/L from 2 days preceding calving until 7 days following calving) showed a higher insulin resistance in the glucose metabolism at their peripheral tissues. In the same study, a higher concentration of NEFAs was significantly correlated with a lower insulin secretion.[46] These findings demonstrate an important role of NEFAs in the development of insulin resistance.

Underlying molecular mechanisms of fatty acid–induced insulin resistance are as yet unstudied in dairy cows but may be extrapolated from human medicine. The first mechanism is called the Randle cycle,[70] or glucose-fatty acid cycle, which involves the biochemical mechanisms that control substrate (glucose or fatty acids) use in skeletal muscle, heart, liver, and pancreas. The Randle cycle postulates that when availability of fatty acids is abundant, the oxidation of the latter inhibits the use of glucose as substrate for the cellular metabolism. This process is mediated by different intracellular pathways: inhibition of pyruvate dehydrogenase, phosphofructokinase activity, and hexokinase activity, and decreased GLUT4 translocation in skeletal muscle.[70] In addition, NEFAs induce the phosphorylation of insulin receptor substrate 1 (IRS-1) on serine residues. The serine phosphorylation of IRS-1 leads to a decrease in insulin-induced tyrosine phosphorylation of IRS-1, which is necessary for normal activation of the insulin signaling cascade.[71]

Besides NEFAs, other (unknown) factors originating from the adipose tissues also affect insulin-stimulated glucose uptake. As demonstrated in obese sheep, insulin sensitivity is decreased despite their NEFA levels being equally as high as those in lean sheep.[72] In human medicine, the metabolic syndrome links visceral obesity, insulin resistance, dyslipidemia, and hypertension.[57] Adipose tissue plays a central role in the development of the metabolic syndrome by increasing the production of proinflammatory adipokines (tumor necrosis factor [TNF]-α, interleukin [IL]-6, monocyte chemoattractant protein [MCP]-1) and decreasing the production of the anti-inflammatory adipokine, adiponectin.[73] The final result of this altered production of adipokines is that obese people are considered to be in a proinflammatory state with the adipose tissue as primary site of inflammation.[73] In dairy cows, the endocrine function of adipose tissue has been confirmed by demonstrating mRNA expression for TNF-α, IL-6, MCP-1, leptin, adiponectin, haptoglobin, visfatin, and resistin.[27,74–78] The effect of these adipokines on insulin-stimulated glucose uptake by the skeletal muscle and adipose tissue is unknown in cattle, with the exception of TNF-α. Prolonged exposure to TNF-α by means of a series of subcutaneous injections induced insulin resistance in young steers and increased triglyceride concentration in the liver of dairy cows.[79–81] Ohtsuka and colleagues[69] concluded that cows suffering from fatty liver had higher serum concentrations of NEFA, were more insulin resistant, and had higher serum TNF-α activity. These observations, together with the study of O'Boyle and colleagues[82] in which it was shown that overconditioned cows have higher plasma TNF-α concentrations, lead the authors to hypothesize that obesity in dairy cows may lead to a state of chronic low-grade inflammation, causing insulin resistance and metabolic disorders, and rendering these cows to hyperinflammatory reactions in cases where infections occur.

Genetic influences on the effect of insulin on glucose metabolism

As in humans, in cattle there also seems to be a genetic component that determines the sensitivity to insulin resistance. Cows with a high genetic merit for milk production (North American cows) are stated to be more insulin resistant than cows with a low genetic merit for milk production (New Zealand cows).[83] In an attempt to identify a gene that may influence the effect of insulin on glucose metabolism, Balogh and colleagues[84] performed IVGTTs in dairy cows 10 to 15 days postpartum. Differences in the growth hormone Alu1 genotype suggested (nonsignificantly) that heterozygous (leucine-valine) dairy cows suffered a higher degree of insulin resistance in comparison with homozygous (leucine-leucine) dairy cows. These studies suggest that the genetic component modulating insulin resistance might be subtle, and may be overwhelmed by other factors contributing to the determination of insulin resistance.

The (epi)genetic determination of insulin sensitivity has been suggested by Bossaert and colleagues.[85] Performing IVGTTs and IVITTs, they demonstrated that female Holstein Friesian calves (bred for milk production) as early as age 15 days had higher insulin secretion and lower glucose clearance in comparison with female Belgian Blue calves (bred for beef production), thus suggesting that Holstein Friesian calves are more insulin resistant than Belgian Blue calves.

The apparent "genetic" differences in insulin resistance for glucose metabolism may be determined by genetic or epigenetic differences between animals. Further investigation is required to define genes that influence insulin resistance and to describe epigenetic effects on these genes.

Release of NEFA from adipose tissue

NEFA release from adipose tissue is the result of the combined effect of lipolysis of triglycerides and reesterification (lipogenesis) of NEFA in the adipocytes.[86] Both pathways are influenced by insulin. In early lactation, blood NEFA levels increase owing to increased lipolysis and decreased lipogenesis, partly mediated by reduced serum insulin concentrations during this time.[86] Faulkner and Pollock[87] and Petterson and colleagues[88] demonstrated a state of insulin resistance of lipid metabolism in pregnant and lactating sheep. Research is limited regarding insulin resistance of lipolytic and lipogenic pathways in the adipose tissue of dairy cows.

Lipolysis and lipogenesis are metabolic pathways influenced by different hormones, and changes in these pathways differ between different fat depots (subcutaneous and abdominal) in the same animal. In sheep, omental adipocytes show higher rates of basal and catecholamine-stimulated lipolysis in comparison with subcutaneous adipose tissue.[89] In dairy cows, subcutaneous adipose tissue shows higher rates of catecholamine-stimulated lipolysis and higher rates of lipogenesis in comparison with omental adipose tissue.[90] This situation might result from a different degree of expression and phosphorylation of hormone-sensitive lipase.[91] On the other hand, Hostens and colleagues[92] recently showed that in cows suffering from left displacement of the abomasum, the fatty acid profile of the circulating NEFAs was more closely associated with the fatty acid profile of the abdominal fat than the subcutaneous fat, suggesting that under these conditions cows preferentially break down the abdominal fat. More research on the metabolic properties and insulin resistance of the different fat depots is needed to quantify the relative contribution of the different fat depots to the NEFA level postpartum, and to identify the locations of fat deposition that are associated with the greatest negative impact on adaptation during the transition period.

Glucose output from the liver

The output of glucose from the liver is the result of 2 metabolic processes: gluconeogenesis and glycogenolysis. Quantitatively, glycogenolysis is of minor importance because glycogen stores in the liver are rather limited and are quickly exhausted in periods of high glucose requirement.[18–20] Gluconeogenesis is by far the most important metabolic pathway in ruminants, and has to be tightly regulated. Regulation occurs through both nutritional (substrate supply) and hormonal factors (insulin, glucagon, somatotropin, cortisol).[8,93]

The net effect of insulin on the liver is a decrease in glucose release into the blood, which results from an inhibitory effect of insulin on glycogenolysis and gluconeogenesis.[40] The inhibitory effect of insulin on gluconeogenesis is due to both direct and indirect effects. Insulin directly inhibits key enzymes in the gluconeogenic pathway while indirectly reducing the availability of glucogenic precursors influencing the peripheral tissues (stimulation of protein synthesis, inhibition of lipolysis).[93]

Insulin decreases gluconeogenesis but increases the proportional use of propionate as substrate for the gluconeogenesis.[94] This process can be explained by the inhibitory effect of insulin on protein, glucose, and triglyceride catabolism, and the stimulatory effect of insulin on protein, glucose, and triglyceride anabolism, thereby decreasing the amount of circulating amino acids, lactate, and glycerol and, thus, decreasing their availability for use in gluconeogenesis. The supply of propionate is mainly regulated by feed intake, so that its availability increases relative to the other substrates.

In humans suffering from type 2 diabetes, the liver is resistant to the inhibitory effect of insulin on hepatic glucose production. This resistance is responsible for the hyperglycemia observed in persons with type 2 diabetes.[40] In lactating dairy cows, such an insulin-resistant state of the hepatic glucose output would not result in hyperglycemia, because of the high glucose uptake by the mammary gland. However, pregnancy and lactation do not alter the insulin response of the hepatic glucose production in sheep and goats.[61,62,87]

Protein metabolism of skeletal muscle, liver, and other peripheral tissues

Insulin influences protein metabolism by stimulation of protein synthesis and inhibition of protein degradation in skeletal muscle and other tissues. Very few studies report on the insulin sensitivity and insulin responsiveness of these metabolic processes. Using the hyperinsulinemic euglycemic euaminoacidemic clamp test in lactating and dry goats, Tesseraud and colleagues[95] found that there was no stimulatory effect of insulin on protein synthesis but that inhibition of protein degradation by insulin was enhanced in early lactation. This observation seems to be in conflict with the findings that peripheral tissues (skeletal muscle) decrease amino acid use and increase amino acid mobilization in early lactation.[11,96] However, early lactation is characterized by low insulin levels, which leads to reduced protein synthesis in skin, skeletal muscle, and other peripheral tissues,[96] and decreased inhibition of protein degradation. The net result is an increased flow of amino acids to the mammary gland and the liver for synthesis of milk protein and hepatic gluconeogenesis.[11]

QUANTITATIVE ASPECTS OF GLUCOSE METABOLISM

The total glucose requirement per day is the result of the combination of:

- Basal glucose requirement (1.57 mol/d)
- Glucose requirement of the gravid uterus (0.10 mol/kg fetus/d)
- Glucose requirement of the mammary gland (0.4 mol/kg milk)

The basal glucose requirement refers to the glucose required for the maintenance of basal functions of tissues in the body (brain, kidneys, intestines, skeletal muscle, heart, adipose tissue, intestines, liver, and so forth) and is minimal in early lactation (predicted average 1.57 mol/d).[93,97] Data from Rose and colleagues[98] indicate that basal glucose availability increases in midlactating dairy cows (calculated at 2.6 mol/d at 205 days in milk [DIM]), probably because of the accretion of energy in adipose tissue.

The glucose requirement of the gravid uterus may be predicted as described by Overton[97] using quantitative data of glucose uptake by the gravid uterus in beef cows.[99] Average glucose uptake by the gravid uterus (total of uterus, placenta, and fetus) was 0.10 mol/kg fetus/d.[99] By using this predicted glucose uptake and the predicted weight of the fetus in dairy cows during the last 90 days of pregnancy as described by Bell and colleagues,[100] it is possible to give a rough estimate of the glucose uptake by the gravid uterus in dairy cows.

The glucose requirement for milk synthesis is much better described in the literature. In vivo estimates of glucose requirements for milk synthesis give values of 72 g glucose per kg milk produced.[34] This figure agrees well with the theoretically predicted value of 68.4 g per kg milk using a conversion efficiency of glucose into lactose from 73% to 74%.[93] It seems that efficiency of glucose conversion does not change with increasing milk production up to 35 kg milk per day.[93]

The predicted total glucose requirement (in grams) per day during the last 30 days before parturition and the first 60 DIM is depicted in **Fig. 3**. Assumptions made to calculate this graph were that basal glucose requirements are the same in the dry period and during the first 60 DIM, and that efficiency of milk production is the same in early lactation and peak lactation.

The glucose requirements increase sharply after parturition as milk yield increases steeply during this time, and are doubled by 7 days after parturition. For a cow producing 42 kg of milk (see **Fig. 3**), glucose requirements are more than 3 kg per day, 90% of this glucose being preserved for lactose production.

This total glucose requirement can be divided into glucose uptake by insulin-sensitive tissues (skeletal muscle, heart, and adipose tissue) and insulin-insensitive tissues (mammary gland, uterus, brain, kidney, and so forth). Only 8% of the total peripheral glucose uptake in midlactating dairy cows producing 26 kg milk is mediated by insulin.[98] In humans, 25% of total glucose uptake is insulin dependent.[40] The large difference between humans and dairy cows is due to the insulin-independent glucose uptake by the mammary gland of the latter.[98]

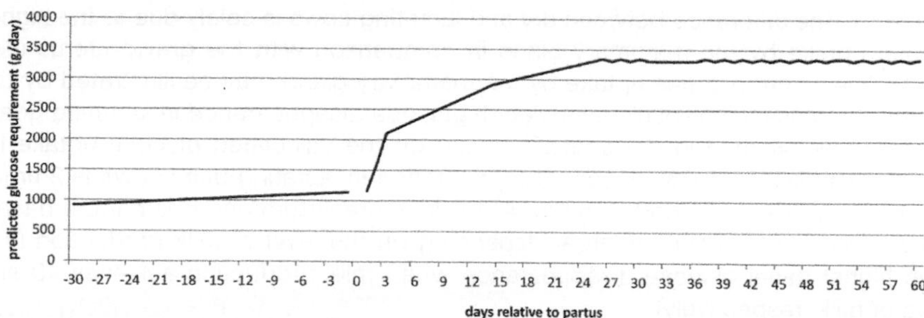

Fig. 3. Predicted total glucose requirement in grams per day during the last 30 days before parturition and the first 60 days in milk (42 kg milk). No prediction was made for the day of parturition because of the lack of data concerning glucose requirement on that day. Glucose requirement was calculated as described by Overton.[97] (*Adapted from* Overton TR. Substrate utilization for hepatic gluconeogenesis in the transition dairy cow. Proceedings of the 1998 Cornell Nutrition Conference for Feed Manufacturers. 1998. p. 237–46.)

HOW TO MEASURE INSULIN RESISTANCE

Important Considerations

To measure insulin sensitivity in cows it is important to keep in mind that in dairy cows, the majority of the glucose disappearance occurs independently of insulin, because of the massive glucose drain to the lactating mammary gland and the gravid uterus. In the basal (ie, non–insulin-stimulated) state, the estimated insulin-independent glucose uptake is 84% and 92% in dry and lactating cows (**Fig. 4**, calculations based on

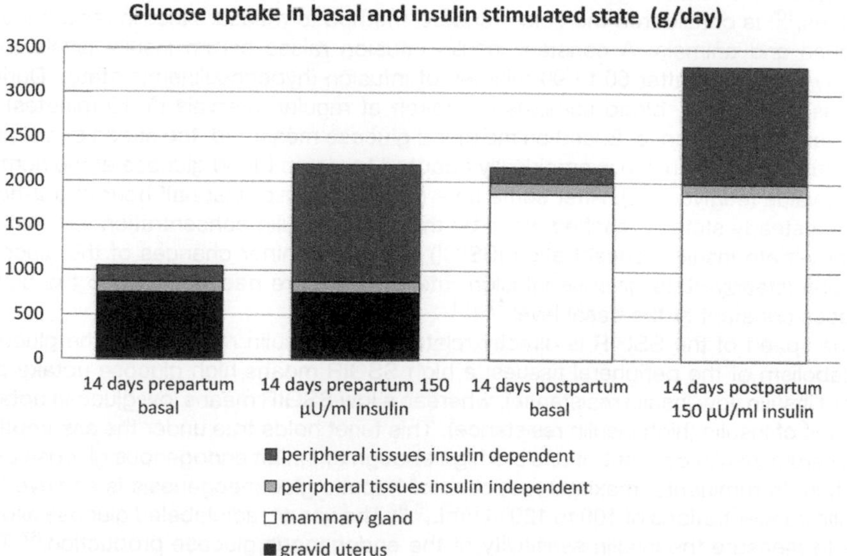

Fig. 4. Estimated glucose uptake (g/d) by different tissues in the basal and insulin-stimulated (150 µU/mL) state in dairy cows 14 days prepartum and 14 days postpartum (26 kg milk) with the same insulin sensitivity (assuming that insulin-dependent glucose uptake is equal in prepartum and postpartum cows), based on calculations as described by Overton[97] and data of Rose and colleagues.[98]

Refs.[97,98]). The difference between dry and lactating cows is solely due to the higher glucose uptake by the mammary gland in comparison with the gravid uterus (see **Fig. 4**). The higher glucose uptake by the mammary gland may be illustrated by the fact that the basal (non–insulin-stimulated) glucose disappearance in lactating goats is 3 times higher than in dry goats.[61] Based on the calculated glucose uptake by the different tissues, basal glucose disappearance in lactating dairy cows is 2 times higher than in the dry period (see **Fig. 4**: 14 days prepartum and postpartum basal). This difference may become larger depending on the level of milk production (3–4 times higher basal glucose disappearance when milk production achieves 40 and 50 kg of milk, respectively).

In **Fig. 4**, the estimated glucose uptake is depicted if one stimulates glucose uptake by an intravenous insulin infusion reaching a serum insulin steady-state concentration of 150 μU/mL, assuming (not necessarily true) that there is no difference in insulin sensitivity in dry versus lactating cows (see **Fig. 4**: in the insulin-stimulated state, the insulin-dependent glucose uptake by the peripheral tissues is of the same order in lactating and dry cows). By infusion of insulin, hepatic and renal gluconeogenesis are inhibited, thus glucose infusion has to take over the body's total glucose provision. This process would lead to a higher infusion rate in lactating cows (see **Fig. 4**: 3300 g/d vs 2200 g/d in dry cows) because basal glucose turnover is higher. To compare insulin sensitivity between dry and lactating cows or lactating cows with different milk yield, it is important to consider this difference in basal glucose disappearance, otherwise the insulin sensitivity of lactating cows may be overestimated. By infusion of radiolabeled glucose in the basal state, it is possible to estimate and correct for this difference in basal glucose disappearance.[61,98]

Hyperinsulinemic Euglycemic Clamp Test

The hyperinsulinemic euglycemic clamp (HEC) test, as described by Defronzo and colleagues,[101] is considered the gold-standard method to measure insulin resistance in humans and animals. A constant insulin infusion raises serum insulin levels to a steady-state level after 60 to 90 minutes of infusion (hyperinsulinemic state). During the insulin infusion, blood samples are taken at regular intervals (5–10 minutes) to measure blood glucose. Based on the blood glucose measured, the speed of a simultaneous glucose infusion is empirically adapted to clamp blood glucose at the normal basal value (euglycemic). After some time (the last hour or last half hour of a 2-hour test), a steady state is reached whereby the serum insulin concentration is constant (steady-state insulin concentration [SSIC]) and no or minor changes of the glucose infusion (steady-state glucose infusion rate [SSGIR]) are needed to keep the blood glucose constant at the basal level.[37,101]

The speed of the SSGIR is directly related to the insulin response of the glucose metabolism of the peripheral tissues: a high SSGIR means high glucose uptake per unit of insulin (low insulin resistance), whereas a low SSGIR means low glucose uptake per unit of insulin (high insulin resistance). This tenet holds true under the assumption that serum insulin concentrations are high enough to inhibit endogenous glucose production. In ruminants, maximal reduction of hepatic gluconeogenesis is achieved at insulin concentrations of 100 to 120 μU/mL.[5,62] The use of radiolabeled glucose allows one to measure the insulin sensitivity of the endogenous glucose production.[37] The assessment of the insulin response may be based on a single insulin infusion, or complete dose-response curves may be generated by using different insulin infusions consecutively.[37] Maximal insulin-stimulated whole-body glucose disposal in dairy cows is achieved with insulin infusions of 5 to 10 mU/kg/min and serum insulin concentrations of 500 to 1000 μU/mL.[102–104] Using data from HEC tests, one may assess insulin sensitivity by calculating an insulin sensitivity index (ISI). Different calculations have been described:

ISI = SSGIR/SSIC[105]

ISI = SSGIR/(steady state glucose concentration $\times$ ΔI)[37]

where ΔI is the difference between SSIC and basal insulin concentration.

Measurements of NEFA during the HEC test may give an idea of the effect of insulin on lipolysis and lipogenesis, and hence may provide an indication of the degree of insulin resistance in adipose tissue.[102]

Major disadvantages of the HEC test are that it is time consuming (several hours for every insulin infusion), very intensive, expensive, and requires some experience to constantly adapt the glucose infusion rate to clamp the blood glucose at the basal level. Another drawback is that insulin response is measured at supraphysiologic insulin levels, limiting the extrapolation to physiologic insulin concentrations. Furthermore, the HEC test is not suitable for performance under field conditions or for use in studies with a large number of animals.[37]

Intravenous Glucose Tolerance Test

The IVGTT is a more practical method to assess insulin resistance in dairy cows. After the intravenous infusion of a glucose bolus, blood samples are taken at regular intervals to determine glucose and insulin concentrations. The amount of glucose infused differs between studies from 150 mg/kg (eg, Ref.[68]), 250 mg/kg (eg, Ref.[65]) to 500 mg/kg (eg, Ref.[46]), as does the time frame of sampling: 180 minutes (eg, Ref.[65]) or 60 minutes (eg, Ref.[44]). The IVGTT is easy to perform in practice, although the interpretation of the obtained data requires some insight into glucose and insulin metabolism.

Blood glucose levels during an IVGTT are derived from the glucose bolus, endogenous glucose production in liver and kidney, glucose uptake by the intestines, renal glucose excretion, glucose uptake by the mammary gland and/or the gravid uterus, and glucose uptake by the insulin-sensitive tissues (skeletal muscle and adipose tissue).[65,85] Blood insulin levels during an IVGTT are the result of insulin secretion by the pancreas in response to the glucose bolus, and the elimination of insulin by the liver. The combination of these physiologic processes results in the typical profile of insulin and glucose concentrations during an IVGTT.

Based on the data obtained during an IVGTT, calculations may be done to identify differences between animals. The following parameters may be calculated[65,85]:

- Clearance rate of glucose and insulin
- Area under the curve for both glucose and insulin
- Time to reach half of the maximal glucose and insulin concentration
- Time to reach the basal glucose and insulin concentration

Insulin resistance can be identified when glucose clearance is low, the area under the curve for glucose is high, and the time to reach half of the maximal glucose concentration and the time to reach basal glucose concentration are high. Exact interpretation of the test implies normal insulin secretion from the pancreas following administration of the glucose bolus, and assumes similar insulin secretion between animals. However, the latter is not always the case. Therefore, a modified IVGTT was developed whereby an additional insulin or tolbutamide bolus is given 20 minutes after the administration of the glucose bolus to evoke an artificial elevation of the blood insulin levels, which increases the comparability between subjects.[37]

Besides the aforementioned calculations, data from the IVGTT may be entered in a mathematical model, the "minimal model" as developed by Bergman and colleagues.[106] The major advantage of this model is that it simultaneously models insulin and glucose concentrations and uses both models to assess the insulin sensitivity.[37] A computer program, MINMOD, has been developed to facilitate calculations.[107] Using this program, the following parameters may be calculated[37,107,108]:

- Si or insulin sensitivity: fractional glucose disappearance per unit insulin
- Sg or glucose effectiveness at zero insulin: the ability of glucose to stimulate its own disappearance and inhibit endogenous glucose production
- AIRg or the acute insulin response to glucose: the increase in insulin after the glucose bolus
- β-cell function: insulin secretory capacity of the pancreatic β-cells
- DI or disposition index: a measure of β-cell function in relation to insulin sensitivity

The IVGTT has been widely used in dairy cows; however, it has only recently been compared with the HEC test in dry cows on a different feeding level before and after fasting. Results indicated good agreement between these methods.[47] The applicability of the minimal model in dairy cows requires some additional investigation.

Intravenous Insulin Tolerance Test

The IVITT consists of an intravenous bolus injection of insulin and subsequent blood sampling at regular intervals for the measurement of blood glucose. In dairy cows, insulin doses of 0.02 U/kg (eg, Ref.[63]), 0.05 U/kg (eg, Ref.[64]) and 0.1 U/kg (eg, Ref.[65]) have been used. The following parameters may be calculated using data obtained from IVITT[65,85]:

- Glucose clearance rate following the administration of the insulin bolus
- Insulin-stimulated reduction in blood glucose (% of basal glucose)
- Area under the curve for glucose following the administration of the insulin bolus

The larger the insulin-stimulated reduction in blood glucose and glucose clearance, the higher the insulin response of the glucose metabolism of the peripheral tissues.

Major disadvantages of the IVITT include the elicited hypoglycemia, which may generate counterregulatory mechanisms that might confound the estimation of insulin sensitivity. Furthermore, potentially dangerous neurologic and cardiovascular side effects of the hypoglycemia may arise if an overdose of insulin is given.[37,109]

Surrogate Indexes for Insulin Resistance

Several surrogate indexes to estimate the level of insulin resistance have been developed in human medicine and have subsequently been copied for use in veterinary medicine. The major purpose of their use is to predict insulin resistance of the peripheral tissues based on a single blood sample after an overnight fast.[37] The following surrogate indexes have been proposed[37,84,110–112]:

$$\text{HOMA-IR} = [\text{glucose (mmol/ml)} \times \text{insulin } (\mu\text{U/ml})]/22.5$$

$$\text{QUICKI} = 1/[\log \text{glucose (mg/dl)} + \log \text{insulin } (\mu\text{U/ml})]$$

$$\text{RQUICKI} = 1/[\log \text{glucose (mg/dl)} + \log \text{insulin } (\mu\text{U/ml}) + \log \text{NEFA (mmol/l)}]$$

$$\text{RQUICKI}_{\text{BHB}} = 1/[\log \text{glucose (mg/dl)} + \log \text{insulin } (\mu\text{U/ml}) + \log \text{NEFA (mmol/l)} + \log \text{BHB (mmol/l)}]$$

$$\text{QUICKI}_{\text{glycerol}} = 1/[\log \text{glucose (mg/dl)} + \log \text{insulin } (\mu\text{U/ml}) + \log \text{glycerol } (\mu\text{mol/l})]$$

HOMA, or homeostasis model assessment, is a mathematical model that predicts the fasting glucose and insulin concentration of an individual using the best possible combination of insulin resistance and insulin secretion. The mathematical model can be simplified to the formula of HOMA-IR, or homeostasis model of insulin resistance, using the formula shown.[37] The lower the HOMA-IR value, the lower the insulin resistance of an individual.

The QUICKIs, or quantitative insulin sensitivity check indexes, are mathematical calculations based on the logarithmic transformation of the fasting glucose and insulin concentrations including some other blood parameters (NEFA, BHB, glycerol). These indexes have been proved to be very useful in human medicine.[37] QUICKI indexes may be interpreted such that lower values are indicative of higher insulin resistance of an individual.

Some of the surrogate indexes have been adopted in veterinary medicine and have been used to predict insulin resistance in dairy cows. However, the applicability of these indexes requires further investigation. Indeed, the fasting state in humans is crucial if one is to obtain reliable information on insulin resistance derived from these surrogate indexes.[37] In dairy cows, with the exception of suckling calves, it is impossible to achieve a fasting state whereby insulin and glucose levels are in a balanced state. In addition, the glucose, insulin, NEFA, BHB, and glycerol levels of dairy cows can change tremendously at the end of pregnancy and during early lactation, thereby reducing the suitability of these indexes to be applied during these periods. Any kind of stress situation during sampling can furthermore lead to important changes in glucose, NEFA, and insulin, which will affect the interpretation of the insulin index.[113] Besides these in vivo considerations regarding the application of surrogate indexes, laboratory techniques may also affect their application. Analysis of insulin concentrations in bovine serum requires the application of analytical procedures specifically developed for bovine insulin. Because cross-reactivity with human insulin is not 100%, it is advised to use these bovine-specific kits to calculate the surrogate indexes for insulin sensitivity and thus allow comparison between different studies.[114]

Nevertheless, some of these indexes have been applied in different studies dealing with dairy cows.[46,47,84,115,116] Some studies reported similar changes in value for QUICKI, RQUICKI, $\text{RQUICKI}_{\text{BHB}}$, and parameters of glucose tolerance tests[84,85,103,104]; others, however, failed to support these observations.[46] The practical application of these techniques requires further validation in dairy cows.

Other Tests

More invasive tests may be used to assess the tissue-specific insulin response in skeletal muscle and adipose tissue.

Vernon and colleagues[59] determined the arteriovenous glucose difference in the hindlimb of lactating and nonlactating sheep using arterial and venous catheters during a HEC test to assess the insulin response of the hindlimb muscles.

Taking muscle biopsies during a HEC test gives the opportunity to study the activation of the intracellular insulin signaling cascade.[117] This approach opens the possibility to identify the signaling molecule that is responsible for inducing insulin resistance.

Besides in vivo testing, in vitro research of biopsies may provide information concerning the insulin response of specific metabolic pathways.

Short-term in vitro cultures of adipose tissue samples may render information about the insulin response of the lipolytic and lipogenic pathways in adipose tissue biopsies, and may provide dose-response curves to assess differences in insulin sensitivity and insulin responsiveness.[118,119]

Performing such studies in dairy cows would provide insight into the insulin response of the different metabolic pathways in the different insulin-sensitive tissues, and may help to identify the underlying pathogenesis of insulin resistance at the molecular level. However, these studies are time consuming, require experience of in vivo and in vitro techniques, and cannot be performed on a large scale.

REFERENCES

1. Aschenbach JR, Kristensen NB, Donkin SS, et al. Gluconeogenesis in dairy cows: the secret of making sweet milk from sour dough. IUBMB Life 2010; 62(12):869–77.
2. Annison EF, White RR. Glucose utilization in sheep. Biochem J 1961;80:162–9.
3. Kaske M, Elmahdi B, von Engelhardt W, et al. Insulin responsiveness of sheep, ponies, miniature pigs and camels: results of hyperinsulinemic clamps using porcine insulin. J Comp Physiol B 2001;171(7):549–56.
4. Hayirli A. The role of exogenous insulin in the complex of hepatic lipidosis and ketosis associated with insulin resistance phenomenon in postpartum dairy cattle. Vet Res Commun 2006;30(7):749–74.
5. Brockman RP, Laarveld B. Hormonal-regulation of metabolism in ruminants—a review. Livest Prod Sci 1986;14(4):313–34.
6. Bell AW, Bauman DE. Adaptations of glucose metabolism during pregnancy and lactation. J Mammary Gland Biol Neoplasia 1997;2(3):265–78.
7. Sasaki S. Mechanism of insulin action on glucose metabolism in ruminants. Anim Sci J 2002;73(6):423–33.
8. Drackley JK, Overton TR, Douglas GN. Adaptations of glucose and long-chain fatty acid metabolism in liver of dairy cows during the periparturient period. J Dairy Sci 2001;84:E100–12.
9. Slyter LL. Influence of acidosis on rumen function. J Anim Sci 1976;43(4): 910–29.
10. Nocek JE. Bovine acidosis: implications on laminitis. J Dairy Sci 1997;80(5): 1005–28.
11. Kuhla B, Nurnberg G, Albrecht D, et al. Involvement of skeletal muscle protein, glycogen, and fat metabolism in the adaptation on early lactation of dairy cows. J Proteome Res 2011;10(9):4252–62.
12. Bell AW. Regulation of organic nutrient metabolism during transition from late pregnancy to early lactation. J Anim Sci 1995;73(9):2804–19.
13. Reynolds CK, Aikman PC, Lupoli B, et al. Splanchnic metabolism of dairy cows during the transition from late gestation through early lactation. J Dairy Sci 2003; 86(4):1201–17.
14. Adewuyi AA, Gruys E, van Eerdenburg FJ. Non esterified fatty acids (NEFA) in dairy cattle. A review. Vet Q 2005;27(3):117–26.
15. Drackley JK. Biology of dairy cows during the transition period: the final frontier? J Dairy Sci 1999;82(11):2259–73.

16. Bell AW, Burhans WS, Overton TR. Protein nutrition in late pregnancy, maternal protein reserves and lactation performance in dairy cows. Proc Nutr Soc 2000; 59(1):119–26.
17. Cox M, Nelson DL. Principles of biochemistry. New York: Palgrave Macmillan; 2004. ISBN-10.
18. Veenhuizen JJ, Drackley JK, Richard MJ, et al. Metabolic changes in blood and liver during development and early treatment of experimental fatty liver and ketosis in cows. J Dairy Sci 1991;74(12):4238–53.
19. Herdt TH. Ruminant adaptation to negative energy balance. Influences on the etiology of ketosis and fatty liver. Vet Clin North Am Food Anim Pract 2000; 16(2):215–30, v.
20. Karcagi RG, Gaal T, Wagner L, et al. Effect of various dietary fat supplementations on liver lipid and glycogen of high-yielding dairy cows in the peripartal period. Acta Vet Hung 2008;56(1):57–70.
21. Shepherd PR, Kahn BB. Mechanisms of disease—glucose transporters and insulin action—implications for insulin resistance and diabetes mellitus. N Engl J Med 1999;341(4):248–57.
22. Zhao FQ, Keating AF. Expression and regulation of glucose transporters in the bovine mammary gland. J Dairy Sci 2007;90(Suppl 1):E76–86.
23. Duhlmeier R, Hacker A, Widdel A, et al. Mechanisms of insulin-dependent glucose transport into porcine and bovine skeletal muscle. Am J Physiol Regul Integr Comp Physiol 2005;289(1):R187–97.
24. Hanson RW, Ballard FJ. The relative significance of acetate and glucose as precursors for lipid synthesis in liver and adipose tissue from ruminants. Biochem J 1967;105(2):529.
25. Komatsu T, Itoh F, Kushibiki S, et al. Changes in gene expression of glucose transporters in lactating and nonlactating cows. J Anim Sci 2005;83(3): 557–64.
26. Ji P, Osorio JS, Drackley JK, et al. Overfeeding a moderate energy diet prepartum does not impair bovine subcutaneous adipose tissue insulin signal transduction and induces marked changes in peripartal gene network expression. J Dairy Sci 2012;95(8):4333–51.
27. Sadri H, Bruckmaier RM, Rahmani HR, et al. Gene expression of tumour necrosis factor and insulin signalling-related factors in subcutaneous adipose tissue during the dry period and in early lactation in dairy cows. J Anim Physiol Anim Nutr (Berl) 2010;94(5):e194–202.
28. Bauman DE, Currie WB. Partitioning of nutrients during pregnancy and lactation—a review of mechanisms involving homeostasis and homeorhesis. J Dairy Sci 1980;63(9):1514–29.
29. Bertolini M, Moyer AL, Mason JB, et al. Evidence of increased substrate availability to in vitro-derived bovine foetuses and association with accelerated conceptus growth. Reproduction 2004;128(3):341–54.
30. Hirayama H, Sawai K, Hirayama M, et al. Prepartum maternal plasma glucose concentrations and placental glucose transporter mRNA expression in cows carrying somatic cell clone fetuses. J Reprod Dev 2011;57(1):57–61.
31. Lucy MC, Green JC, Meyer JP, et al. Short communication: glucose and fructose concentrations and expression of glucose transporters in 4-to 6-week pregnancies collected from Holstein cows that were either lactating or not lactating. J Dairy Sci 2012;95(9):5095–101.
32. Hay WW Jr. Placental-fetal glucose exchange and fetal glucose metabolism. Trans Am Clin Climatol Assoc 2006;117:321.

33. Lemosquet S, Raggio G, Lobley GE, et al. Whole-body glucose metabolism and mammary energetic nutrient metabolism in lactating dairy cows receiving digestive infusions of casein and propionic acid. J Dairy Sci 2009;92(12): 6068–82.
34. Kronfeld DS. Major metabolic determinants of milk volume, mammary efficiency, and spontaneous ketosis in dairy-cows. J Dairy Sci 1982;65(11):2204–12.
35. Hocquette JF, Balage M, Ferre P. Facilitative glucose transporters in ruminants. Proc Nutr Soc 1996;55(1B):221–36.
36. Kahn CR. Insulin resistance, insulin insensitivity, and insulin unresponsiveness: a necessary distinction. Metabolism 1978;27(12 Suppl 2):1893–902.
37. Muniyappa R, Lee S, Chen H, et al. Current approaches for assessing insulin sensitivity and resistance in vivo: advantages, limitations, and appropriate usage. Am J Physiol Endocrinol Metab 2008;294(1):E15–26.
38. Bauman DE. Regulation of nutrient partitioning during lactation: homeostasis and homeorhesis revisited. Ruminant Physiology 2000;311–28.
39. American Diabetes Association. Diagnosis and classification of diabetes mellitus. Diabetes Care 2004;27(Suppl 1):S5–10.
40. DeFronzo RA. Pathogenesis of type 2 diabetes mellitus. Med Clin North Am 2004;88(4):787–835, ix.
41. Kahn SE. The relative contributions of insulin resistance and beta-cell dysfunction to the pathophysiology of type 2 diabetes. Diabetologia 2003; 46(1):3–19.
42. Taniyama H, Shirakawa T, Furuoka H, et al. Spontaneous diabetes-mellitus in young cattle—histologic, immunohistochemical, and electron-microscopic studies of the islets of Langerhans. Vet Pathol 1993;30(1):46–54.
43. Nazifi S, Karimi T, Ghasrodashti AR. Diabetes mellitus and fatty liver in a cow: case report. Comp Clin Pathol 2004;13(2):82–5.
44. Bossaert P, Leroy JL, De Vliegher S, et al. Interrelations between glucose-induced insulin response, metabolic indicators, and time of first ovulation in high-yielding dairy cows. J Dairy Sci 2008;91(9):3363–71.
45. Hove K. Insulin secretion in lactating cows: responses to glucose infused intravenously in normal, ketonemic, and starved animals. J Dairy Sci 1978;61(10): 1407–13.
46. Kerestes M, Faigl V, Kulcsar M, et al. Periparturient insulin secretion and whole-body insulin responsiveness in dairy cows showing various forms of ketone pattern with or without puerperal metritis. Domest Anim Endocrinol 2009; 37(4):250–61.
47. Schoenberg KM, Ehrhardt RM, Overton TR. Effects of plane of nutrition and feed deprivation on insulin responses in dairy cattle during late gestation. J Dairy Sci 2012;95(2):670–82.
48. Opsomer G, Wensing T, Laevens H, et al. Insulin resistance: the link between metabolic disorders and cystic ovarian disease in high yielding dairy cows? Anim Reprod Sci 1999;56(3–4):211–22.
49. Andersen JB, Mashek DG, Larsen T, et al. Effects of hyperinsulinaemia under euglycaemic condition on liver fat metabolism in dairy cows in early and mid-lactation. J Vet Med A Physiol Pathol Clin Med 2002;49(2):65–71.
50. Sjaastad ØV, Sand O, Hove K. Physiology of domestic animals. 2nd edition. Oslo, Scandinavian Veterinary Press: 2010.
51. Bossaert P, De Cock H, Leroy JL, et al. Immunohistochemical visualization of insulin receptors in formalin-fixed bovine ovaries post mortem and in granulosa cells collected in vivo. Theriogenology 2010;73(9):1210–9.

52. Sinclair KD. Declining fertility, insulin resistance and fatty acid metabolism in dairy cows: developmental consequences for the oocyte and pre-implantation embryo. Acta Scientiae Veterinariae 2010;38(Suppl 2):s545–57.
53. Vanholder T, Leroy JL, Dewulf J, et al. Hormonal and metabolic profiles of high-yielding dairy cows prior to ovarian cyst formation or first ovulation post partum. Reprod Domest Anim 2005;40(5):460–7.
54. Stanley K, Fraser R, Bruce C. Physiological changes in insulin resistance in human pregnancy: longitudinal study with the hyperinsulinaemic euglycaemic clamp technique. Br J Obstet Gynaecol 1998;105(7):756–9.
55. Barbour LA, McCurdy CE, Hernandez TL, et al. Cellular mechanisms for insulin resistance in normal pregnancy and gestational diabetes. Diabetes Care 2007;30:S112–9.
56. Stolic M, Russell A, Hutley L, et al. Glucose uptake and insulin action in human adipose tissue—influence of BMI, anatomical depot and body fat distribution. Int J Obes Relat Metab Disord 2002;26(1):17–23.
57. Cornier MA, Dabelea D, Hernandez TL, et al. The metabolic syndrome. Endocr Rev 2008;29(7):777–822.
58. De Koster J, Opsomer G. Are modern dairy cows suffering from modern diseases? Vlaams Diergen Tijds 2012;81(2):71–80.
59. Vernon RG, Faulkner A, Hay WW, et al. Insulin resistance of hindlimb tissues in vivo in lactating sheep. Biochem J 1990;270(3):783–6.
60. Vernon RG, Taylor E. Insulin, dexamethasone and their interactions in the control of glucose-metabolism in adipose-tissue from lactating and non-lactating sheep. Biochem J 1988;256(2):509–14.
61. Debras E, Grizard J, Aina E, et al. Insulin sensitivity and responsiveness during lactation and dry period in goats. Am J Phys 1989;256(2):E295–302.
62. Petterson JA, Dunshea FR, Ehrhardt RA, et al. Pregnancy and undernutrition alter glucose metabolic responses to insulin in sheep. J Nutr 1993;123(7):1286–95.
63. McCann JP, Reimers TJ. Glucose response to exogenous insulin and kinetics of insulin metabolism in obese and lean heifers. J Anim Sci 1985;61(3):612–8.
64. Oikawa S, Oetzel GR. Decreased insulin response in dairy cows following a four-day fast to induce hepatic lipidosis. J Dairy Sci 2006;89(8):2999–3005.
65. Pires JA, Souza AH, Grummer RR. Induction of hyperlipidemia by intravenous infusion of tallow emulsion causes insulin resistance in Holstein cows. J Dairy Sci 2007;90(6):2735–44.
66. Pires JA, Pescara JB, Grummer RR. Reduction of plasma NEFA concentration by nicotinic acid enhances the response to insulin in feed-restricted Holstein cows. J Dairy Sci 2007;90(10):4635–42.
67. Agenas S, Burstedt E, Holtenius K. Effects of feeding intensity during the dry period. 1. Feed intake, body weight, and milk production. J Dairy Sci 2003;86(3):870–82.
68. Holtenius K, Agenas S, Delavaud C, et al. Effects of feeding intensity during the dry period. 2. Metabolic and hormonal responses. J Dairy Sci 2003;86(3):883–91.
69. Ohtsuka H, Koiwa M, Hatsugaya A, et al. Relationship between serum TNF activity and insulin resistance in dairy cows affected with naturally occurring fatty liver. J Vet Med Sci 2001;63(9):1021.
70. Hue L, Taegtmeyer H. The Randle cycle revisited: a new head for an old hat. Am J Physiol Endocrinol Metab 2009;297(3):E578–91.

71. LeMarchand-Brustel Y, Gual P, Gremeaux T, et al. Fatty acid-induced insulin resistance: role of insulin receptor substrate 1 serine phosphorylation in the retroregulation of insulin signalling. Biochem Soc Trans 2003;31:1152–6.
72. Bergman EN, Reulein SS, Corlett RE. Effects of obesity on insulin sensitivity and responsiveness in sheep. Am J Physiol 1989;257(5 Pt 1):E772–81.
73. Gustafson B, Hammarstedt A, Andersson CX, et al. Inflamed adipose tissue—a culprit underlying the metabolic syndrome and atherosclerosis. Arterioscler Thromb Vasc Biol 2007;27(11):2276–83.
74. Ingvartsen KL, Boisclair YR. Leptin and the regulation of food intake, energy homeostasis and immunity with special focus on periparturient ruminants. Domest Anim Endocrinol 2001;21(4):215–50.
75. Komatsu T, Itoh F, Mikawa S, et al. Gene expression of resistin in adipose tissue and mammary gland of lactating and non-lactating cows. J Endocrinol 2003; 178(3):R1–5.
76. Lemor A, Hosseini A, Sauerwein H, et al. Transition period-related changes in the abundance of the mRNAs of adiponectin and its receptors, of visfatin, and of fatty acid binding receptors in adipose tissue of high-yielding dairy cows. Domest Anim Endocrinol 2009;37(1):37–44.
77. Mukesh M, Bionaz M, Graugnard DE, et al. Adipose tissue depots of Holstein cows are immune responsive: inflammatory gene expression in vitro. Domest Anim Endocrinol 2010;38(3):168–78.
78. Saremi B, Al-Dawood A, Winand S, et al. Bovine haptoglobin as an adipokine: serum concentrations and tissue expression in dairy cows receiving a conjugated linoleic acids supplement throughout lactation. Vet Immunol Immunopathol 2012;146(3–4):201–11.
79. Kushibiki S, Hodate K, Shingu H, et al. Effects of long-term administration of recombinant bovine tumor necrosis factor-alpha on glucose metabolism and growth hormone secretion in steers. Am J Vet Res 2001;62(5):794–8.
80. Kushibiki S, Hodate K, Shingu H, et al. Insulin resistance induced in dairy steers by tumor necrosis factor alpha is partially reversed by 2,4-thiazolidinedione. Domest Anim Endocrinol 2001;21(1):25–37.
81. Bradford BJ, Mamedova LK, Minton JE, et al. Daily injection of tumor necrosis factor-alpha increases hepatic triglycerides and alters transcript abundance of metabolic genes in lactating dairy cattle. J Nutr 2009;139(8):1451–6.
82. O'Boyle N, Corl CM, Gandy JC, et al. Relationship of body condition score and oxidant stress to tumor necrosis factor expression in dairy cattle. Vet Immunol Immunopathol 2006;113(3–4):297–304.
83. Chagas LM, Lucy MC, Back PJ, et al. Insulin resistance in divergent strains of Holstein-Friesian dairy cows offered fresh pasture and increasing amounts of concentrate in early lactation. J Dairy Sci 2009;92(1):216–22.
84. Balogh O, Szepes O, Kovacs K, et al. Interrelationships of growth hormone AluI polymorphism, insulin resistance, milk production and reproductive performance in Holstein-Friesian cows. Vet Med 2008;53(11):604–16.
85. Bossaert P, Leroy JL, De Campeneere S, et al. Differences in the glucose-induced insulin response and the peripheral insulin responsiveness between neonatal calves of the Belgian Blue, Holstein-Friesian, and East Flemish breeds. J Dairy Sci 2009;92(9):4404–11.
86. Chilliard Y, Ferlay A, Faulconnier Y, et al. Adipose tissue metabolism and its role in adaptations to undernutrition in ruminants. Proc Nutr Soc 2000;59(1):127–34.
87. Faulkner A, Pollock HT. Metabolic responses to euglycaemic hyperinsulinaemia in lactating and non-lactating sheep in vivo. J Endocrinol 1990;124(1):59–66.

88. Petterson JA, Slepetis R, Ehrhardt RA, et al. Pregnancy but not moderate undernutrition attenuates insulin suppression of fat mobilization in sheep. J Nutr 1994; 124(12):2431–6.
89. Vernon RG, Doris R, Finley E, et al. Effects of lactation on the signal-transduction systems regulating lipolysis in sheep subcutaneous and omental adipose-tissue. Biochem J 1995;308:291–6.
90. Smith RW, Walsh A. Effects of pregnancy and lactation on the metabolism of bovine adipose-tissue. Res Vet Sci 1988;44(3):349–53.
91. Locher LF, Meyer N, Weber EM, et al. Hormone-sensitive lipase protein expression and extent of phosphorylation in subcutaneous and retroperitoneal adipose tissues in the periparturient dairy cow. J Dairy Sci 2011;94(9):4514–23.
92. Hostens M, Fievez V, Leroy JL, et al. The fatty acid profile of subcutaneous and abdominal fat in dairy cows with left displacement of the abomasum. J Dairy Sci 2012;95(7):3756–65.
93. Danfaer A. Nutrient metabolism and utilization in the liver. Livest Prod Sci 1994; 39(1):115–27.
94. Brockman RP. Effect of insulin on the utilization of propionate in gluconeogenesis in sheep. Br J Nutr 1990;64(1):95–101.
95. Tesseraud S, Grizard J, Debras E, et al. Leucine metabolism in lactating and dry goats—effect of insulin and substrate availability. Am J Phys 1993;265(3): E402–13.
96. Baracos VE, Brunbellut J, Marie M. Tissue protein-synthesis in lactating and dry goats. Br J Nutr 1991;66(3):451–65.
97. Overton TR. Substrate utilization for hepatic gluconeogenesis in the transition dairy cow. Proceedings of the 1998 Cornell Nutrition Conference for Feed Manufacturers. 1998. p. 237–46.
98. Rose MT, Obara Y, Itoh F, et al. Non-insulin- and insulin-mediated glucose uptake in dairy cows. J Dairy Res 1997;64(3):341–53.
99. Ferrell CL. Maternal and fetal influences on uterine and conceptus development in the cow. 2. Blood-flow and nutrient flux. J Anim Sci 1991;69(5):1954–65.
100. Bell AW, Slepetis R, Ehrhardt RA. Growth and accretion of energy and protein in the gravid uterus during late pregnancy in Holstein cows. J Dairy Sci 1995; 78(9):1954–61.
101. Defronzo RA, Tobin JD, Andres R. Glucose clamp technique—method for quantifying insulin-secretion and resistance. Am J Phys 1979;237(3):E214–23.
102. Kräft S. Charakterisierung der peripheren Insulin-response und Insulin-sensitivität bei trockenstehenden, laktierenden und leberverfetteten Milchkühe ohne und mit Ketose mittels hyperinsulinämischer, euglycämischer Clamps [dissertation]. Hannover (Germany): Klinik für Rinder der Tierärtzlichen Hochschule Hannover; 2004.
103. Kusenda M. Insulin-Sensitivität und Insulin-Response nach einer einmaligen Dexamethasonbehandlung bie Milchkühen in der Frühlaktation. Hannover (Germany): Klinik für Rinder, Tierärtzliche Hochschule Hannover; 2010.
104. Haarstrich D. Insulinsensitivität und Insulinresponse nach einer Langzeit-Supplementation von konjugierten Linolsäuren bei laktierenden Milchkühen. Hannover (Germany): Klinik fürRinder, Tierärztliche Hochschule Hannover; 2011.
105. Mitrakou A, Vuorinenmarkkola H, Raptis G, et al. Simultaneous assessment of insulin-secretion and insulin sensitivity using a hyperglycemic clamp. J Clin Endocrinol Metab 1992;75(2):379–82.
106. Bergman RN, Ider YZ, Bowden CR, et al. Quantitative estimation of insulin sensitivity. Am J Physiol 1979;236(6):E667–77.

107. Boston RC, Stefanovski D, Moate PJ, et al. MINMOD Millennium: a computer program to calculate glucose effectiveness and insulin sensitivity from the frequently sampled intravenous glucose tolerance test. Diabetes Technol Ther 2003;5(6):1003–15.
108. Cnop M, Vidal J, Hull RL, et al. Progressive loss of beta-cell function leads to worsening glucose tolerance in first-degree relatives of subjects with type 2 diabetes. Diabetes Care 2007;30(3):677–82.
109. Ferrannini E, Mari A. How to measure insulin sensitivity. J Hypertens 1998;16(7): 895–906.
110. Katz A, Nambi SS, Mather K, et al. Quantitative insulin sensitivity check index: a simple, accurate method for assessing insulin sensitivity in humans. J Clin Endocrinol Metab 2000;85(7):2402–10.
111. Perseghin G, Caumo A, Caloni M, et al. Incorporation of the fasting plasma FFA concentration into QUICKI improves its association with insulin sensitivity in non-obese individuals. J Clin Endocrinol Metab 2001;86(10):4776–81.
112. Rabasa-Lhoret R, Bastard JP, Jan V, et al. Modified quantitative insulin sensitivity check index is better correlated to hyperinsulinemic glucose clamp than other fasting-based index of insulin sensitivity in different insulin-resistant states. J Clin Endocrinol Metab 2003;88(10):4917–23.
113. Leroy JL, Bossaert P, Opsomer G, et al. The effect of animal handling procedures on the blood non-esterified fatty acid and glucose concentrations of lactating dairy cows. Vet J 2011;187(1):81–4.
114. Abuelo A, De Koster J, Hernandez J, et al. Quantifying bovine insulin: conversion of units. Vet Clin Pathol 2012;41(3):308–10.
115. Holtenius P, Holtenius K. A model to estimate insulin sensitivity in dairy cows. Acta Vet Scand 2007;49:29.
116. Schoenberg KM, Perfield KL, Farney JK, et al. Effects of prepartum 2,4-thiazolidinedione on insulin sensitivity, plasma concentrations of tumor necrosis factor-alpha and leptin, and adipose tissue gene expression. J Dairy Sci 2011;94(11): 5523–32.
117. Kruszynska YT, Worrall DS, Ofrecio J, et al. Fatty acid-induced insulin resistance: decreased muscle PI3K activation but unchanged Akt phosphorylation. J Clin Endocrinol Metab 2002;87(1):226–34.
118. Green A, Newsholme EA. Sensitivity of glucose-uptake and lipolysis of white adipocytes of the rat to insulin and effects of some metabolites. Biochem J 1979;180(2):365–70.
119. Arner P. Regional adiposity in man. J Endocrinol 1997;155(2):191–2.

Assessing and Managing Body Condition Score for the Prevention of Metabolic Disease in Dairy Cows

John R. Roche, PhD[a,*], Jane K. Kay, PhD[b], Nic C. Friggens, PhD[c], Juan J. Loor, PhD[d,e], Donagh P. Berry, PhD[f]

KEYWORDS

• Body condition score • Dairy • Review • Health

KEY POINTS

- Genetic selection for increased milk production has resulted in cows that lose more BCS in early lactation and that, consequently, are more susceptible to health disorders after calving.
- Excessive BCS at calving results in greater BCS loss after calving, increasing the risk of milk fever, ketosis, and fatty liver.
- Recent experiments during the transition period highlight benefits from controlling (ie, high-dietary roughage) energy intake precalving, with restricted cows being less prone to ketosis, fatty liver, and milk fever.
- The collective data indicate that a calving BCS of 3.0 for mature cows and 3.25 for heifers with a moderate energy restriction precalving will minimize the risk of BCS-related health disorders around calving.

INTRODUCTION

Reserves of adipose tissue are stringently maintained by peripherally and centrally produced hormones in accordance with the "lipostatic" theory.[1] The provision of nutrients for the neonate mammal is facilitated by the catabolism of fat and muscle for a period of time postpartum. A dairy cow exhibits this mammalian tendency to

[a] Animal Science, DairyNZ, Private Bag 3221, Hamilton 3240, New Zealand; [b] Dairy Cow Nutrition, DairyNZ, Private Bag 3221, Hamilton 3240, New Zealand; [c] Modélisation Systémique Appliquée aux Ruminants (Systemic Modelling Applied to Ruminants), 16 rue Claude Bernard, Paris 75231, France; [d] Animal Sciences, University of Illinois, 498 Animal Sciences Laboratory, Urbana, IL 61801, USA; [e] Nutritional Sciences, University of Illinois, 1207 W. Gregory, Urbana, IL 61801, USA; [f] Animal Genetics, Teagasc, Moorepark Dairy Production Research Centre, Fermoy, County Cork, Ireland

* Corresponding author.

E-mail address: John.roche@dairynz.co.nz

Vet Clin Food Anim 29 (2013) 323–336

http://dx.doi.org/10.1016/j.cvfa.2013.03.003

vetfood.theclinics.com

nurture the neonate from her tissue stores,[2] losing "condition" for approximately 40 to 100 days after calving before replenishing lost tissue reserves.[3–6] What makes dairy cows distinctly unique from all other mammalian species has been the intense trans-generational genetic selection for early lactation and total milk production during the last 50 years,[7] which has resulted in many physiologic changes that facilitate greater mobilization of energetically important tissues in dairy cows in comparison with other mammals.[6,8] Such selection pressures have also resulted in a reduction in the health of dairy cows.[9,10]

This article reviews the assessment of cow condition and determines the importance of body condition score (BCS) for cow health, giving due consideration to optimum BCS management strategies that may be used to minimize the likelihood of periparturient health problems.

ASSESSING COW CONDITION

Although it was probably evident for centuries that cows lost and gained condition during the lactation cycle, there was no simple measure of a cow's stored energy reserves until the 1970s.[11] Body weight (BW) alone is not a good indicator of body reserves, as the relationship is affected by factors such as parity, stage of lactation, frame size, gestation, and breed.[11,12] In addition, because tissue mobilization in early lactation occurs as feed intake is increasing,[4,5,13,14] actual decreases in weight of body tissue can be masked by enhanced gastrointestinal fill, such that BW changes do not accurately reflect changes in adipose and weight of lean tissue. Recent work[15] indicates that providing very frequent BW measurements (eg, at every milking) may help overcome some of these issues, but that for accurate assessment of adipose and lean tissue, measurements of body condition are needed.

Body condition was defined by Murray[16] as the ratio of body fat to nonfat components in the body of a live animal. However, large-scale direct measurements of body adiposity were (and remain) difficult and expensive. As a result, multiple systems to subjectively appraise the stored energy reserves of dairy cattle were introduced in the 1970s and 1980s, and scores were assigned to reflect the degree of apparent adiposity of the cow; these scores were termed "body condition scores." Lowman and colleagues[17] were the first to introduce a BCS scale (0–5-point system) for dairy cows, adapting a scoring system used to rank beef cattle. Further BCS systems evolved independently across the world, with a 6-point scale further refined for the United Kingdom (0–5),[18] an 8-point scale developed in Australia (1–8),[19] a 5-point system established in the United States (1–5),[20] and a 10-point scale introduced in New Zealand (1–10).[21,22] Throughout this review, the scale of 1 to 5[20] is reported. Equations to convert between scales were reported by Roche and colleagues.[22]

As the importance of body condition to milk production, reproduction, and health of cows became better established, the BCS scales became more precise and the assessment method expanded to encompass more body regions. For example, the anatomy considered in the original scale proposed by Lowman and colleagues[17] included only the spinous process of the lumbar vertebrae, the hip bones, the tail head, and the "second" thigh; most systems now include the thoracic and vertebral region of the spinal column (chine, loin, and rump), the ribs, the spinous processes (loin), the tuber sacrale (hip or hook bones), the tuber ischii (pin bones), the anterior coccygeal vertebrae (tail head), and the thigh region.[22] These additional measurement sites ensure the important points identified by Lowman and colleagues[17] are retained, and expand the assessment to provide a more complete picture of the energy-reserve status of the cow.

Irrespective of the scale used, low values reflect emaciation and high values equate to obesity. The effectiveness of BCS in estimating available energy reserves was outlined by Wright and Russel[23] and Otto and colleagues,[24] who reported a strong positive relationship (r = 0.75–0.93) between BCS and the proportion of physically dissected fat in Friesian cows. Waltner and colleagues[25] also evaluated several methods for estimating "body adiposity" against recorded body-fat depots (perirenal, mesenteric, omental, subcutaneous), and reported a strong correlation between BCS and body fat (r = 0.83), with only the diameter of the fat cells in the abdominal depot (r = 0.88) superseding BCS as a method of estimating body fat.

Accuracy of BCS Assessment

Although modern BCS systems are more definitive than the early versions proposed, limitations of these scoring systems must still be recognized. BCS assesses the level of subcutaneous fat possessed by a cow with reasonable accuracy (r^2 = 0.75–0.93 for Friesian cows),[23,24] but poorly predicts intermuscular and intramuscular fat (r^2 = 0.43).[23] The latter stores are major depot regions containing 35% to 45% of body fat. These data, therefore, imply that BCS may be less accurate in cows with little subcutaneous fat, although changes in body fatness in these subcutaneous and "internal" depots are generally proportional, such that BCS correlates strongly with total chemical content of body fat.

To aid consistent BCS assessment, several teams have independently produced BCS educational material.[21,26–28] All materials tend to be a mix of pictures and text, which detail changes in the conformation of anatomic locations regarded as important with BCS change.[22] Edmonson and colleagues[28] evaluated one such tool and reported consistent BCS predictions with little interassessor variability, no significant cow-assessor interaction, and no significant effect of assessor experience. However, Kristensen and colleagues[29] reported improved BCS assessment and reduced interassessor variability when veterinarians were first trained by expert assessors.

PHYSIOLOGY OF LIPID METABOLISM

Changes in a cow's condition, measured over several weeks, provide gross information about the cow's nutrient intake relative to its requirements during that time. Although protein and mineral stores are also used by the cow in early lactation, the most important reserve is adipose tissue. A greater understanding of factors affecting lipid metabolism therefore results in a better understanding of the factors influencing BCS mobilization and replenishment.

Homeostatic and Homeorhetic Mechanisms

During periods of chronic energy deficit, key hormones and tissue responsiveness are altered to change lipid metabolism, increasing long-chain fatty acid (LCFA) mobilization into blood (ie, nonesterified fatty acids [NEFA]) to maintain physiologic equilibrium.[2] This condition is known as homeostasis, the net result of which is the mobilization of adipose tissue reserves in response to the energy deficit.

Homeostatic control implies that if the nutritional environment is adequate, the lactating dairy cow can meet its energy demands from dry-matter intake (DMI), and tissue mobilization will be minimized. Thus, if homeostatic controls were the only regulator of lipid metabolism during early lactation, an increased energy intake should, in theory, abolish mobilization of body lipids. However, attempts to reduce body-lipid mobilization in early lactation (weeks 1–4 postpartum) by feeding energy-rich diets or decreasing energy output have generally not been successful,[4,30–32] and severe feed restrictions during the same period have not increased BCS mobilization[32]; these data imply that another mechanism is involved in BCS mobilization during this early lactation period. This finding is consistent with reported effects of genetic merit for milk production and energy intake on the activity of key lipolytic and lipogenic enzymes.[8,33] These data led to the conclusion that early-lactation lipolysis was largely genetically controlled, whereas enzymes involved in lipogenesis were primarily regulated by energy intake. More recent studies[4] indicate a potential cow genotype by diet interaction in lipogenesis, but concur with the lack of effect of diet on the homeorhesis-regulated lipolysis initiated around parturition.

There are characteristic changes in lipid metabolism during pregnancy and lactation in most mammals. Endocrine profiles change and lipid metabolism is altered to increase lipid reserves during pregnancy; these reserves are subsequently used at the initiation of lactation.[34,35] These changes occur not as a function of a changing nutritional environment, but rather as a function of physiology (ie, stage of lactation); this is homeorhetic control of lipid metabolism.[2] The implication behind the concept of homeorhesis is that the animal has a genetic drive to safeguard important biological functions, such as survival of the neonate (through provision of milk) or reproduction. This drive can only be fulfilled if the necessary resources are partitioned to these functions/processes by "orchestrated or coordinated changes in metabolism of body tissue, necessary to support a dominant physiologic state."[2]

Thus, lipid metabolism is regulated by both homeostatic and homeorhetic mechanisms. Homeostatic regulators of lipid metabolism are nutritionally sensitive, whereas homeorhetic regulators are, for the most part, nutritionally insensitive, instead being a function of a physiologic state. Regulation and coordination of energy intake and post-absorptive nutrient partitioning, in particular lipid metabolism, are key components of the periparturient homeorhetic adaptations in the dairy cow.

Lipid Metabolism

Adipose tissue represents the body's predominant energy reserve and consists of triacylglycerol (TAG)-filled cells known as adipocytes, within which lipolysis and lipogenesis are continuously occurring, resulting in constant degradation and resynthesis of intracellular TAG (**Fig. 1**).

Lipogenesis

Lipogenesis occurs in ruminant adipocytes via 2 pathways: de novo synthesis and uptake of preformed LCFA from circulation. Compared with monogastric animals, who use glucose for lipogenesis, ruminants use acetate derived from rumen fermentation as the predominant carbon source for de novo fatty acid (FA) synthesis. Acetyl–coenzyme A (CoA) carboxylase, the rate-limiting enzyme in this process,[36] catalyzes the formation of malonyl-CoA, the committed step in FA synthesis. Malonyl-CoA is then condensed with acetyl-CoA by FA synthase to produce the first 4-carbon acyl unit, butyrate. Additional malonyl-CoA (produced by acetyl-CoA carboxylase) are condensed with the growing acyl chain (via FA synthase) to produce longer-chain FA, resulting in palmitate as the primary product (C16:0).[36]

In the case of FA uptake from circulating chylomicron or very low-density lipoproteins (VLDL), endothelial lipoprotein lipase hydrolyzes plasma TAG, producing NEFA and monoacylglycerol.[37] Uptake of NEFA can occur via free diffusion (known as unsaturable transport), particularly at high local concentrations, or via the membrane-bound proteins FA translocase (CD36) and FA transport protein (known as saturable transport).[38] Intracellular activation to acyl-CoA or transport of the "free" LCFA is

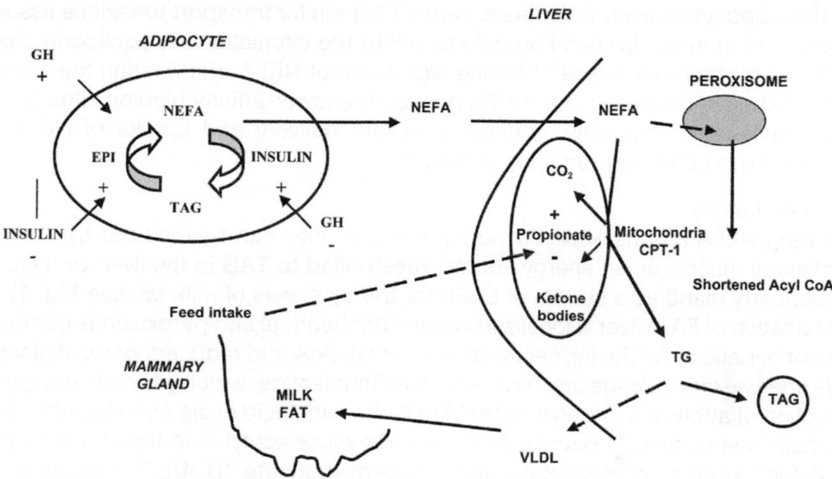

Fig. 1. Lipid metabolism in the transition dairy cow. Positive signs (+) indicate stimulation, and negative signs (–) indicate inhibition. Dashed lines are processes that occur at low rates or only during certain physiologic states. CoA, coenzyme A; CPT-1, carnitine palmitoyltransferase I; EPI, epinephrine; GH, growth hormone; NEFA, nonesterified fatty acids; TAG, triacylglycerol; TG, triglyceride; VLDL, very low-density lipoproteins. (*Adapted from* Drackley JK. Biology of dairy cows during the transition period: the final frontier. J Dairy Sci 1999;82:2262; with permission.)

mediated by acyl-CoA synthases and binding proteins.[38] There are several isotypes of the FA transport and acyl-CoA synthases and their expression, and that of the LCFA translocase changes in adipose tissue and mammary gland of dairy cows during the transition from pregnancy to lactation (eg, decrease in adipose and increase in the mammary gland).[39–41] Esterification of LCFA to TAG in adipose tissue occurs through either the phosphatidic pathway or the monoacylglycerol pathway, depending on the availability of glycerol-3-phosphate and monoacylglycerol.[42] Because adipose tissue lacks glycerol kinase, the main source of glycerol-3-phosphate for TAG synthesis is glyceroneogenesis, likely from exogenous lactate.[43] The key enzyme in this process is cytosolic phosphoenolpyruvate carboxykinase, whose expression in adipose decreases markedly after parturition[41] in line with the catabolic signals.

Lipolysis

During basal lipolysis, adipose triglyceride lipase catalyzes the hydrolysis of TAG to diacylglycerol and FA.[44,45] The FA is then recycled to TAG rather than being exported out of the adipocyte. During stimulated lipolysis, as in states of chronic energy deficit, hormone-sensitive lipase (HSL) acts as a catalyst to FA hydrolysis at the sn-1 and sn-3 positions.[46] Activation of HSL by lipolytic hormones is mediated by reversible phosphorylation via cyclic adenosine monophosphate–dependent protein kinase A, which also phosphorylates perilipin, a hydrophobic protein that is a component of the lipid droplet membrane. Both steps are crucial for sustained lipolysis because phosphorylated perilipin is partly dissociated from the lipid droplet membrane, thus providing access for HSL to the TAG core. Monoacylglycerol lipase hydrolyzes the remaining FA at the sn-2 position, and the overall process generates 3 NEFA and a glycerol backbone.[46] Even during periods of active lipolysis, a major portion of the hydrolyzed LCFA are reesterified within the adipocyte.[43] The portion of NEFA that is released from the adipocyte quickly attaches to serum albumin for transport to various tissues. Glycerol and monoacylglycerol are released into the circulation via aquaporin channels in the plasma membrane.[45] During high rates of NEFA mobilization the ratio of NEFA to albumin increases, and NEFA occupy the lower-affinity binding sites on the albumin molecule. This weak connection favors delivery and uptake of NEFA by energy-requiring and lipid-requiring tissues.[46]

NEFA metabolism

Circulating NEFA are metabolized via 3 pathways: they can be oxidized by the liver and skeletal muscle as an energy source, reesterified to TAG in the liver, or used by the mammary gland as a source of LCFA for the synthesis of milk fat (see **Fig. 1**).

β-Oxidation of FA in liver is localized in the mitochondrial and peroxisomal compartments of hepatic cells; the former produces acetyl-CoA and reduced forms of nicotinamide adenine dinucleotide and flavin adenine dinucleotide, which generate energy via production of adenosine triphosphate (ATP) in the citric acid cycle and electron transport chain, respectively.[46] Hepatic cells convert excess acetyl-CoA from β-oxidization into ketone bodies (acetoacetate and β-hydroxybutyrate [BHB]).[47] Ketosis is an important energy-providing mechanism for dairy cows in early lactation, even though acetyl-CoA conversion to ketone bodies, rather than complete β-oxidation, is less energetically efficient.[46] During early lactation, the majority (>80%) of available glucose is partitioned to the mammary gland, and because vital organs (eg, the brain) cannot metabolize FA as an energy source, ketone-body oxidation becomes essential for survival.[46] The rate of ketone-body formation is directly proportional to lipolytic and FA oxidation rates.

An alternative pathway to hepatic NEFA oxidation is via peroxisomes, subcellular organelles present in most organs of the body.[48] Compared with mitochondrial β-oxidation, which generates energy in the form of reduced nicotinamide adenine dinucleotide in addition to acetyl-CoA, peroxisomal β-oxidation produces hydrogen peroxide (via catalase) and, more importantly, shorter acyl-CoA, which can then be transported to the mitochondria for further oxidation. Because peroxisomes do not contain a respiratory chain linked to ATP formation, it is proposed that the less energy-efficient peroxisomal β-oxidation may play a role as an overflow pathway to oxidize FA only during extensive NEFA mobilization (see **Fig. 1**).

Nonesterified FA that do not undergo hepatic β-oxidization are reesterified to TAG and released into the circulation as VLDL (see **Fig. 1**). During periods of negative energy balance, the hepatic capacity for FA reesterification increases. However, the VLDL export rate from the liver remains low,[49] possibly because of the bovine's reduced capacity to generate apoprotein B, one key component controlling the overall rate of VLDL synthesis and secretion.[50] Thus, increased hepatic NEFA uptake and reesterification combined with an inherently low rate of VLDL synthesis and release can result in hepatocyte TAG accumulation, a phenomenon often referred to as fatty liver.

BCS AND HEALTH

The relationship among BCS and variables of cow health[51–55] is less consistent than that reported for BCS and milk or BCS and fertility.[6] Nevertheless, Uribe and colleagues[10] and Ingvartsen and colleagues[9] reported a negative genetic correlation between milk production and health in Holstein-Friesian cows, implying that selection for milk production alone has resulted in increased morbidity. If this is true, one would expect an increased risk of a health problem in thin cows or those that lose excessive BCS in early lactation. Although this is consistent with the increasing public perception that thin cows are welfare compromised, there is little research to either support or refute this hypothesis.

If a relationship between a cow's energy balance/status and health exists, it could manifest in 2 ways:

1. Thin cows or cows in severe negative energy balance may be more susceptible to infection (causal relationship).
2. "Unhealthy" animals may have a reduced DMI, and a resultant greater body-tissue mobilization to satisfy the drive to produce milk (associative relationship).

BCS and Periparturient Metabolic Diseases

Metabolic diseases are complex disorders that occur when the cow's ability to adjust to a major physiologic change (eg, calving) is compromised. Such diseases have been a persistent problem for farmers for centuries, with milk fever first described in Germany in 1793[56] and ketosis reported in the United States as early as 1849.[57] The majority of cases of metabolic and infectious diseases occur during the transition period around calving, and much of the effort during this time is aimed at prevention of these diseases.

Most metabolic diseases stem from excessive BCS loss, nutritional inadequacy, or failure to prime metabolic processes for the change from gestational to lactational demands. There is also increasing evidence of a link between nutritional and management factors that contributes to immune dysfunction and nonclassic metabolic disorders (eg, milk fever that occurs before the drain on calcium following the first milking) and infectious diseases.[58–60]

Fatty liver

Fatty liver disease, or hepatic lipidosis, is probably the metabolic disorder most associated with excessive BCS during the transition period. Excessive TAG accumulation in liver occurs when the hepatic uptake of NEFA exceeds their oxidation and secretion, and occurs primarily at some point during the first 4 weeks postpartum.[61] Fatty liver occurs often in cows that are overconditioned at parturition and results in dramatic decreases in DMI, a greater incidence of downer cows, and negative health effects that may be irreversible.[60,62,63] However, fatty liver can also occur in cows that are not overconditioned, with reports of up to 50% of dairy cows affected during early lactation.[64]

From a biochemical standpoint, the bovine liver can esterify NEFA in vitro at a rate similar to that in simple-stomached species such as rat, pig, and chicken, but the rates of TAG export in VLDL from ruminant liver is markedly lower than those of other species.[49] This feature is partly responsible for the consistent increase in liver TAG during the first few weeks postpartum.[60]

Milk fever

Roche and Berry[55] reported a nonlinear association between BCS and the incidence of milk fever. The odds of a cow succumbing to milk fever were 13% and 30% greater at a calving BCS of less than 2.5 and greater than 3.5, respectively, compared with a calving BCS of 3.0. The investigators hypothesized that the relationship between fatter cows at calving and milk fever is probably a result of both attenuated postcalving DMI[6] in cows with excessive BCS (>3.5) and an increased milk production supported by catabolism of tissue reserves.[65,66] The reason for increased milk fever in very thin (BCS <2.5) cows at calving is unclear, as cows in negative energy balance precalving retain periparturient eucalcemia more effectively than well-fed cows.[32,65] Such an association may, instead, reflect a general malaise in thin cows and an inability to maintain eucalcemia (associative relationship), rather than an effect of low BCS on eucalcemia per se. For example, cows succumbing to postparturient disorders have been reported to reduce DMI before calving.[67,68]

Ketosis

Roche and colleagues[69] reported a moderate correlation ($r = 0.51$) between calving BCS and BCS loss postcalving, implying that overconditioned cows at calving mobilize more fat in early lactation. Combined with a lower DMI associated with greater BCS[6] and an increase in lactose requirements for milk production (and therefore hepatic gluconeogenesis), hepatic oxaloacetate would likely become limiting for FA oxidation, and FA and ketone bodies would accumulate. Consistent with this hypothesis, Gillund and colleagues[52] reported a doubling of the risk of ketosis in dairy cows with a calving BCS of greater than 3.5 compared with those calving at BCS 3.25. These conclusions are consistent with the metabolic profiles presented by Roche.[32] This study reported an interaction between calving BCS (precalving level of feeding) and postcalving level of feeding on circulating ketone-body concentrations; plasma concentrations of BHB were between 50% and 100% greater in cows that calved at BCS 3.0 and underwent a feed restriction postpartum (type I ketosis) than in cows that calved at BCS 2.85 and underwent the same feed restriction. These data, and the doubling of the odds of ketosis with only a 0.25 BCS increase in calving BCS,[52] highlight the sensitivity of periparturient dairy cows to small differences in BCS with regard to ketosis.

BCS and Infectious Diseases

There are only limited data evaluating the association between energy balance and the risk of infectious diseases. Uterine infections have been associated with both precalving and early-lactation BCS loss,[54,70] implicating overconditioning in the risk of infectious disease. Similarly, Berry and colleagues[51] reported greater odds of clinical mastitis during lactation in cows with greater BCS at calving. In direct contrast, however, Heuer and colleagues[53] and Hoedemaker and colleagues[71] reported a greater risk of metritis in thin cows, suggesting that the association between BCS and the risk of infectious diseases is nonlinear, with a greater risk in extreme BCS cows.

It is unclear why fatter or heavier cows in early lactation should be more prone to high somatic cell count (SCC) and clinical mastitis, but the relationship may be merely associative. Ketosis is a disorder that occurs more frequently in overconditioned cows at calving,[52] and it has been reported to predispose cows to clinical mastitis.[72]

There is also an association between the prevalence of subclinical disease and BCS, although the relationship is complicated by parity. Berry and colleagues[51] reported that first-parity and second-parity cows exhibited a negative relationship between early-lactation BCS and SCC, whereas cows in their third lactation or greater presented with a positive relationship (ie, SCC increased with increasing BCS postpartum). This finding is similar to the interaction between calving BCS and the incidence of subclinical endometritis, with increased numbers of polymorphonuclear cells in uterine samples 28 and 42 days postcalving in low BCS first-lactation and second-lactation cows, but no such relationships in older cows.[73]

In summary, the published data indicate that "thinness" of mature cows does not predispose them to a greater risk of intramammary infection, although younger cows may be more susceptible to infection when thin. By comparison, overconditioning at calving (BCS >3.5) may predispose cows to a greater risk of mastitis, through associated metabolic disorders.

BCS at calving and the rate of BCS loss after calving contribute to the probability of both infectious and metabolic diseases. The lack of consensus in the literature on the effect of BCS on health probably relates to differences in the diseases investigated and the methods of diagnosis. Periparturient metabolic disorders are more associated with elevated calving BCS than thinness, probably as a result of increased BCS loss after calving and a lower DMI after calving. The negative association between BCS and the risk of infection (uterine or mammary) is parity dependent, with data indicating that younger cows (first and second parity) will benefit from a greater calving BCS (~3.25) than mature cows.[6]

MANAGEMENT OF TRANSITION COW AND BCS TO OPTIMIZE HEALTH

As well as adhering to best management practice around mineral and vitamin nutrition and dry cow management, there are 2 practical approaches to minimize the risk of cows developing BCS-related metabolic diseases after calving:

- Ensure cows are not excessively fat at calving
- Limit energy intake in the 2 weeks preceding calving

The positive association between calving BCS and the incidence of metabolic diseases is well established.[6] However, this must be considered within the context of favorable associations between calving BCS and milk production and BCS and reproduction, and the association between low BCS and infectious diseases in young cows. Recognizing this quadratic response to BCS, Roche and colleagues[6] recommended a calving BCS of 3.0 (5-point scale), therein finding a middle ground for system optimization.

In addition to managing peripartum BCS, recent research has highlighted the importance of transition cow nutrition in optimizing cow health. Traditionally, epidemiologic and metabolic research results were interpreted to support the long-held recommendation of "priming" or "steaming up" the cow several weeks before calving.[74] This practice was based on a positive association between precalving plasma NEFA and the incidence of postpartum metabolic disease,[75] and a negative association between prepartum energy intake and postpartum TAG accumulation in the liver.[76] However, experiments investigating the effect of prepartum energy balance on postpartum metabolism and health[32,62,65,77] do not agree with these recommendations, instead reporting that increasing plasma NEFA concentrations through controlled energy intake precalving improves peripartum and postpartum health and physiologic function; a moderate restriction in energy intake precalving resulted in improved postpartum energy balance, lower liver TAG and blood BHB, increased hepatic gluconeogenesis and β-oxidation, and greater DMI.[32,62,65,77]

Recent experiments in periparturient cow behavior and physiology help explain these apparent inconsistencies. Huzzey and colleagues[68] and Goldhawk and colleagues[67] highlighted that cows that succumb to either ketosis or metritis after calving have a lower DMI precalving, well before metabolic evidence of disease. Similarly, Burke and colleagues[58] reported an increase in subclinical uterine inflammation 28 to 42 days after calving in cows that had lower concentrations of blood albumin precalving than their nonaffected counterparts, implying liver dysfunction before uterine inflammation. Thus, Huzzey and colleagues[68] and Burke and colleagues[58] identified changes to animal behavior and physiology before evident pathology, indicating that the relationship between prepartum NEFA and postpartum health were associative rather than causative.

As a result of this greater understanding of peripartum physiologic dysfunction and its relationship with metabolic diseases, management recommendations for the transition cow have changed. It is now recommended that cows achieve a BCS of 3.0 to 3.25 1 month before calving and then consume 80% to 100% of their energy requirements in the month before calving. For a complete review, see Roche and colleagues.[60]

SUMMARY

Genetic selection for increased milk production has resulted in cows that lose more BCS in early lactation and, consequently, are more susceptible to postcalving health disorders. Excessive BCS at calving results in greater BCS loss after calving, increasing the risk of milk fever, ketosis, and fatty liver. By comparison, the immune system of thin cows is less effective at calving, predisposing these cows to infectious diseases, particularly the younger cohort. Recent experiments during the transition period highlight benefits from controlling (ie, high-dietary roughage) energy intake precalving, with restricted cows being less prone to ketosis, fatty liver, and milk fever. The collective data indicate that a calving BCS of 3.0 for mature cows and 3.25 for heifers with a moderate energy restriction precalving will minimize the risk of BCS-related health disorders around calving.

REFERENCES

1. Roche JR, Blache D, Kay JK, et al. Neuroendocrine and physiological regulation of intake, with particular reference to domesticated ruminant animals. Nutr Res Rev 2008;21:207–34.
2. Bauman DE, Currie WB. Partitioning of nutrients during pregnancy and lactation: a review of mechanisms involving homeostasis and homeorhesis. J Dairy Sci 1980;63:1514–29.
3. Friggens NC, Ingvartsen KL, Emmans GC. Prediction of body lipid change in pregnancy and lactation. J Dairy Sci 2004;87:988–1000.
4. Roche JR, Berry DP, Kolver ES. Holstein-Friesian strain and feed effects on milk production, body weight, and body condition score profiles in grazing dairy cows. J Dairy Sci 2006;89:3532–43.
5. Roche JR, Berry DP, Lee JM, et al. Describing the body condition score change between successive calvings: a novel strategy generalizable to diverse cohorts. J Dairy Sci 2007;90:4378–96.
6. Roche JR, Friggens NC, Kay JK, et al. Invited review: body condition score and its association with dairy cow productivity, health, and welfare. J Dairy Sci 2009;92:5769–801.
7. Dillon P. A comparison of different dairy cow breeds on a seasonal grass-based system of milk production. 2. Reproduction and survival. Livest Prod Sci 2006;83:35–42.
8. McNamara JP, Hillers JK. Regulation of bovine adipose tissue metabolism during lactation. 1. Lipid synthesis in response to increased milk production and decreased energy intake. J Dairy Sci 1986;69:3032–41.
9. Ingvartsen KL, Dewhurst RJ, Friggens NC. On the relationship between lactational performance and health: is it yield or metabolic imbalance that cause production diseases in dairy cattle? A position paper. Livest Prod Sci 2003;83:277–308.
10. Uribe HA, Kennedy BW, Martin SW, et al. Genetic parameters for common health disorders of Holstein cows. J Dairy Sci 1995;78:421–30.
11. Stockdale CR. Body condition at calving and the performance of dairy cows in early lactation under Australian conditions: a review. Aust J Exp Agr 2001;41:823–9.

12. Berry DP, Macdonald KA, Penno JW, et al. Association between body condition score and live weight in pasture-based Holstein-Friesian dairy cows. J Dairy Res 2006;73:487–91.
13. Berry DP, Veerkamp RF, Dillon P. Phenotypic profiles for body weight, body condition score, energy intake, and energy balance across different parities and concentrate feeding levels. Livest Sci 2006;104:1–12.
14. Ingvartsen KL, Andersen JB. Integration of metabolism and intake regulation: a review focusing on periparturient animals. J Dairy Sci 2000;83:1573–97.
15. Thorup VM, Edwards D, Friggens NC. On-farm estimation of energy balance in dairy cows using only frequent body weight measurements and body condition score. J Dairy Sci 2012;95:1784–93.
16. Murray JA. Meat production. Cambridge. J Agric Sci 1919;9:174–81.
17. Lowman BG, Scott N, Somerville S. Condition scoring of cattle. Bulletin No. 6. Edinburgh (United Kingdom): East of Scotland College of Agriculture; 1973.
18. Mulvaney P. Dairy cow condition scoring. Handout No. 4468. Reading (United Kingdom): National Institute for Research in Dairying; 1977.
19. Earle DF. A guide to scoring dairy cow condition. J Agric (Victoria) 1976;74: 228–31.
20. Wildman EE, Jones GM, Wagner PE, et al. A dairy cow body condition scoring system and its relationship to selected production characteristics. J Dairy Sci 1982;65:495–501.
21. Macdonald KA, Roche JR. Condition scoring made easy. Condition scoring dairy herds. 1st edition. Hamilton (New Zealand): Dexcel Ltd; 2004. ISBN 0-476-00217-6.
22. Roche JR, Dillon PG, Stockdale CR, et al. Relationships among international body condition scoring systems. J Dairy Sci 2004;87:3076–9.
23. Wright IA, Russel AJ. Partition of fat, body composition and body condition score in mature cows. Anim Prod 1984;38:23–32.
24. Otto KL, Ferguson JD, Fox DG, et al. Relationship between body condition score and composition of ninth to eleventh rib tissue in Holstein dairy cows. J Dairy Sci 1991;74:852–9.
25. Waltner SS, McNamara JP, Hillers JK, et al. Validation of indirect measures of body fat in lactating cows. J Dairy Sci 1994;77:2570–9.
26. DEFRA. Condition scoring of dairy cows. Publication PB6492. London: Department for Environment, Food and Rural Affairs; 2001.
27. DNRE. The condition magician. Body condition scoring in dairy herds. Victoria (Australia): Department of Natural Resources and Environment; 2002. ISBN 0 7311 49831.
28. Edmonson AJ, Lean IJ, Weaver LD, et al. A body condition scoring chart for Holstein dairy cows. J Dairy Sci 1989;72:68–78.
29. Kristensen E, Dueholm L, Vink D, et al. Within- and across-person uniformity of body condition scoring in Danish Holstein cattle. J Dairy Sci 2006;89: 3721–8.
30. Grummer RR, Hoffman PC, Luck ML, et al. Effect of prepartum and postpartum dietary energy on growth and lactation of primiparous cows. J Dairy Sci 1995; 78:172–80.
31. Pedernera M, García SC, Horagadoga A, et al. Energy balance and reproduction on dairy cows fed to achieve low or high milk production on a pasture-based system. J Dairy Sci 2008;91:3896–907.
32. Roche JR. Milk production responses to pre- and post-calving dry matter intake in grazing dairy cows. Livest Sci 2007;110:12–24.

33. McNamara JP, Hillers JK. Regulation of bovine adipose tissue metabolism during lactation. 2. Lipolysis response to milk production and energy intake. J Dairy Sci 1986;69:3042–50.
34. Friggens NC. Body lipid reserves and the reproductive cycle: towards a better understanding. Livest Prod Sci 2003;83:219–26.
35. Pond CM. In: Peaker M, Vernon RG, Knight CH, editors. Physiological strategies in lactation. London: The Zoological Society of London; 1984. p. 1–29.
36. Bauman DE, Davis CL. Biosynthesis of milk fat. In: Larson BL, Smith VR, editors. Lactation: a comprehensive treatise, vol. 2. New York: Academic Press; 1974. p. 31–75.
37. Fielding BA, Frayn KN. Lipoprotein lipase and the disposition of dietary fatty acids. Br J Nutr 1998;80:495–502.
38. Glatz JF, Luiken JJ, Bonen A. Membrane fatty acid transporters as regulators of lipid metabolism: implications for metabolic disease. Physiol Rev 2010;90: 367–417.
39. Bionaz M, Loor JJ. ACSL1, AGPAT6, FABP3, LPIN1, and SLC27A6 are the most abundant isoforms in bovine mammary tissue and their expression is affected by stage of lactation. J Nutr 2008;138:1019–24.
40. Bionaz M, Loor JJ. Gene networks driving bovine milk fat synthesis during the lactation cycle. BMC Genomics 2008;9:366.
41. Ji P, Osorio JS, Drackley JK, et al. Overfeeding a moderate energy diet prepartum does not impair bovine subcutaneous adipose tissue insulin signal transduction and induces marked changes in peripartal gene network expression. J Dairy Sci 2012;95:4333–51.
42. Lehner R, Kuksis A. Biosynthesis of triacylglycerols. Prog Lipid Res 1996;35: 169–201.
43. Nye C, Kim J, Kalhan SC, et al. Reassessing triglyceride synthesis in adipose tissue. Trends Endocrinol Metab 2008;19:356–61.
44. Ahmadian M, Duncan RE, Sul HS. The skinny on fat: lipolysis and fatty acid utilization in adipocytes. Trends Endocrinol Metab 2009;20:424–8.
45. Duncan RE, Ahmadian M, Jaworski K, et al. Regulation of lipolysis in adipocytes. Annu Rev Nutr 2007;27:79–101.
46. Stipanuk MH. Biochemical and physiological aspects of human nutrition. Philadelphia: W. B. Saunders; 2000.
47. Herdt TH. Ruminant adaptation to negative energy balance: influences on the etiology of ketosis and fatty liver. Vet Clin North Am Food Anim Pract 2000;16: 215–30.
48. Singh I. Biochemistry of peroxisomes in health and disease. Mol Cell Biochem 1997;167:1–29.
49. Bauchart D. Lipid absorption and transport in ruminants. J Dairy Sci 1993;76: 3864–81.
50. Drackley JK. Biology of dairy cows during the transition period: the final frontier. J Dairy Sci 1999;82:2259–73.
51. Berry DP, Lee JM, Macdonald KA, et al. Associations between body condition score, bodyweight and somatic cell count and clinical mastitis in seasonally calving dairy cattle. J Dairy Sci 2007;90:637–48.
52. Gillund P, Reksen O, Grohn YT, et al. Body condition related to ketosis and reproductive performance in Norwegian dairy cows. J Dairy Sci 2001;84:1390–6.
53. Heuer C, Schukken YH, Dobbelaar P. Postpartum body condition score and results from first test day milk as predictors of disease, fertility, yield, and culling in commercial dairy herds. J Dairy Sci 1999;82:295–304.

54. Markusfeld O, Gallon N, Ezra E. Body condition score, health, yield and fertility in dairy cows. Vet Rec 1997;141:67–72.
55. Roche JR, Berry DP. Periparturient climatic, animal, and management factors influencing the incidence of milk fever in grazing systems. J Dairy Sci 2006; 89:2775–83.
56. Schultz LH. Milk fever and ketosis. In: Church DC, editor. Digestive physiology and the nutrition of ruminants. 1971.
57. Udall DH. The practice of veterinary medicine. 4th edition. Ithaca (NY): 1943.
58. Burke C, Meier S, McDougall S, et al. Relationships between endometritis and metabolic state during the transition period in pasture-grazed dairy cows. J Dairy Sci 2010;93:5363–73.
59. Loor JJ, Bertoni G, Hosseini A, et al. Invited review. Functional welfare—using biochemical and molecular technologies to understand an animal's welfare state better. Anim Prod Sci, in press.
60. Roche JR, Bell AW, Overton TR, et al. Invited review. Nutritional management of the transition cow in the 21st century—a paradigm shift in thinking. Anim Prod Sci, in press.
61. Bobe G, Young JW, Beitz DC. Invited review: pathology, etiology, prevention, and treatment of fatty liver in dairy cows. J Dairy Sci 2004;87:3105–24.
62. Loor JJ, Dann HM, Janovick Guretzky NA, et al. Plane of nutrition prepartum alters hepatic gene expression and function in dairy cows as assessed by longitudinal transcript and metabolic profiling. Physiol Genomics 2006;27:29–41.
63. Morrow DA. Fat cow syndrome. J Dairy Sci 1976;59:1625–9.
64. Jorritsma R, Jorritsma H, Schukken YH, et al. Prevalence and indicators of post partum fatty infiltration of the liver in nine commercial dairy herds in The Netherlands. Livest Prod Sci 2001;68:53–60.
65. Roche JR, Kolver ES, Kay JK. Influence of precalving feed allowance on periparturient metabolic and hormonal responses and milk production in grazing dairy cows. J Dairy Sci 2005;88:677–89.
66. Roche JR, Lee JM, Macdonald KA, et al. Relationships among body condition score, body weight, and milk production variables in pasture-based dairy cows. J Dairy Sci 2007;90:3802–15.
67. Goldhawk C, Chapinal N, Veira DM, et al. Prepartum feeding behavior is an early indicator of subclinical ketosis. J Dairy Sci 2009;92:4971–7.
68. Huzzey JM, Veira DM, Weary DM, et al. Prepartum behavior and dry matter intake identify dairy cows at risk for metritis. J Dairy Sci 2007;90:3220–33.
69. Roche JR, Macdonald KA, Burke CR, et al. Associations among body condition score, body weight, and reproductive performance in seasonal-calving dairy cattle. J Dairy Sci 2007;90:376–91.
70. Butler WR, Smith RD. Interrelationships between energy balance and postpartum reproductive function in dairy cattle. J Dairy Sci 1989;72:767–83.
71. Hoedemaker M, Prange D, Gundelach Y. Body condition change ante- and postpartum, health and reproductive performance in German Holstein cows. Reprod Domest Anim 2009;44:167–73.
72. Oltenacu PA, Ekesbo I. Epidemiological study of clinical mastitis in dairy cattle. Vet Res 1994;25:208–17.
73. McDougall S, Hussein H, Aberdein D, et al. Relationships between cytology, bacteriology and vaginal discharge scores and reproductive performance in dairy cattle. Theriogenology 2011;76:229–40.
74. Boutflour RB. Limiting factors in the feeding and management of milk cows. In: Report from World's Dairy Congress. 1928. p. 15–20.

75. Dyk PB. The association of prepartum non-esterified fatty acids and body condition with peripartum health problems of 95 Michigan dairy farms [MS Thesis]. East Lansing (MI): Michigan State University; 1995.
76. Bertics SJ, Grummer RR, Cadorniga-Valino C, et al. Effect of prepartum dry matter intake on liver triglyceride concentration and early lactation. J Dairy Sci 1992; 75:1914–22.
77. Douglas GN, Overton TR, Bateman HG, et al. Prepartal plane of nutrition, regardless of dietary energy source, affects periparturient metabolism and dry matter intake in Holstein cows. J Dairy Sci 2006;89:2141–57.

Energy and Protein Nutrition Management of Transition Dairy Cows

Ian J. Lean, BVSc, DVSc, PhD, MANZCVS[a,*],
Robert Van Saun, DVM, MS, PhD[b], Peter J. DeGaris, BVSc (Hons), PhD[c]

KEYWORDS

- Transition • Protein • Skeleton • Antioxidant • Vitamins

KEY POINTS

- The periparturient or transition period in the 4 weeks before and 4 weeks after calving is characterized by greatly increased risk of disease.
- The last 3 to 4 weeks of gestation are characterized by a period of rapid fetal growth, colostrogenesis and mammary development, and metabolic adjustments favoring mobilization of fat and other nutrients; all in combination with declining dry matter intake (DMI).
- The first 3 to 4 weeks after parturition features slowly increasing DMI in conjunction with rapidly increasing nutrient losses in support of milk production.

INTRODUCTION

The aims of this article and a companion article in this issue are to briefly review some of the underlying physiology of changes that occur around calving, examine the potential to control the risk of disease in this period, increase milk production, and improve reproductive performance through better nutritional management. Practical guidelines for veterinarians and advisors are provided.

The periparturient or transition period in the 4 weeks before and 4 weeks after calving is characterized by greatly increased risk of disease.[1–3] The last 3 to 4 weeks of gestation are characterized by a period of rapid fetal growth, colostrogenesis and mammary development, and metabolic adjustments favoring mobilization of fat and other nutrients; all in combination with declining dry matter intake (DMI). The first 3 to 4 weeks after parturition features slowly increasing DMI in conjunction with rapidly

[a] SBScibus, PO Box 660, Camden, New South Wales 2570, Australia; [b] Department of Veterinary & Biomedical Sciences, Pennsylvania State University, University Park, PA 16802, USA; [c] Tarwin Veterinary Group, 32 Anderson St, Leongatha, Victoria 3953, Australia
* Corresponding author.
E-mail address: ianl@sbscibus.com.au

Vet Clin Food Anim 29 (2013) 337–366
http://dx.doi.org/10.1016/j.cvfa.2013.03.005 vetfood.theclinics.com
0749-0720/13/$ – see front matter

increasing nutrient losses in support of milk production. During this time rapid mammary tissue growth continues as well as hypertrophy of key metabolic and digestive organs. Metabolically, the cow is in a state of nutrient reserve mobilization, primarily adipose and labile protein but also bone. A critical adaptation is to stabilize homeostatic control mechanisms of key nutrients including glucose and calcium in support of lactation. These adaptations to the demands of the fetus and lactation are a process termed homeorhesis.[4] Homeorhetic processes are the long-term adaptations to a change in state such as from being nonlactating to lactating or nonruminant to ruminant and involve an orchestrated series of changes in metabolism that allow an animal to adapt to the challenges of the altered state.

Diseases that result from disordered homeorhetic change reflect disorders in homeostasis, in other words, these are failures to adapt that result in shortages of nutrients that are vital for existence. These conditions are often interrelated[2,5,6] and include

- Hypocalcemia and downer cows
- Hypomagnesemia
- Ketosis, fatty liver, and pregnancy toxemia
- Udder edema
- Abomasal displacement
- Retained fetal membranes/metritis
- Poor fertility and poor production

Although in the past, there has been a tendency to look at metabolic systems in isolation, metabolic processes within the body are intricately linked. This concept reflects a need for effective homeostatic control of metabolism. A failure of one metabolic process inevitably affects the efficiency of others. As research progresses, homeostatic links between metabolic processes once believed to be distant and unrelated are continually uncovered. As a result of the increased understanding of homeostatic processes, the concept of transition feeding has evolved from one focused only on control of milk fever to an integrated nutritional approach that addresses optimization:

- Calcium and bone metabolism
- Energy metabolism
- Protein metabolism
- Immune function
- Rumen function

Addressing any one of these areas in isolation would be of some benefit, but developing integrated nutritional strategies based on an understanding of the homoeostatic and homeorhetic processes involved in the transition from a nonlactating to lactating animal would have substantial benefits.

Grummer[7] stated that "If transition feeding is important, then perturbations in nutrition during this period should affect lactation, health and reproductive performance." There is now a substantial body of evidence clearly confirming that the transition period represents a brief but critically important period of time in a cow's life when careful manipulation of diet can have a substantial impact on subsequent health and productivity. The aims of transition can be summarized in the establishment of 4 freedoms from the disorders outlined in **Table 1**.[8]

By achieving these goals, minimizing the loss of body protein before calving, and enhancing mammary development in the periparturient period, milk production will increase in the subsequent lactation. Although transition cow nutrition research results are not consistent across studies, milk production responses relative to controls are in

Table 1
Defining the 4 freedoms

Condition	Detail
Macromineral deficiency	Mainly refers to calcium, magnesium, and phosphorus. Milk fever and grass tetany (hypomagnesemia) can result from a conditioned deficiency whereby excess potassium reduces the capacity of the cow to maintain stable blood concentrations of calcium and magnesium
Lipid mobilization disorders	Includes ketosis, fatty liver, and pregnancy toxemia; diseases that are largely influenced by a failure to provide sufficient or effective energy sources around calving
Immune suppression	Often associated with lack of energy or protein intake; micronutrients are often involved including copper, selenium, zinc, and vitamins A, E, and D
Ruminal disruption	Cows are vulnerable to changes in diet resulting from lower feed intake, poor quality silages, and rapid introduction of concentrates after calving

the order of 500 to 1000 kg of milk per lactation with improved transition cow nutrition and management. Targets for the various disease conditions encountered during transition are outlined in **Table 2** and a framework for understanding the effects of transition and longer-term nutrition on reproduction is provided in **Fig. 1**.

This article takes a slightly different approach to providing suggestions regarding dietary requirements for the transition. In particular, the different sources of nonstructural carbohydrates are examined separately and fats are not treated generically. There is an increasing body of evidence that these are biologically active substances with marked differences in action. This article addresses aspects of lipid mobilization disorders and ruminal disruption. The focus is on meeting energy and protein needs while maintaining stable rumen function.

Definition: Negative energy balance refers to deficits in energy requirements that are estimated. A negative nutrient balance refers to the loss of body tissue consisting of fat, glycogen, protein, minerals, and vitamins that occurs around calving.

WHAT IS THE NATURE OF METABOLIC CHANGE AROUND CALVING?

Changes in hormone metabolism before calving have been well described.[4,9] Bauman and Currie[4] noted the following adaptive changes to lactation: increased lipolysis, decreased lipogenesis, increased gluconeogenesis, increased glycogenolysis, increased use of lipids and decreased glucose use as an energy source, increased mobilization of protein reserves, increased absorption of minerals and mobilization of mineral reserves, increased food consumption, and increased absorptive capacity for nutrients. Examining the homeorhetic and homeostatic responses to lactation assists understanding of the factors influencing the risk of disease. These responses can be exaggerated or perturbed by release of inflammatory mediators from lipid mobilization, environmental stressors, or subclinical disease conditions increasing postparturient disease risks.[10–14]

In brief, the following hormones influence the initiation of lactation and are associated with profound changes in metabolism. The precipitous decrease in plasma

Table 2
Achievable targets for cow health problems (expressed as the percentage of cases of calving cows within 14 days of calving)

Disease	Target (%)	Alarm Level (%)
Milk fever	1 (2 in old cows >8 y)	>3
Clinical ketosis	<1	>2
Subclinical ketosis >1 mmol/L (enzymatic assay week 1 after calving)	<10	>10
Retained placenta >6 h	<5	>7
Lameness >2 Specher et al locomotion score (1–5)	<4 when score >2	>4 when score >2
Clinical mastitis	<5 cases/100 cows in first 30 d	>5
Hypomagnesemia	0	Any
Calvings requiring assistance	<2	>3
Displaced abomasums (%)	<1	>2
Clinical acidosis (%)	<1	>1

progesterone levels that occurs at parturition is a key stimulus for lactogenesis. Estrogen levels increase rapidly in the last week of gestation and may play an important role in the initiation of lactation. Prolactin is important to the development of the mammary gland before lactation in cows. However, in dairy cattle, prolactin does not seem to play an important role in the maintenance of lactation. Glucocorticoids are important in the initiation and maintenance of lactation. Plasma cortisol levels increase in the immediate periparturient period and are associated with a transient hyperglycemia at calving.

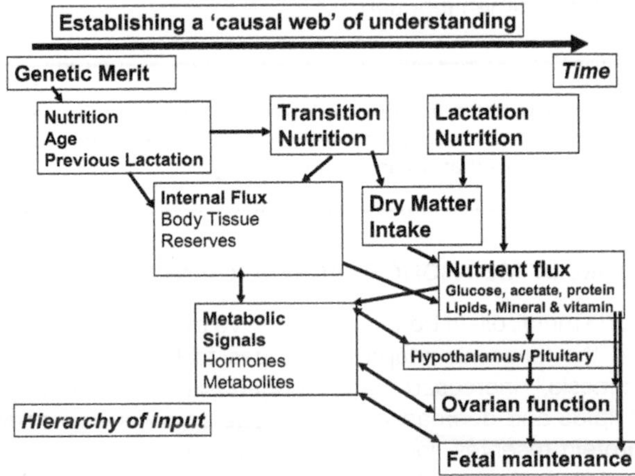

Fig. 1. A causal web to develop a model of metabolic subfertility in dairy cattle. The web shows a hierarchy of inputs and factors influencing subfertility. Nutrition before the dry period or initial calving and transition nutrition determine the nutrient stores available from body tissue reserves and those from lactation nutrition influence the nutrients available at any given time. These inputs, genetics, age, and environment determine reproductive responses. (*From* Lean IJ, Rabiee A. Quantitative metabolic and epidemiologic approaches to fertility of the dairy cow. In: Proceedings of the Dairy Cattle Reproduction Council. Denver (CO): 2007. p. 115–32.)

Insulin and glucagon play a central role in the homeostatic control of glucose. There is evidence, however, of insensitivity of cows to insulin in early lactation. The transitory hyperglycemia that occurs at calving does not seem to stimulate insulin. The insulin responses in hypoglycemic and ketonemic cows were less for glucose infusions and feeding than in normal cows, suggesting marked insulin resistance. Metz and van den Bergh[15] found that the response of adipose tissue to insulin in the periparturient cow was altered, because insulin addition did not reduce rates of lipolysis in vitro. Lipogenic activities of adipocytes are reduced by about one-third after calving. Glucagon plays a gluconeogenic role in the bovine, but may not stimulate lipolysis to the same extent as in nonruminant species. Thyroid hormone has a lactogenic function either when supplied orally or when injected and has been used in experimental protocols to induce ketosis.[16] However, thyroxine levels either decrease or are unchanged after calving.

Somatotropin plays a key lactogenic role in cattle as shown by milk production responses to exogenous somatotropin (rBST) and positive relationships between production and somatotropin levels in comparisons of high-yielding and low-yielding cattle. Somatotropin is possibly the most important hormonal determinant of increased milk yield in cattle. There is evidence that treatment with rBST may improve the health of periparturient cows, indicating the potential for somatotropin to positively integrate metabolism (see later discussion).

Fetal Demand for Nutrients

Bell[9] reviewed studies examining the nutrient demands of the fetus in late gestation. The fetal requirements for energy, although modest, are demanding in that the requirement for glucose is 4 times greater than that for acetate.

This demand highlights problems with the low energy density/low energy intake of dry cow diets recommended in the past. The fetus may even have an a priori demand for glucose as plasma glucose concentrations decreased in cows treated with sodium monensin before calving, despite the glucogenic action of monensin.[17]

The fetus also has significant requirements for amino acids, which are used for tissue deposition and oxidation. The fetal requirement for amino acids seems to be 3 times greater than the net requirement for fetal growth[9] because of significant oxidation of amino acids in the fetus.

In summary, fetal demands increase markedly in the last 4 weeks of gestation. There is an increased demand for glucose, an approximately 3-fold increase in demand for glucose immediately after calving, a doubling of the amino acid requirement, a 5-fold increase in fatty acid requirements, and a doubling of calcium needs in lactation compared with the needs of the cow and fetus.

CHALLENGES TO SUCCESSFUL ADAPTATION

Reduced Dry Matter Intake

Periparturient disease conditions are associated with decreased DMI, and feed intake is a critical determinant of health and productivity in the dry period. Feed intake and nutrient density of the diet determine the availability of nutrients to the cow and rapidly developing fetus. Grant and Albright[18] reviewed the feeding behavior and management factors during the transition period for dairy cattle and found that feed intake decreased by about 30% during the week before calving.

Factors that influence feed intake include social dominance, digestibility of the diet, access to feed, and palatability of the feed.[18] Cows and sheep with higher body condition scores have lower DMI after parturition,[19,20] and lower DMI has been noted immediately after calving and before calving[21] for cows with clinical ketosis.

Stephenson and colleagues[17] found that plasma 3-hydroxybutyrate (BHB) concentrations increased from 35 days before calving, in association with increased plasma free fatty acid concentrations (NEFA). Similar increases have been observed in other studies. It is unclear whether BHB and nonesterified fatty acid (NEFA) levels increase as a result of lower DMI, changes in the nutrient density of the diet, or increased fetal demand.

Providing access to feed for more than 8 hours per day and maintaining adequate availability and nutrient density of feed, controlling dominance behavior by grouping and providing adequate feed access and controlling body condition to an ideal of approximately 3.5 on the 5 point scale[22] reduce the risk of inadequate nutrient intake. In particular, the use of more digestible forages with lower slowly digestible fiber content allows greater DMI. Considerations around grouping of cattle need to be tempered with an understanding that movement of cattle between groups results in activity to establish new social hierarchies.[23–25]

The effect of greater DMI was demonstrated by force feeding periparturient cows through a ruminal fistula.[26] Cows that received more feed had less hepatic lipid accumulation and higher milk production after calving. The higher milk production resulted from greater postpartum feed intake and a highly significant positive correlation between precalving and postcalving feed intake was identified.[26] DMI before calving seems to be an important determinant of production after calving.

Impact of Lipid Mobilization on Liver Function

Reynolds and colleagues[27] measured glucose flux across portal-drained viscera over the transition period, finding minimal net change but a 267% increase in total splanchnic tissue output of glucose. This dramatic increase was almost exclusively a result of increased hepatic gluconeogenesis. Increased hepatic protein synthesis[9] and greater oxygen consumption[27] during transition are consistent with increased hepatic gluconeogenesis. The liver seems to be able to better synthesize glucose from propionate at 21 days postpartum compared with 1 day postpartum or 21 days prepartum.[28] The volatile fatty acid (VFA), propionate, is the primary source (50%–60%), of glucose but other substrates must be used to maintain glucose production, including lactate (15%–20%) from placental metabolism and skeletal muscle glycolysis, amino acids (20%–30%) from skeletal muscle catabolism and dietary absorption, and glycerol (2%–4%) released from adipose tissue lipolysis.[27,29]

Overton[30] examined the effects of lipid mobilization on liver function. Increased tissue mobilization increases the flux of NEFAs to the liver for oxidation and increases the need to export some of these back to peripheral tissues as ketones. The liver may not be able to reexport sufficient of these and accumulates fat in hepatocytes. The implications of this accumulation are that the rates of both gluconeogenesis and ureagenesis may be impaired.[31] Strang and colleagues[31] found that hepatic ureagenesis was reduced 40% through exposure of liver cells to NEFAs, which resulted in increased triglyceride accumulation similar to that of cows after calving. Triglyceride accumulation in the liver around the time of calving has been recognized for many years.[7,32]

Excessive lipolysis results in a greatly increased blood NEFA concentration and greater hepatic triglyceride accumulation and is associated with a higher risk of 1 or more periparturient diseases.[7,33–36] Any factor resulting in greater energy demand (eg, twin pregnancy, cold stress), lower energy intake (eg, poor feed quality, reduced feed availability, heat stress) or both decreases energy balance and ultimately blood NEFA concentration.[7]

In summary, maternal tissues reduce their use of glucose to meet energy needs over the transition, and increase hepatic gluconeogenesis to provide sufficient endogenous glucogenic substrate to account for lower nutrient intake. Failure to adapt to the demand for glucose increases mobilization of lipids and lipid-related disorders, such as hepatic lipidosis, ketosis, and pregnancy toxemia, the most severe of these.

ENERGY AND PROTEIN METABOLISM: OPPORTUNITIES AND LIMITATIONS TO IMPROVING PERFORMANCE

The demands for amino acids and glucose by the fetoplacental unit, and amino acids, glucose, and fatty acids by the mammary gland, particularly during stage 2 lactogenesis,[9,37] combine with a lowered potential DMI immediately before calving[38] to place the cow at great risk of mobilizing significant amounts of body fat and protein.

Energy Reserves: Body Condition

The body condition score (BCS) is a major determinant of the calving to first estrus interval; cows in higher body condition display estrus earlier.[19] Improved prepartum nutrition to increase BCS to moderate or better at calving was generally associated with increased milk production in dairy cows.[39–41] Excessive BCS (>3.75, scale of 1 to 5) in late pregnancy induces lower DMI during late pregnancy and early lactation resulting in greater negative energy balance in early lactation, as shown by excessive reduction in BCS (>1).[42] Westwood and colleagues[43] identified several factors that significantly influenced the display of estrus at first and second ovulation. Higher body weight of cattle before calving and postcalving appetite were significant factors that increased estrus display. Measures of metabolites in blood that reflected a better energy balance, including cholesterol concentrations and the ratio of glucose to 3-hydroxybutyrate, were also associated with greater display of estrus at ovulation.

In summary, improved BCS to approximately 3.75/5 is associated with better fertility, but greater increases are probably detrimental. The relationship between BCS and fertility may be better understood once the tissue components (fat, protein, glycogen) included in the BCS can be evaluated.

Energy Intake: Carbohydrates

The estimated energy balance after calving improves with increased energy density of the prepartum ration.[44–46] These improvements have been associated with trends toward increased milk production, lowered milk fat percentage, and significant increases in protein percentage and yield.[45] The effect of increased energy density of the prepartum diet, in particular increased fermentable carbohydrate concentration, may in part be mediated through increased development of rumen papillae in response to increased VFA production.[47] The increased absorptive capacity of the rumen may have reduced the risk of VFA accumulation and depression of rumen pH and the subsequent risk of acidosis in response to the feeding of high concentrate diets postpartum. Because adaptation and development of rumen papillae takes between 3 and 6 weeks,[48,49] the benefit of increasing exposure to a prepartum diet high in fermentable carbohydrate is likely to be curvilinear. There are also likely to be benefits associated with the prepartum adaptation of the rumen microflora to postpartum diets high in concentrates.[2] However, there is a challenge in controlling the risks of metabolic disease, particularly lipid mobilization disorders should cows become overconditioned. Overconditioning, however, is more a function of lactation diets than those in the dry period.

Acidosis

Part of the challenge is to provide diets appropriate to preparing the rumen for feeds of greater energy density, but controlling weight, particularly lipid, gain. Adaptation to feeds of higher energy density is important; in almost all production systems, there is a marked increase in exposure to starches and sugars at the time of calving. These increase the risk of acidosis, a relatively poorly understood condition. There are significant recent reviews and articles that advance our understanding of acidosis and the definition of acidosis. Although measures of rumen pH are often used for diagnosis, inconsistencies in cut-off thresholds that define acidosis severity have created confusion in the definition of acidosis.[50–52] Studies and definitions of acidosis based on area under the curve estimates of pH are likely sound; these have largely been conducted on limited numbers of fistulated cattle, therefore production outcomes such as milk production, weight gain for beef cattle, or lameness have not been associated with the cut-off points. There is a lack of studies that relate ruminal conditions to outcomes of acidosis or risk factors for acidosis, apart from diets deliberately designed to challenge rumen function; however, a few studies have provided a more detailed examination of acidosis based on large numbers of cattle. Bramley and colleagues,[53] Morgante and colleagues,[54] and O'Grady and colleagues[55] sampled 800, 120, and 144 head of dairy cattle, respectively, and investigated associations between diets and outcomes. All 3 studies provided similar findings of associations between low ruminal pH and a ruminal environment in which the levels of total VFA were increased, but propionate and valerate were particularly increased. Bramley and colleagues[53] found that approximately 10% of cows were in the group characterized by high ruminal concentrations of propionate, acetate, butyrate, valerate, and lactic acid, and low ammonia and pH, compared with other groups of cows. The least predictive variables for this group were pH and lactic acid concentrations and the most predictive were propionate and valerate concentrations. These cows had lower milk fat percentages and herds with a high prevalence of acidotic cows had a higher prevalence of lameness and diets lower in neutral detergent fiber and higher in nonfiber carbohydrates, suggesting that the categorization of these cows was sound.

It is unsurprising that pH was a poor predictive variable for acidosis in the field; the rumen is not homogeneous. Samples obtained by stomach tube, probably from the dorsal sac of the rumen, differ from those obtained using rumenocentesis by approximately 0.5 pH and are poorly related with r^2 of 0.2.[53] Golder and colleagues[56] examined the cut-off points for optimal sensitivity and specificity of use of rumen pH obtained using stomach tube or rumenocentesis in predicting acidosis. The optimal cut-off points for prediction of acidosis were less than 6.6 and less than 6.0 for stomach tube and rumenocentesis pH, respectively; however, neither provided a satisfactory test for acidosis, which was defined using the method of Bramley and colleagues.[53] The stomach tube pH had a sensitivity of 0.80 and a specificity of 0.76 and rumenocentesis pH had a sensitivity of 0.74 and a specificity of 0.79. It is likely, however, that testing groups of cows for pH less than 5.5, as advocated by Garrett and colleagues,[57] provides a satisfactory indicator of acidosis at the herd level.

The authors hypothesize that acidosis occurs along a continuum of ruminal conditions from subacute to peracute with different expressions of risk of acidosis reflecting the substrates available to the rumen. Similarly, it can be hypothesized that the risk of acidosis will vary depending on the length of exposure to rapidly fermentable diets, preformed acids in silage, and the type of fermentable substrate.

There are marked substrate differences in the risk of lactic acid generation and VFA production.[51,56] Simply, VFA and lactic acid formation is much more influenced by rapidly fermented substrates such as sugars rather than starches. Therefore, inclusion rates for starch and sugars should be considered separately; however, the recommendations in **Table 3** are preliminary.

Protein Reserves: Body Condition

The importance of mobilized tissue protein as a source of amino acids for mammary metabolism and gluconeogenesis may be relatively small over the period from calving to peak lactation,[58] but is important in the first 1 to 2 weeks of lactation.[9] A reduction in skeletal muscle fiber diameter of 25% was observed immediately after calving[59] and a decline in the ratio of muscle protein to DNA was found in ewes during early lactation.[60] These findings support the concept that skeletal muscle is an important source of endogenous amino acids in early lactation. This hypothesis that improved protein and energy balance improves subsequent production is supported to some extent by the trend toward proportionally higher milk and protein yields in response to increasing days of exposure to a BioChlor-based (Church and Dwight, NJ) prepartum transition diet in younger cows, which are likely to have a greater energy and protein requirement to support growth (DeGaris, personal communication, 2010).

Table 3
Targets for diets: far off, transition, and fresh cows (first 40 days)

Diet Composition (% Dry Matter)	Dry Cows	Transition Cows	Fresh Cows
DMI[a]	1.75–2	2%–2.5%	3 to 4+
Neutral detergent fiber (NDF) (%)	>36	>36	>32
Physically effective NDF (%)	30	25–30	>19
Crude protein (CP) (%)	>12	14–16	16–19
Degradability of CP (%)	80	65–70	65–70
Estimated energy MCal (Nel)/kg MJ (ME)/kg	1.5 (1.33)[a] 10 (9)[a]	1.65 11	1.73–1.8 11.5–12
Estimated Nel (MCal/lb)	0.66 (0.60)	0.73	0.76–0.79
Starch (%)	Up to 18	16–20	24–26
Sugar (%)	Up to 4	4–6	6–8
Ether extract (%)	3	4–5	4–5
Calcium (%)	0.4	0.4–0.5	0.8–1.0
Phosphorus (%)	0.25	0.25	0.4
Magnesium (%)	0.3	0.45	0.3
DCAD (mEq/100 g)	0–25	−10	25–40
Selenium (mg/kg)	3	3	3
Copper (mg/kg)	10	15	20
Zinc (mg/kg)	40	48	48
Manganese (mg/kg)	12	15	15
Iodine (mg/kg)	0.6	0.6	0.6
Vitamin A (IU/kg)	2000	3200	3200
Vitamin D (IU/kg)	1000	2500	2500
Vitamin E (IU/kg)	15	30	15

Abbreviations: DCAD, dietary cation-anion difference; ME, metabolizable energy; Nel, net energy at lactation.

[a] Energy intake and content that is desirable varies with body condition.

Estimates of body protein reserves mobilized at calving are 25% to 27% of total body protein in a dairy cow, approximately 10 to 17 kg total.[61–63] Belyea and colleagues[61] noted that there was a significant variation in the abilities of cows to mobilize protein. Bell[9] estimated that a metabolizable protein (MP) deficit over 23 days after calving would be nearly 7 kg without accounting for gluconeogenic costs, and 12.5 kg with gluconeogenic costs included. These values seem consistent with previous studies. If 10 kg of protein was lost from muscle, this would equate to a loss of around 60 kg of muscle mass.

The proteins and ultimately amino acids mobilized are used for mammary milk protein synthesis and for gluconeogenesis in the liver to support lactation. It seems that the rates of mobilization of fat and protein are similar,[64,65] but there has been little recent work on the amounts of labile fat and protein in body tissue despite this being an important area of physiology. Given the amounts of body weight lost after calving, especially in cows of high body condition, we can be confident that the lipid reserves of these cows exceed the protein reserves. Vandehaar and St Pierre[66] highlighted the partitioning of energy to body weight observed by Oba and Allen[67] when lower neutral detergent fiber (NDF) diets were fed. It can be hypothesized that cattle exposed to such diets and achieving higher BCS will have greater start-up milk, but the internal flux of nutrients provided from tissue mobilization has a higher ratio, and almost certainly greater amounts of lipid compared with protein.

In summary, it is likely that the amount of labile protein is an important determinant of health. We can use a working assumption that diets that do not meet the MP needs of cattle and exceed energy needs in a previous lactation may place cows at greater risk of metabolic disorder.

Protein Intake Before Calving

Studies investigating optimal concentrations of dietary protein in prepartum diets have focused on crude protein (CP) content,[68–71] rumen degradable or rumen undegradable fractions in the diet,[69–72] but have not considered in depth the potential for ruminal microbial protein synthesis or MP balance. It has been suggested that by increasing prepartum protein body tissue reserves, the transition cow can better use these reserves after calving to support lactation and minimize metabolic disorders,[7,73] an effect possibly mediated through increased labile protein reserves. To examine the data in a systematic way, the authors conducted a meta-analysis of studies that have altered the protein content of feeds before calving. Briefly, a literature search of databases was conducted and the diets from 11 studies containing 26 comparisons were extracted. The following information was extracted: authors, year of publication, journal, study design, control and test protein levels, days before calving that the trial started and days in milk at trial end, rumen undegradable percentages, breed, number of milkings per day, feeding type, housing, parity, number of cows in control and treatment groups, DMI, milk yield (kg/cow/d), milk fat yield (kg/cow/d), milk fat percentage, milk protein yield (kg/cow/d), milk protein percentage, fat corrected milk and level corrected for energy corrected milk, average body weight, and measures of variance (standard error).

Fig. 2 displays a Forest plot of milk production results. In this plot, studies are identified and the size of the box is proportional to the weighting of the study within the meta-analysis. The extremities of the horizontal lines represent the 95% confidence intervals of the results for each comparison and diamonds represent the overall estimates using a fixed effect model using the inverse variance method (I-V Overall), and a random effects model using the inverse variance method of DerSimonan and Laird (D + L Overall). The results were homogeneous but were not significant, indicating that milk production was not increased with increased CP in the precalving diet. Further work is needed to evaluate these responses in terms of MP. A preliminary meta-analysis[8] found no relationship between MP yield and subsequent milk production, however the current database is larger and this matter will be revisited. A key consideration is that simply increasing CP may not increase MP and increasing the fermentability of the diet with starch may yield more MP than perhaps that achieved by increasing CP or even undegradable protein.

Nonetheless, prepartum diets with positive MP and energy balances may increase subsequent milk production by providing adequate substrate for fetal and mammary development. McNeil and colleagues[74] fed ewes in late gestation diets to meet estimated energy requirements and variable CP content (8%, 12%, and 15% CP). Ewes fed the low CP diet had fetuses nearly 20% less in weight compared with ewes fed the higher CP diet. Fetal weights were not different between the 12% and 15% CP diets, yet the ewes receiving the 12% CP diet lost maternal skeletal protein similar to the ewes fed the 8% CP diet. These data suggest some capacity exists for the placenta to sustain amino acid delivery to the fetus, but it is not unlimited in the face of more severe or sustained dietary protein insufficiency. Mammary development was greater in ewes on the higher CP diets. Similarly, increased BCS at calving, reflecting improved body tissue reserves, increased subsequent milk production.[19,75]

Data on the effect of prepartum protein on subsequent reproduction and health is scant. Overconditioned (>3.75 BCS) mature Holstein cows fed additional protein prepartum from animal protein bypass sources had decreased prevalence of ketosis and less health disorders.[76] These supplemented cows also had improved reproductive performance, similar to the effects seen in primiparous cows supplemented with additional bypass protein.[77] Better health was also observed in cows fed additional bypass protein or supplementation with rumen-protected methionine and lysine supplements prepartum until early lactation.[78] Increasing time exposure to a prepartum transition diet was found to improve the reproductive performance and health of cows in a grazing system.[79] Improved reproduction may result directly from protein status effects on oocyte development or quality, or may be secondary to decreased postpartum disease events or improved body condition and protein reserve status.

Mature cows fed a higher protein diet (14% CP) prepartum with supplemental methionine lost less body protein and had increased body fat in early lactation compared with cows consuming a diet with lower protein (11% CP).[80] Insulin is the primary mediator of nutrient use and its status and tissue sensitivity have been implicated in both disease risk and impaired reproduction. The revised quantitative insulin sensitivity check index (RQUICKI) calculation is a function of insulin, glucose, and NEFA concentrations and is inversely related to BCS.[81] Feeding additional bypass protein to dry mature cows increased RQUICKI values relative to BCS or score change[82] and values increased for mature cows fed balanced protein fractions in the diet compared with cows consuming a diet high in degradable protein.[83] Not all studies supplementing protein in prepartum diets have observed effects on health or reproduction; differences in dietary treatments, exposure time, protein source and amino acid balance, management factors, and many other interactions may have influences on this outcome.

Despite many anecdotal observations of increased calf birth weight and dystocia problems with increasing prepartum protein supplementation, controlled studies do not support a cause-and-effect response.[84] No differences in calf birth weights were seen when dairy heifers were fed protein in excess of prepartum NRC (National Research Council) recommendations.[77] Feeding additional protein (12% vs 14% CP) during the dry period did not increase calf birth weight (44.5 vs 42.2 kg) in mature Holstein cows.[76] However, heavier birth weights (47.1 kg) were observed in another

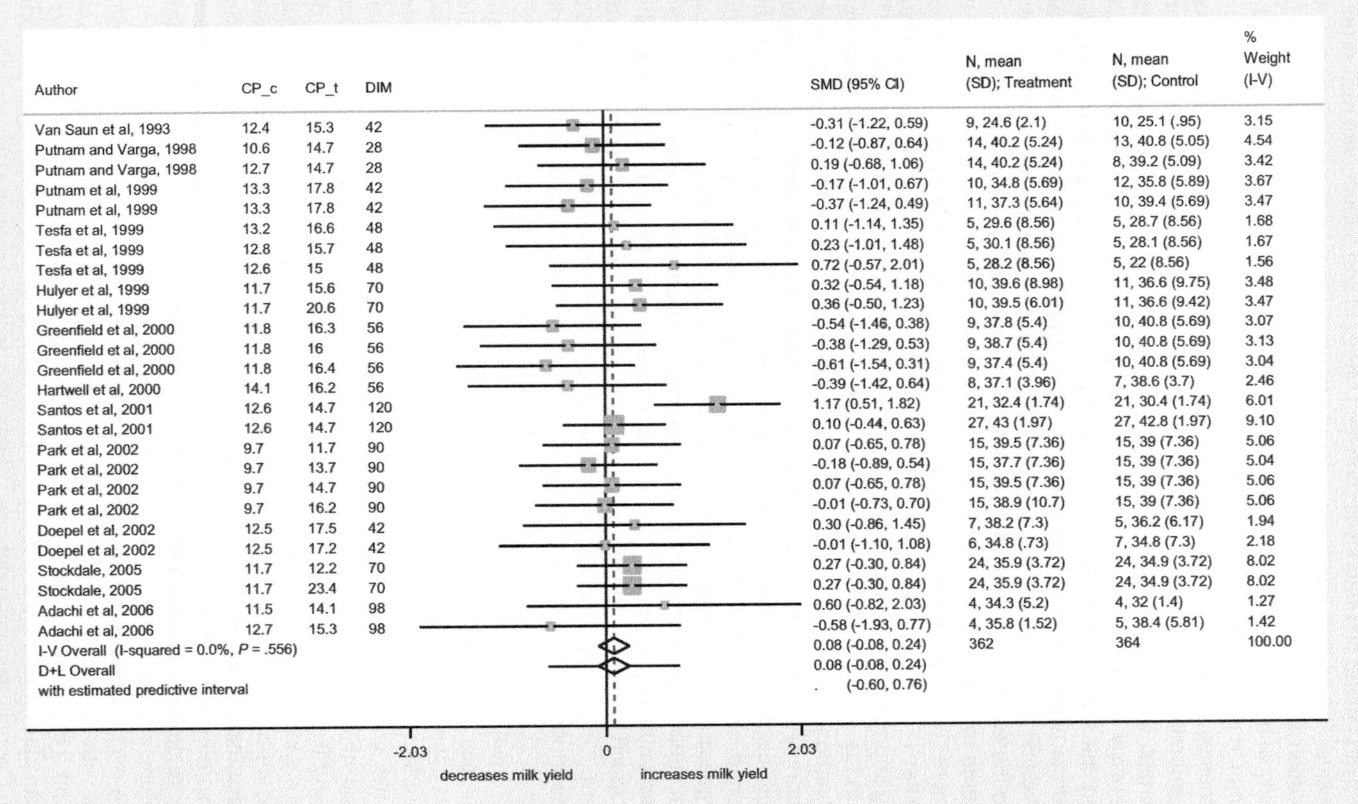
Author CP_c CP_t DIM SMD (95% CI) N, mean (SD); Treatment N, mean (SD); Control % Weight (I-V)
Van Saun et al, 1993 12.4 15.3 42 -0.31 (-1.22, 0.59) 9, 24.6 (2.1) 10, 25.1 (.95) 3.15
Putnam and Varga, 1998 10.6 14.7 28 -0.12 (-0.87, 0.64) 14, 40.2 (5.24) 13, 40.8 (5.05) 4.54
Putnam and Varga, 1998 12.7 14.7 28 0.19 (-0.68, 1.06) 14, 40.2 (5.24) 8, 39.2 (5.09) 3.42
Putnam et al, 1999 13.3 17.8 42 -0.17 (-1.01, 0.67) 10, 34.8 (5.69) 12, 35.8 (5.89) 3.67
Putnam et al, 1999 13.3 17.8 42 -0.37 (-1.24, 0.49) 11, 37.3 (5.64) 10, 39.4 (5.69) 3.47
Tesfa et al, 1999 13.2 16.6 48 0.11 (-1.14, 1.35) 5, 29.6 (8.56) 5, 28.7 (8.56) 1.68
Tesfa et al, 1999 12.8 15.7 48 0.23 (-1.01, 1.48) 5, 30.1 (8.56) 5, 28.1 (8.56) 1.67
Tesfa et al, 1999 12.6 15 48 0.72 (-0.57, 2.01) 5, 28.2 (8.56) 5, 22 (8.56) 1.56
Hulyer et al, 1999 11.7 15.6 70 0.32 (-0.54, 1.18) 10, 39.6 (8.98) 11, 36.6 (9.75) 3.48
Hulyer et al, 1999 11.7 20.6 70 0.36 (-0.50, 1.23) 10, 39.5 (6.01) 11, 36.6 (9.42) 3.47
Greenfield et al, 2000 11.8 16.3 56 -0.54 (-1.46, 0.38) 9, 37.8 (5.4) 10, 40.8 (5.69) 3.07
Greenfield et al, 2000 11.8 16 56 -0.38 (-1.29, 0.53) 9, 38.7 (5.4) 10, 40.8 (5.69) 3.13
Greenfield et al, 2000 11.8 16.4 56 -0.61 (-1.54, 0.31) 9, 37.4 (5.4) 10, 40.8 (5.69) 3.04
Hartwell et al, 2000 14.1 16.2 56 -0.39 (-1.42, 0.64) 8, 37.1 (3.96) 7, 38.6 (3.7) 2.46
Santos et al, 2001 12.6 14.7 120 1.17 (0.51, 1.82) 21, 32.4 (1.74) 21, 30.4 (1.74) 6.01
Santos et al, 2001 12.6 14.7 120 0.10 (-0.44, 0.63) 27, 43 (1.97) 27, 42.8 (1.97) 9.10
Park et al, 2002 9.7 11.7 90 0.07 (-0.65, 0.78) 15, 39.5 (7.36) 15, 39 (7.36) 5.06
Park et al, 2002 9.7 13.7 90 -0.18 (-0.89, 0.54) 15, 37.7 (7.36) 15, 39 (7.36) 5.04
Park et al, 2002 9.7 14.7 90 0.07 (-0.65, 0.78) 15, 39.5 (7.36) 15, 39 (7.36) 5.06
Park et al, 2002 9.7 16.2 90 -0.01 (-0.73, 0.70) 15, 38.9 (10.7) 15, 39 (7.36) 5.06
Doepel et al, 2002 12.5 17.5 42 0.30 (-0.86, 1.45) 7, 38.2 (7.3) 5, 36.2 (6.17) 1.94
Doepel et al, 2002 12.5 17.2 42 -0.01 (-1.10, 1.08) 6, 34.8 (.73) 7, 34.8 (7.3) 2.18
Stockdale, 2005 11.7 12.2 70 0.27 (-0.30, 0.84) 24, 35.9 (3.72) 24, 34.9 (3.72) 8.02
Stockdale, 2005 11.7 23.4 70 0.27 (-0.30, 0.84) 24, 35.9 (3.72) 24, 34.9 (3.72) 8.02
Adachi et al, 2006 11.5 14.1 98 0.60 (-0.82, 2.03) 4, 34.3 (5.2) 4, 32 (1.4) 1.27
Adachi et al, 2006 12.7 15.3 98 -0.58 (-1.93, 0.77) 4, 35.8 (1.52) 5, 38.4 (5.81) 1.42
I-V Overall (I-squared = 0.0%, P = .556) 0.08 (-0.08, 0.24) 362 364 100.00
D+L Overall 0.08 (-0.08, 0.24)
with estimated predictive interval . (-0.60, 0.76)
-2.03
0
2.03
decreases milk yield
increases milk yield

group of mature Holstein cows with prolonged dry periods (>75 days) fed a low protein (9% CP) diet initially followed by a high protein (15% CP) diet during the last 4 weeks of gestation.[76] Sheep studies suggest that mid-gestation nutrition has greater potential to alter calf birth weight.[85]

Few studies have found prepartum dietary effects on colostrum quality. Greater immunoglobulin concentration in colostrum was observed in cows fed moderate (12% CP) or higher (14% CP) protein diets that contained animal product bypass protein sources compared with cows consuming a prepartum diet without supplemental bypass sources.[76] These immunoglobulin concentration differences in colostrum were the opposite of immunoglobulin concentrations measured in maternal serum over the last 4 weeks before calving. These observations might suggest an amino acid role in the transfer of immunoglobulins from maternal serum to colostrum.

In summary, excellent physiologic data suggest a need for diets that contain good levels of MP. The authors formulate diets that meet or exceed the MP requirements of CPM Dairy (Version 3.09). These diets require 14% to 16% CP and adequate starch and sugar as defined later (see **Table 3**).

Amino Acids

The balance and ratios of specific absorbed amino acids are of importance to production.[86,87] Methionine and lysine are often considered the first rate-limiting amino acids in support of lactation across a range of diets for dairy cows.[88] It is often assumed that methionine and lysine are also limiting amino acids for pregnancy, although no studies have validated this hypothesis. Methionine was added for the last 2 weeks of pregnancy for cows on high protein diets with bypass protein (39.6% CP) from animal sources and improved methionine availability to peripheral tissues was observed.[89] The investigators suggested that high bypass protein diets fed prepartum may restrict the contribution of microbial protein to MP. Histidine has been identified as a limiting amino acid, especially when most of the MP is derived from microbial protein.[90] Typical formulations for prepartum diets coupled with declining intake would result in microbial protein supplying more than 60% of MP delivered to the intestine.

Fig. 2. Forrest plot of the standardized mean difference of the effect of prepartum CP levels on postpartum milk production. Box size is proportional to the inverse variance of the estimates. The orange dot is the standardized mean difference or effect size of the trial. The horizontal lines represent the 95% confidence interval for the effect size. The solid vertical gray line represents a mean difference of zero or no effect. The diamonds represent the summary estimates using the fixed effect model (I-V overall) and the random effects model (D+L overall). The estimated predictive interval is of a future trial using the estimate of heterogeneity from the inverse variance effects. The figure shows that there was a positive but nonsignificant effect of changes in CP percentage in the diet fed before calving on postcalving milk production. Author refers to the first author and year of the publication. CP-c and CP-t refer to the CP content of rations in the control and treatment groups. DIM refers to days in milk. SMD is the standardized mean difference (standardized using the z-statistic). Thus, points to the left of the line represent a reduction in the parameter, whereas points to the right of the line indicate an increase. Each square represents the mean effect size for that study. The upper and lower limit of the line connected to the square represents the upper and lower 95% confidence interval for the effect size. The size of the square reflects the relative weighting of the study to the overall effect size estimate with larger squares representing greater weight. The dotted vertical line represents the overall effect size estimate. The diamond at the bottom represents the 95% confidence interval for the overall estimate. The solid vertical line represents a mean difference of zero or no effect.

The role of amino acid balance in peripartum diets has been studied intensively, although most emphasis has been placed on postpartum dietary effects relative to milk yield and component responses. Responses to rumen-protected methionine, lysine, or both in postpartum diets have been variable.[91] Modest milk yield and true protein yield responses are more often associated with methionine supplementation and in diets that may be marginal in meeting MP requirements.[92,93] The methionine response may be a result of its ability to support gluconeogenesis and liver fat transport compared with lysine. Variability in study findings may be attributed to confounding effects of dietary energy density (ie, microbial protein contribution), prepartum and postpartum protein content, DMI, and their interactions relative to potential response to amino acid supplementation. Study design can influence interpretation; the results of short-term Latin Square studies may be influenced by the cow's ability to mobilize body protein to mask treatment effects. Longer-term supplementation trials may minimize this impact. This effect is further complicated by prepartum dietary protein content and its effect on labile protein availability after calving. Higher prepartum protein diets lessened the impact of dietary protein manipulations after calving,[94] whereas lower prepartum protein diets accentuated the amino acid response.[72] In formulating postpartum diets, emphasis should be placed on providing sufficient MP with a balanced amino acid profile.

In summary, cows require amino acids. The balance needed is determined by their physiologic state. There is evidence for balancing diets for amino acids in support of early lactation, but less evidence for diets before calving. We recommend that prepartum diets should be formulated to meet or exceed MP requirements (CPM Version 3.09). The use of supplemental amino acids requires further study.

An alternative prepartum nutritional strategy

Although study results from Bertrics and colleagues[26] suggested that greater feed intake could reduce NEFA mobilization and decrease the risk for hepatic fatty infiltration, other studies indicated moderate feed intake could also show similar positive postpartum responses.[44,95–97] Cows moderately restricted in feed intake (80% of energy requirement) had lower NEFA concentrations precalving, less hepatic fat content, and greater postpartum intake. Ensuing studies suggested that energy consumption in the early dry period (>30 days before expected calving) also had significant effects on postpartum health and lactational performance.[96,98–101] Excessive energy intake may predispose the cow to greater maternal tissue insulin insensitivity coupled with the decline in physiologic insulin concentration that occurs just before calving, thus permitting more exaggerated NEFA mobilization and subsequent metabolic derangements. From these observations, a feeding management approach controlling total energy consumed and moderately restricting intake throughout the prepartum period has been advocated.[102]

The aim of these diets is to provide sufficient energy to meet daily needs and not supply excessive energy intake relative to NRC (2001) requirements.[88] Cereal straw forage or mature grass hay is used to dilute dietary energy provided from other more energy dense ingredients. These diets are typically corn silage based. Use of lactation-diet feed ingredients can be achieved by the dilution, allowing for easy adaptation to postpartum diets. Wheat straw is preferred because of its consistency and better NDF digestibility compared with other straw products. The bulking ingredient is used to allow for ad libitum intake rather than management attempting restricted intake. To be successful, the bulking ingredient should be properly incorporated into the diet and not fed separately. To ensure intake and to minimize sorting, the hay or straw should be chopped to achieve a consistent particle size of 4 to 6 cm (1.5–2 in). The straw or hay should be of high quality and palatable. An important aspect of the success of a controlled energy diet is ensuring adequate protein intake. Drackley and Janovick[102] recommend supplying more than 1000 g of MP, which can be achieved in diets formulated for 12% to 14% CP. To achieve postruminal delivery of this amount of MP, some bypass product sources of bypass protein will need to be included in the diet.

Use of controlled energy diets should be perceived as a complete dry cow program.[102] The use of straw typically controls dietary potassium concentration, thus reducing the risk of disrupted calcium homeostasis. Application of these diets in the field supports the contention that these diets can be successfully fed as single dry cow group systems, thus reducing some pen changes during transition. Research and field experience with these diets suggests reduced postpartum disease problems and potentially improved reproductive performance.[96,98,101,103] Similar health and production responses were seen in a series of studies using grass hay or wheat straw feeding either ad libitum or restricted.[104] Van Saun[76] used similarly formulated high fiber diets, but in a 2 group dry cow feeding program. Diets were formulated to provide either 1100 or 1300 g of MP per day to multiparous cows. Although the study cows were generally overconditioned (BCS >3.75/5), similar positive effects on health and reproduction were observed.

In summary, a key factor with prepartum DMI is to optimize intake in an effort to minimize any dramatic decline in intake just before calving. Significant intake declines stimulate greater NEFA mobilization, which adversely affects critical metabolic adaptations to lactation. Differing dry cow diet feeding strategies have been applied in the field with similar success, suggesting that other factors beyond nutrient content need to be considered. Grouping strategies, pen movements, environmental stressors, and feeding management play significant roles in the success or failure of any given dry cow feeding strategy.

Intake of Fats

Perhaps the most rapidly developing area of ruminant nutrition is that of fat nutrition. Recent understandings of the role of fats in metabolism open new avenues to improving metabolism, health, and reproduction in cattle. Studies have identified substantial potential for milk fats, including the conjugated linoleic acids (CLA), to positively influence human health[105] and along with this, increased understanding of the mechanisms by which different specific fatty acids in milk are generated. Critically, there is an increased awareness of the potential for specific dietary fats to improve health production and fertility. Vast differences (up to 15 standard deviations) in milk production and composition responses to different commonly used fats are observed.[106]

Lean and Rabiee[107] noted that there is a striking difference in the ration of lipid intake to milk yield for North American cows compared with Australasian cows; it can be estimated that lipid intake for North American cattle is about 15.5 g/L versus 20 to 22 g/L for the Australasian cows. Furthermore, for essential fatty acid (C18:2 and C18:3) intake at the duodenum, ratios are 0.7 g/L versus 1.4 to 1.6 g/L, respectively, or approximately half. These findings suggest support for the numerous pivotal roles identified for lipids in reproductive metabolism.[108,109]

Linoleic (C18:2) and linolenic fatty acids (C18:3) are classified as essential fatty acids and must be supplied in the diet, because the double bonds between the Δ-9-carbon and the terminal methyl group of the fatty acids cannot be produced by cattle. Roles for fatty acids include precursors for reproductive hormones (eg, prostaglandins), in membrane structures as phospholipids, and in immune function. The optimal requirement for 15% to 25% of energy being supplied as lipogenic precursors (or about 8% long-chain fatty acids in the diet) for efficient milk production was described.[110]

Although feeding fats during the prepartum and immediate postpartum period has not traditionally been recommended[111] because of the potential to reduce DMI, particularly in heifers,[42] there are now many studies in which beneficial effects have been observed.[112–115] These included a reduction in liver triglyceride accumulation[112] and levels of NEFA[113] in the immediate postpartum period and improved pregnancy rates.[116] Inclusion of fat in the diet may increase serum cholesterol concentrations,[117,118] a factor associated with better fertility. Westwood and colleagues[43] found that higher concentrations of plasma cholesterol were associated with a shorter interval from calving to conception, with greater probabilities of conception and successful pregnancy by day 150 of lactation, a finding consistent with those of Kappel and colleagues[119] and Ruegg and colleagues,[120] who found associations between cholesterol concentrations and fertility measures. Similarly, Moss[121] found that low blood cholesterol concentrations at mating were strongly associated with conception failure. However, fat feeding has a variable impact on the reproductive performance of lactating dairy cows with some positive[122–126] and some negative reports.[123,127,128] Reviews[109,129] have indicated that the effect of supplemental C18:2 from oil seeds and CaLCFA on fertility varied significantly, but suggest that supply of C18:2, C18:3, eicosapentaenoic acid (C20:5), and docosahexaenoic acid (C22:6) in forms that reach the lower gut, may have more profound effects on fertility.

Von Soosten and colleagues[130] elegantly explored the effects of protected CLA compared with a stearic acid–based fat supplement on tissue mobilization in a serial slaughter study. Overall, a trend for decreased body mass mobilization suggested a protective effect of CLA supplementation on the use of body reserves within 42 days in milk (DIM). Continuous CLA supplementation until 105 DIM increased body protein accretion. These effects suggested a more efficient use of metabolizable energy in CLA-supplemented early lactation dairy cows; an effect of ruminally protected fats not based solely on palm oil was identified independently in the meta-analysis of Rabiee and colleagues.[106]

The fat and fertility data require more research studies and meta-analytical evaluation that will include an evaluation of fat sources used and amounts and ratios of specific fats fed to elucidate the optimal approaches. However, de Veth and colleagues[115] demonstrated marked improvements (median time to conception was decreased by 34 days to 117 vs 151 DIM) in the fertility of cattle fed a ruminally protected CLA compared with cows not receiving the fat. Thatcher and colleagues[109] also found positive effects of supplementation with ruminally protected CLA and palm fatty acids on reproduction and health. Linolenic acid (C18:3) predominates in forage lipids,[131] however, concentrations of linoleic acid (C18:2) are also high in some pastures. It is possible that this and high digesta flow rates for cows on high-quality pasture diets may, in part, explain some of the differences in reproductive performance achieved in well-fed and well-managed pastured herds compared with NA (North American) herds. Data from Kay and colleagues[132] show that around 90% of *cis*-9, *trans*-11 CLA in milk is derived by endogenous synthesis of fats in fresh pasture. Studies in Ireland[133] found positive trends to a lower services per conception, but little overall effect of supplementation with protected CLA on fertility in cows on pasture, a finding consistent with the suggestions of Lean and Rabiee[107] that at least some of the differences in fertility of cows on pasture-based diets and those on total mixed ration diets may reflect the CLA generated from pasture.

In summary, fat supplements can improve energy balance, reduce the risk of metabolic diseases such as ketosis, and crucially allow energy density to be maintained in diets without increased dependence on rapidly fermentable carbohydrates. Evidence is increasing of a positive role for CLA, fed either as protected fats or derived from pasture in retaining body tissue after calving and improving fertility. Feeding fats in transition is an essential component of an integrated response to the challenges of needing to control tissue mobilization.

OTHER INTERVENTIONS

Somatotropin

Two actions of somatotropin increase the potential for rBST to improve periparturient health. The diabetogenic action of somatotropin, which decreases the sensitivity of peripheral tissues to insulin and increases blood glucose concentrations, increases the potential for treatment precalving to reduce the risk of ketosis. Administration of rBST to lactating cows is associated with insulin release[134] and liver function is also altered in cows treated with rBST resulting in increased gluconeogenesis.[135] Putnam and colleagues[70] fed cows 2 rations that differed in CP concentration (13.3% vs 17.8%) and treated cows with rBST every 14 days from 28 days before anticipated calving until parturition in a factorial study. Glucose concentrations tended to increase ($P = .08$) and the point directions were toward a decrease in NEFA and BHB concentrations for the rBST-treated cows both before and after calving. The rBST treatment significantly decreased concentrations of BHB before calving. Gulay and colleagues[136,137] found similar increases in glucose concentrations but NEFA concentrations were increased in cows treated with low doses of rBST before and after calving.

A second action is altered partitioning of nutrients in cows treated during a previous lactation. Lean and colleagues[138] treated 3 groups of cattle with different doses of rBST (17.2, 51.6 and 86 mg/d, respectively) during a previous lactation and found higher blood glucose, lower BHB, and lower NEFA concentrations in the treated cattle after calving. There are limited data to support routine use of rBST precalving to prevent lipid-related disorders but fundamental modes of action suggest a potential for benefit. Changes in body composition from rBST treatment in a previous lactation seem to be positive for health.

Methyl Donors

Hepatic fatty infiltration is an expected consequence of body lipid mobilization around the time of calving.[59,139] Excessive hepatic lipidosis results from an interaction between negative energy balance and acute phase inflammatory response, which reduces apoprotein synthesis, and is a significant precondition for many periparturient disease entities.[140] A limited supply of methionine and lysine may reduce production of very low density lipoprotein (VLDL) and predispose to hepatic lipidosis.[141,142] Choline and methionine metabolism are closely related and a significant percentage of methionine is used for choline synthesis.[143] Choline, a methyl donor and constituent of phosphatidylcholine, facilitates hepatic lipid export by increasing VLDL formation. Choline and methionine have interchangeable functions as methyl donors and may partially replace or spare the other.[144] Another methyl donor intermediate is betaine, an oxidative product of choline; recent research has not shown a beneficial response to its use in replacing methionine.[145]

Cows afflicted with either ketosis or hepatic lipidosis had lower serum apoproteins associated with VLDL structures, suggesting an inability of the liver to export triglycerides.[146] Similar to niacin, choline is readily degraded in the rumen, therefore a rumen-protected form is necessary for it to be efficacious when administered orally.[147] Early studies feeding increasing amounts of rumen-protected choline (treatments ranged from 0 to 20 g choline/d) showed a modest to no impact of choline on energy balance and liver triglyceride measurements.[148,149] In a controlled fatty liver induction study, feeding 15 g of choline per day during the induction phase reduced blood NEFA and liver triglyceride levels.[150] Feeding 15 g choline per day after induction of fatty liver tended to increase liver triglyceride clearance, which could contribute to improved performance[151] and health.[152,153] Liver triglyceride levels were reduced and glycogen content increased when choline was fed at 25 and 50 g/d prepartum (21 days) and postpartum (60 days), respectively.[154] Other recent preliminary studies found no response to choline supplementation, possibly attributed to lower BCSs and a lesser risk for negative energy balance.[155,156]

There is growing evidence suggesting that choline is a limiting nutrient for the high-producing dairy cow, especially around the time of calving.[144,157] However, the time frame of supplementation, dosage, BCS, dietary methionine status, and other factors may influence the response observed. A pooled study of choline supplementation before and after calving showed improved DMI and milk yield,[157] whereas a pooled analysis that included studies with only postpartum choline supplementation showed minimal effects on intake, milk yield, and composition.[158] There was no consistent finding of choline response measures of energy balance or any mechanism to explain the observed improvement in intake. If choline supplementation (15 g/d) starting prepartum can improve hepatic VLDL export and reduce fat accumulation, then improvement in hepatic function should reduce disease risk and increase performance.

Rumen Modifiers

There are few data available that specifically address the use of rumen modifiers, apart from monensin, in the transition period. The ionophore, sodium monensin, is widely used in dairy cattle production in the United States, Canada, Australasia, South America, South Africa. The effects of sodium monensin are primarily to increase ruminal propionate production, reflecting an increase in propionate-producing bacteria compared with those producing formate, acetate, lactate, and butyrate. There is a concomitant decrease in methane production from the rumen and a sparing effect on ruminal protein digestion.[159–162] The effects of monensin on blood metabolites, production, reproduction, and health were examined in a series of meta-analyses.[163–165] Data were obtained from up 59 articles and, in some cases, nearly 10,000 cows to provide more precise estimates of effect and to understand the sources of variance in the effects of this intervention. Monensin use in lactating dairy cattle significantly reduced blood concentrations of BHB by 13%, acetoacetate by 14%, and NEFA by 7%. Monensin increased blood glucose by 3% and urea by 6% but had no significant effect on cholesterol, calcium, milk urea, or insulin.

Monensin use in lactating dairy cattle significantly decreased DMI by 0.3 kg but increased milk yield by 0.7 kg and improved milk production efficiency by 2.5%. Monensin decreased milk fat percentage 0.13% but had no effect on milk fat yield; however, there was significant heterogeneity between studies for both of these responses. The percentage of milk protein was decreased by 0.03% but protein yield increased by 0.016 kg/d with treatment. Monensin increased the BCS by 0.03 and improved body weight change similarly (0.06 kg/d). These findings indicate a benefit of monensin for improving milk production efficiency while maintaining body condition. The effect of monensin on the percentage of milk fat and yield was influenced by diet.

Over all the trials analyzed,[163] monensin decreased the risk of ketosis (relative risk [RR] = 0.75), displaced abomasums (RR = 0.75), and mastitis (RR = 0.91). No significant effects of monensin were found for milk fever, lameness, dystocia, retained placenta, or metritis. Monensin had no effect on first-service conception risk (RR = 0.97) or days to pregnancy (hazard ratio = 0.93). However, the effect of monensin on dystocia, retained placenta, and metritis was variable. The causes of the variation were explored with meta-regression, indicating that longer periods of treatment with monensin before calving increased the risk of dystocia. Similarly, longer days of treatment before calving also increased the risk of retained placenta. Improvements in ketosis, displaced abomasums, and mastitis were achieved with monensin.

In summary, monensin use increased milk and milk protein production and the efficiency of production and reduced the risk of ketosis. Exposure to prolonged treatment in the dry period with monensin may increase the risk of dystocia and retained placenta, but treatment periods of around 3 weeks reduce the risk of these disorders. Monensin use reduces the risks of lipid mobilization disorders.

TOXINS

Endophyte Alkaloids and Other Mycotoxins

The effects of mycotoxins on cattle health in general have been documented and reviewed[166,167] but there are limited data on their effects specifically during the transition period when there is the potential for exacerbation of many of the challenges to successful adaptation to lactation.[168] The key effects of mycotoxins that may exacerbate the challenges faced during the transition period are altered rumen function, reduction in DMI, immunosuppression, and hepatotoxicity.

The rumen microflora and fauna provide an important first line of defense against some mycotoxins.[169] Orachatoxin, deoxynivalenol (DON), and, to a lesser extent, aflatoxin are metabolized to less toxic compounds in the rumen. Other mycotoxins seem to be unaffected by the rumen environment; fumonsins pass through the rumen virtually unchanged.[170] In contrast, zearalenone is metabolized to the more toxic α-zearalenol in the rumen.[169] Any alteration in rumen function is likely to increase the rate of ruminal bypass and intestinal absorption of mycotoxins usually detoxified by the rumen microbial flora and fauna.

Several mycotoxins have the ability to directly damage the rumen microbial mass. Patullin has an antibiotic activity against gram-positive and gram-negative bacteria as well as protozoa and has been shown to reduce cellulolysis of alfalfa hay, VFA production, and microbial protein synthesis.[171,172] The fusarium toxins, beauvericin and enniatin, also have an antibiotic effect against gram-positive bacteria and *Mycoplasma* spp.[173]

Ruminal acidosis may reduce the ability of the rumen to detoxify some mycotoxins. Sheep fed grain-based diets are less able to detoxify orachatoxin than those fed hay-based diets,[174] and cattle with subacute ruminal acidosis may be less able to detoxify DON.[168]

Any mycotoxicosis resulting in reduced rumen function or systemic disease will likely reduce DMI. Feed refusal of moldy feeds because of taste aversion is likely caused by contamination with microbial volatile organic compounds,[168] consisting of a wide range of volatile chemicals that are unpalatable to most species. The aerobic deterioration of ensiled feeds poses a particular risk. Bolsen and colleagues[175] demonstrated significant decreases in DMI as well as apparent digestibility of dry matter, organic matter, and NDF in cattle fed silage that consisted of 25% aerobically surface-spoiled silage. In addition, the investigators noted that rumen fiber mats in treated cattle were either partially or totally destroyed.

The immunosuppressive effects of many of the mycotoxins have long been recognized with even subclinical doses impairing the activity of B and T lymphocytes, antibody production, and macrophage and neutrophil function. Aflatoxins and trichothecenes can inhibit chemotaxis and phagocytosis of bovine neutrophils and macrophages,[176] and aflatoxins inhibit lymphoid cell proliferation and associated cytokines.[167] There is also evidence of synergistic inhibition of the immune system between aflatoxin and T-2 toxin.[177]

Several mycotoxins have been shown to be hepatotoxic. Sporodesmin, produced by *Pithomyces chartarum* growing in dead and decaying pastures during late summer and early autumn, causes facial eczema. This disease, mainly seen in the southern hemisphere, is characterized by hepatic photosensitization, reduced milk production, reproductive failure, and increased culling, particularly in cattle affected in the late dry period or early lactation. A negative effect on milk yield has been demonstrated in cattle treated with subclinical doses of sporodesmin.[178]

Perennial rye grasses may be high in the endophyte alkaloids ergovaline and lolitreme (and others). The presence of these alkaloids at increased levels may have extensive effects on production, reproduction, and the health of dairy cattle.[179] Although no studies have examined the effect of these alkaloids on cattle when fed specifically during the peripartum period, there are many potential pathways whereby a negative effect on subsequent productivity may be exerted. Random surveys of pastures in southwest Victoria, Australia, found levels of alkaloids in excess of those required to cause disease in cattle in approximately 30% of samples.[180]

In summary, despite the lack of specific data pertaining to the transition period, many mycotoxins have the potential to increase the risk of a poor transition. The authors, therefore, stress the need for careful attention to the state of silages used in the transition and the avoidance of poor feed quality. Even brief periods of inappetance pose a substantial health risk during transition.

RECOMMENDATIONS AND SUMMARY

Our recommendations for the diets are outlined in **Table 3** and in the companion article on minerals in this issue. Some of our recommendations will be refined by more work, particularly with regard to the role of protein nutrition over the gestation interval. There is a need to review the role of MP intake in the dry period on production, fertility, and health. The recent work on fat nutrition is clearly showing that fats are both powerful and different in their actions. The recommendations on these will be refined, as will specific recommendation for fiber and intake of nonfiber carbohydrate fractions.

In summary, dietary strategies should

- Ensure good protein stores (indicator BCS at calving >3.35/5)
- Avoid excessive adiposity (indicator BCS at calving <3.5) and
- Avoid abrupt dietary change to starch and sugars (starch 16%–20% before calving, 24%–26% after calving; sugars 4% before calving and 8% after calving)
- Provide high-quality proteins before and after calving (ie, positive MP diets)
- Avoid feed sources with spoilage (eg, silages that can put cows off feed)
- Use fats in transition diets, particularly ruminally protected CLA, unless pasture intakes are high

When combined with sensible mineral and dietary cation-anion difference strategies, these recommendations should result in better outcomes for cows and farmers.

ACKNOWLEDGMENTS

The authors thank Ms Veiss Harvey and Dr Ahmad Rabiee for the meta-analysis information provided.

REFERENCES

1. Shanks L. Postpartum distribution of costs and disorders of health. J Dairy Sci 1981;64:683–8.

2. Curtis CR, Erb EH, Sniffen CJ, et al. Path analysis of dry period nutrition, postpartum metabolic and reproductive disorders, and mastitis in Holstein cows. J Dairy Sci 1985;68:2347–60.
3. Stevenson MA, Lean IJ. Culling in eight New South Wales dairy herds: part 1. Descriptive epidemiology. Aust Vet J 1998;76:482–8.
4. Bauman DE, Currie WB. Partitioning of nutrients during pregnancy and lactation: a review of mechanism involving homeostasis and homeorhesis. J Dairy Sci 1980;63:1514–29.
5. Curtis CR, Erb EH, Sniffen CJ. Association of parturient hypocalcemia with eight periparturient disorders in Holstein cows. J Am Vet Med Assoc 1983;183:559–61.
6. Curtis MA. Epidemiology of uterine infections in dairy cows. Antioxidant and metabolic investigations. PhD thesis. Sydney: University of Sydney; 1997.
7. Grummer RR. Impact of changes in organic nutrient metabolism on feeding the transition dairy cow. J Anim Sci 1995;73:2828–33.
8. Lean IJ, DeGaris PJ, Wade LK, et al. Transition management of dairy cows: 2003. In: Parkinson TJ, editor. Proceedings of the Australian & New Zealand Combined Dairy Veterinarians' Conference. Taupo (New Zealand): Foundation for Continuing Education of the N.Z. Veterinary Association; 2003. p. 221–48.
9. Bell AW. Regulation of organic nutrient metabolism during transition from late pregnancy to early lactation. J Anim Sci 1995;73:2804–19.
10. Bernabucci U, Ronchi B, Lacetera N, et al. Influence of body condition score on relationships between metabolic status and oxidative stress in periparturient cows. J Dairy Sci 2005;88:2017–26.
11. Bertoni G, Trevisi E, Han X, et al. Effects of inflammatory conditions on liver activity in puerperium period and consequences for performance in dairy cows. J Dairy Sci 2008;91:3300–10.
12. Trevisi E, Amadori M, Cogrossi S, et al. Metabolic stress and inflammatory response in high-yielding periparturient dairy cows. Res Vet Sci 2012;93:695–704.
13. Zebeli Q, Sivaraman S, Dunn SM, et al. Intermittent parenteral administration of endotoxin triggers metabolic and immunological alterations typically associated with displaced abomasum and retained placenta in periparturient dairy cows. J Dairy Sci 2011;94:4968–83.
14. Bradford BJ, Mamedova LK, Minton E, et al. Daily injection of tumor necrosis factor-alpha increases hepatic triglycerides and alters transcript abundance of metabolic genes in lactating dairy cattle. J Nutr 2009;139:1451–6.
15. Metz SH, Van Den Bergh SG. Regulation of fat mobilization in adipose tissue of dairy cows in the period around parturition. Neth J Agr Sci 1977;25:198–211.
16. Hibbitt KG. The induction of ketosis in the lactating dairy cow. J Dairy Res 1966;33:291–8.
17. Stephenson KA, Lean IJ, Hyde ML, et al. Effects of monensin on the metabolism of periparturient dairy cows. J Dairy Sci 1997;80:830–7.
18. Grant RJ, Albright JL. Feeding behavior and management factors during the transition period in dairy cattle. J Anim Sci 1996;73:2791–803.
19. Garnsworthy PC, Topps JH. The effect of body condition of dairy cows at calving on their food intake and performance when given complete diets. Anim Prod 1982;35:113–9.
20. Cowan RT, Robinson JJ, McDonald I, et al. Effects of body fatness at lambing and diet in lactation on body tissue loss, feed intake and milk yield of ewes in early lactation. J Agr Sci 1980;95:497–514.

21. Lean IJ, Bruss ML, Trout HF, et al. Bovine ketosis and somatotropin: risk factors for ketosis and effects of ketosis on health and production. Res Vet Sci 1994;57:200–9.
22. Edmondson AJ, Lean IJ, Weaver LD, et al. A body condition scoring chart for Holstein dairy cows. J Dairy Sci 1989;72:68–78.
23. Cook NB, Nordlund KV. Behavioral needs of the transition cow and considerations for special needs facility design. Vet Clin North Am Food Anim Pract 2004;20:495–520.
24. Hosseinkhani A, DeVries TJ, Proudfoot KL, et al. The effects of feed bunk competition on the feed sorting behavior of close-up dry cows. J Dairy Sci 2008;91:1115–21.
25. Proudfoot KL, Veira DM, Weary DM, et al. Competition at the feed bunk changes the feeding, standing, and social behavior of transition dairy cows. J Dairy Sci 2009;92:3116–23.
26. Bertics SJ, Grummer RR, Cadorniga-Valino C, et al. Effect of prepartum dry matter intake on liver triglyceride concentration and early lactation. J Dairy Sci 1992; 75:1914–22.
27. Reynolds CK, Aikman PC, Lupoli B, et al. Splanchnic metabolism of dairy cows during the transition from late gestation through early lactation. J Dairy Sci 2003; 86:1201–17.
28. Drackley JK, Overton TR, Douglas GN. Adaptations of glucose and long-chain fatty acid metabolism in liver of dairy cows during the periparturient period. J Dairy Sci 2001;84:E100–12.
29. Overton TR, Waldron MR. Nutritional management of transition dairy cows: strategies to optimize metabolic health. J Dairy Sci 2004;87(Suppl E):E105–19.
30. Overton TR, Piepenbrink MS. Managing metabolism of transition cows through nutrition. In: Proceedings of the 36th Pacific Northwest Animal Nutrition Conference. Seattle (WA), 2001.
31. Strang BD, Bertics SJ, Grummer RR, et al. Effect of long-chain fatty acids on triglyceride accumulation, gluconeogenesis, and ureagenesis in bovine hepatocyctes. J Dairy Sci 1998;81:728–39.
32. Roberts CJ, Reid IM, Rowlands GJ, et al. A fat mobilisation syndrome in dairy cows in early lactation. Vet Rec 1981;108:7–9.
33. Holtenius P, Hjort M. Studies on the pathogenesis of fatty liver in cows. Bov Pract 1990;25:91.
34. Dyke PB, Emery RS, Liesman JL, et al. Prepartum nonesterified fatty acids in plasma are higher in cows developing periparturient health problems [abstract]. J Dairy Sci 1995;78(Suppl 1):264.
35. Kaneene JB, Miller RA, Herdt TH, et al. The association of serum nonesterified fatty acids and cholesterol, management and feeding practices with peripartum disease in dairy cows. Prev Vet Med 1997;31:59–72.
36. LeBlanc SJ, Leslie KE, Duffield TF. Metabolic predictors of displaced abomasum in dairy cattle. J Dairy Sci 2005;88:159–70.
37. Tucker HA. Endocrine and neural control of the mammary gland. In: Larson BL, editor. Lactation. Ames: Iowa State University Press; 1985. p. 39.
38. Marquardt JP, Horst RL, Jorgensen NA. Effect of parity on dry matter intake at parturition in dairy cattle. J Dairy Sci 1977;60:929–34.
39. Rogers GL, Grainger C, Earle DF. Effect of nutrition of dairy cows in late pregnancy on milk production. Aust J Exp Agric Anim Husb 1979;19:7–12.
40. Domecq JJ, Skidmore AL, Lloyd JW, et al. Relationships between body condition scores and milk yield in a large dairy herd of high yielding Holstein cows. J Dairy Sci 1997;80:101–12.

41. Waltner SS, McNamara JP, Hillers JK. Relationships of body condition score to production variables in high producing Holstein dairy cattle. J Dairy Sci 1993; 76:3410–9.
42. Hayirli A, Grummer RR, Nordheim EV, et al. Animal and dietary factors affecting feed intake during the prefresh transition period in Holsteins. J Dairy Sci 2002; 85:3430–43.
43. Westwood CT, Lean IJ, Garvin JK. Factors influencing fertility of Holstein dairy cows: a multivariate description. J Dairy Sci 2002;85:3225–37.
44. Holcomb CS, Van Horn HH, Head HH, et al. Effects of prepartum dry matter intake and forage percentage on postpartum performance of lactating dairy cows. J Dairy Sci 2001;84:2051–8.
45. Minor DJ, Trower SL, Strang BD, et al. Effect of nonfibre carboydrate and niacin on periparturient metabolic status and lactation of dairy cows. J Dairy Sci 1998; 81:189–200.
46. Grum DE, Drackley JK, Younker RS, et al. Nutrition during the dry period and hepatic lipid metabolism of periparturient dairy cows. J Dairy Sci 1996;79: 1850–64.
47. Dirksen G, Liebich HG, Mayer K. Adaptive changes of the ruminal mucosa and functional and clinical significance. Bov Pract 1985;20:116–20.
48. Kauffold P, Voiqt J, Piatkowski B. Studies of the influence of nutritional factors on the ruminal mucosa. 1. Structure and functional state of the ruminal mucosa after feeding of extreme rations and abrupt change in nutrition. Arch Tierernahr 1975;25:247–56 [in German].
49. Dirksen G, Dori S, Arbel SA, et al. The rumen mucosa - its importance as a metabolic organ of the high producing dairy cow. Israel J Vet Sci 1997;52:73–9.
50. Kleen JL, Hooijer GA, Rehage J, et al. Subacute ruminal acidosis (SARA): a review. J Vet Med A Physiol Pathol Clin Med 2003;50:406–14.
51. Nagaraja TG, Titgemeyer EC. Ruminal acidosis in beef cattle: the current microbiological and nutritional outlook. J Dairy Sci 2007;90:E17–38.
52. Plaizier JC, Krause DO, Gozho GN, et al. Subacute ruminal acidosis in dairy cows: the physiological causes, incidence and consequences. Vet J 2008; 176:21–31.
53. Bramley E, Lean IJ, Fulkerson WJ, et al. The definition of acidosis in dairy herds predominantly fed on pasture and concentrates. J Dairy Sci 2008;91:308–21.
54. Morgante M, Stelletta C, Berzaghi P, et al. Subacute rumen acidosis in lactating cows: an investigation in intensive Italian dairy herds. J Anim Physiol Anim Nutr 2007;91:226–34.
55. O'Grady L, Doherty ML, Mulligan FJ. Subacute ruminal acidosis (SARA) in grazing Irish dairy cows. Vet J 2008;176:44–9.
56. Golder HM, Celi P, Rabiee AR, et al. Effects of grain, fructose, and histidine on ruminal pH and fermentation products during an induced subacute acidosis protocol. J Dairy Sci 2012;95:1971–82.
57. Garrett EF, Pereira MN, Nordlund KV, et al. Diagnostic methods for the detection of subacute ruminal acidosis in dairy cows. J Dairy Sci 1999;82:1170–8.
58. Bauman DE, Elliot JM. Control of nutrient partitioning in lactating ruminants. In: Mepham TB, editor. Biochemistry of lactation. Amsterdam: Elsevier; 1983. p. 437.
59. Reid IM, Roberts CJ, Baird GD. The effects of underfeeding during pregnancy and lactation on structure and chemistry of bovine liver and muscle. J Agr Sci 1980;94:239–45.
60. Smith RW, Knight KA, Walsh A. Effects of lactation on the concentration of protein, lipids and nucleic acids in ovine skeletal muscle. Res Vet Sci 1981;30:253–4.

61. Belyea RL, Frost GR, Martz FA, et al. Body composition of dairy cattle by potassium-40 scintillation detection. J Dairy Sci 1978;61:206–11.
62. Botts RL, Hemken RW, Bull LS. Protein reserves in the lactating cow. J Dairy Sci 1979;62:433–40.
63. Parquay R, De Baere R, Lousse A. The capacity of the mature cow to lose and recover nitrogen and the significance of protein reserves. Br J Nutr 1972;27: 27–37.
64. Oldham JD, Emmans GC. Prediction of responses to protein and energy yielding nutrients. In: Nutrition and lactation in the dairy cow. Proceedings of the 46th University of Nottingham Easter School in Agricultural Sciences. London, 1988. p. 76–96.
65. Baldwin RL, France J, Gill M. Metabolism of the lactating cow. I. Animal elements of a mechanistic model. J Dairy Res 1987;54:77–105.
66. VandeHaar MJ, St-Pierre N. Major advances in nutrition: relevance to the sustainability of the dairy industry. J Dairy Sci 2006;89:1280–91.
67. Oba M, Allen MS. Effects of brown midrib 3 mutation in corn silage on productivity of dairy cows fed two concentrations of dietary neutral detergent fiber: 1. Feeding behavior and nutrient utilization. J Dairy Sci 2000;83:1333–41.
68. Putnam DE, Varga GA. Protein density and its influence on metabolite concentration and nitrogen retention by Holstein cows in late gestation. J Dairy Sci 1998;81:1608–18.
69. Huyler MT, Kincaid RL, Dostal DF. Metabolic and yield responses of multiparous Holstein cows to prepartum rumen-undegradable protein. J Dairy Sci 1999;82: 527–36.
70. Putnam DE, Varga GA, Dann HM. Metabolic and production responses to dietary protein and exogenous somatotropin in late gestation dairy cows. J Dairy Sci 1999;82:982–95.
71. Greenfield RB, Cecava MJ, Johnson TR, et al. Impact of dietary protein amount and rumen degradability on intake, prepartum liver triglyceride, plasma metabolites and milk production in transition dairy cattle. J Dairy Sci 2000;83:703–10.
72. Wu Z, Fisher RJ, Polan CE, et al. Lactation performance of cows fed low or high ruminally undegradable protein prepartum and supplemental methionine and lysine postpartum. J Dairy Sci 1997;80:722–9.
73. Van Saun RJ. Dry cow nutrition: the key to improved fresh cow performance. Vet Clin North Am Food Anim Pract 1991;7:599–620.
74. McNeill DM, Ehrhardt RA, Slepetis R, et al. Protein requirement of sheep in late pregnancy: partitioning of nitrogen between conceptus and maternal tissues. J Anim Sci 1997;75:809–81.
75. Boisclair Y, Grieve DG, Stone JB, et al. Effect of prepartum energy, body condition and sodium bicarbonate on production of cows in early lactation. J Dairy Sci 1986;69:2636–47.
76. Van Saun RJ. Effects of undegradable protein fed prepartum on subsequent lactation, reproduction, and health in Holstein dairy cattle. PhD thesis. Ithaca: Cornell University; 1993.
77. Van Saun RJ, Idleman SC, Sniffen CJ. Effect of undegradable protein amount fed prepartum on postpartum production in first lactation Holstein cows. J Dairy Sci 1993;76:236–44.
78. Xu S, Harrison JH, Chalupa WH, et al. The effect of ruminal bypass lysine and methionine on milk yield and composition of lactating cows. J Dairy Sci 1998; 81:1062–77.

79. DeGaris PJ, Lean IJ, Rabiee AR, et al. Effects of increasing days of exposure to pre-partum diets on reproduction and health in dairy cows. Aust Vet J 2010;88: 84–92.
80. Philips GJ, Citron TL, Sage JS, et al. Adaptations in body muscle and fat in transition dairy cattle fed differing amounts of protein and methionine hydroxy analog. J Dairy Sci 2003;86:3634–47.
81. Holtenius P, Holtenius K. A model to estimate insulin sensitivity in dairy cows. Acta Vet Scand 2007;49:29–31.
82. Van Saun RJ. Insulin sensitivity measures in dry dairy cows and relationship to body condition score. In: Proceedings of the 14th International Congress of Production Diseases in Farm Animals. Ghent (Belgium): 2010.
83. Van Saun RJ. Insulin sensitivity measures in lactating dairy cows and relationship to body condition score. In: Proceedings of the 26th World Buiatrics Congress Santiago. Chile: 2010.
84. Rice LE. Dystocia-related risk factors. Vet Clin North Am Food Anim Pract 1994; 10:53–68.
85. Bell AW. Influence of maternal nutrition and other factors on calf birth weight. In: Proceedings of the Cornell Nutrition Conference for Feed Manufacturers. Syracuse (NY): 2004. p. 159–65.
86. Rulquin J, Verite R. Amino acid nutrition of dairy cows: production effects and animal requirements. In: Garnsworthy PC, Cole DJ, editors. Recent advances in animal nutrition. Nottingham (United Kingdom): University Press; 1993. p. 55.
87. Sniffen CJ, Chalupa WH, Ueda T, et al. Amino acid nutrition of the lactating dairy cow. In. Proceedings of the Cornell Nutrition Conference. Rochester: 2001. p. 188–97.
88. Board on Agriculture and Natural Resources. Nutrient requirements of dairy cattle. 7th edition. Washington, DC: National Academy Press; 2001.
89. Bach A, Huntington GB, Stern MD. Response of nitrogen metabolism in preparturient dairy cows to methionine supplementation. J Dairy Sci 2000;78:742–9.
90. Lee C, Hristov AN, Cassidy TW, et al. Rumen-protected lysine, methionine, and histidine increase milk protein yield in dairy cows fed a metabolizable protein-deficient diet. J Dairy Sci 2012;95:6042–56.
91. Robinson PH. Impacts of manipulating ration metabolizable lysine and methionine levels on the performance of lactating dairy cows: a systematic review of the literature. Livest Sci 2010;127:115–26.
92. Patton RA. Effect of rumen-protected methionine on feed intake, milk production, true milk protein concentration, and true milk protein yield, and the factors that influence these effects: a meta-analysis. J Dairy Sci 2010;93: 2105–18.
93. Ordway RS, Boucher SE, Whitehouse NL, et al. Effects of providing two forms of supplemental methionine to periparturient Holstein dairy cows on feed intake and lactational performance. J Dairy Sci 2009;92:5154–66.
94. Socha MT, Putnam DE, Garthwaite BD, et al. Improving intestinal amino acid supply of pre- and postpartum dairy cows with rumen-protected methionine and lysine. J Dairy Sci 2005;88:1113–26.
95. Grum DE, Drackley JK, Younker RS, et al. Production, digestion, and hepatic lipid metabolism of dairy cows fed increased energy from fat or concentrate. J Dairy Sci 1996;79:1836–49.
96. Douglas GN, Overton TR, Bateman HG, et al. Prepartal plane of nutrition, regardless of dietary energy source, affects periparturient metabolism and dry matter intake in Holstein cows. J Dairy Sci 2006;89:2141–57.

97. Agenas A, Burstedt E, Holtenius K. Effects of feeding intensity during the dry period. 1. Feed intake, body weight, and milk production. J Dairy Sci 2003; 86:870–82.
98. Dann HM, Morin DE, Murphy MR, et al. Prepartum intake, postpartum induction of ketosis, and periparturient disorders affect the metabolic status of dairy cows. J Dairy Sci 2005;88:3249–64.
99. Dann HM, Litherland NB, Underwood JP, et al. Diets during far-off and close-up dry periods affect periparturient metabolism and lactation in multiparous cows. J Dairy Sci 2006;89:3563–77.
100. Janovick NA, Drackley JK. Prepartum dietary management of energy intake affects postpartum intake and lactation performance by primiparous and multiparous Holstein cows. J Dairy Sci 2010;93:3086–102.
101. Janovick NA, Boisclair YR, Drackley JK. Prepartum dietary energy intake affects metabolism and health during the periparturient period in primiparous and multiparous Holstein cows. J Dairy Sci 2011;94:1385–400.
102. Drackley JK, Janovick NA. Controlled energy diets for dry cows. In: Proceedings of the Western Dairy Management Conference. Reno. (NV): 2007. p. 7–16.
103. Beever DE. The impact of controlled nutrition during the dry period on dairy cow health, fertility and performance. Anim Reprod Sci 2006;96:212–26.
104. Litherland NB, Weich WD, Lobao D, et al. Prepartum feeding strategies for greater postpartum success. In: Proceedings of the Minnesota Nutrition Conference. Owatonna (MN): 2012. p. 18–9.
105. Parodi PW. Conjugated linoleic acid and other anticarcinogenic agents of bovine milk fat. J Dairy Sci 1999;82:1339–49.
106. Rabiee AR, Breinhild K, Scott W, et al. Effect of fat additions to diets of dairy cattle on milk production and components: a meta-analysis and meta-regression. J Dairy Sci 2012;95:3225–47.
107. Lean IJ, Rabiee A. Quantitative metabolic and epidemiological approaches to fertility of the dairy cow. In: Proceedings of the Dairy Cattle Reproduction Council. Denver (CO): 2007. p. 115–32.
108. Staples CR, Burke JM, Thatcher WW. Influence of supplemental fats on reproductive tissues and performance of lactating cows. J Dairy Sci 1998;81:856–71.
109. Thatcher WW, Bilby TR, Bartolome JA, et al. Strategies for improving fertility in the modern dairy cow. Theriogenology 2006;65:30–44.
110. Kronfeld DS. The potential importance of the proportions of glucogenic, lipogenic and aminogenic nutrients in regard to the health and productivity of dairy cows. Fortschr Tierphysiol Tierernahr 1976;(7):3–26.
111. Santos JE, Juchem SO, Galvao KN, et al. Transition cow management to reduce metabolic disease and improve reproductive management. Adv Dairy Tech 2003;15:287–304.
112. Selberg KT, Staples CR, Badinga L. Production and metabolic responses to dietary conjugated linoleic acid (CLA) and trans-octadecenoic acid isomers in periparturient dairy cows [abstract]. J Dairy Sci 2002;85(Suppl 1):19.
113. Doepel L, Lapierre H, Kennelly JJ. Peripartum performance and metabolism of dairy cows in response to prepartum energy and protein intake. J Dairy Sci 2002;85:2315–34.
114. Jones B, Fish RD, Martin A, et al. Case study: effects of supplemental linoleic and linolenic acids on reproduction in Holstein cows. Prof Anim Sci 2008;24:500–5.
115. De Veth MJ, Bauman DE, Koch W, et al. Efficacy of conjugated linoleic acid for improving reproduction: a multi-study analysis in early-lactation dairy cows. J Dairy Sci 2009;92:2662–9.

116. Frajblat M. Metabolic state and follicular development in the post-partum lactating dairy cow. PhD thesis. Ithaca: Cornell University; 2000.
117. Grummer RR, Carroll DJ. A review of lipoprotein cholesterol metabolism: importance to ovarian function. J Anim Sci 1988;66:3160–73.
118. Chilliard Y. Dietary fat and adipose tissue metabolism in ruminants, pigs, and rodents: a review. J Dairy Sci 1993;76:3897–931.
119. Kappel LC, Ingraham RH, Morgan EB, et al. Relationship between fertility and blood glucose and cholesterol concentrations in Holstein cows. Am J Vet Res 1984;45:2607–12.
120. Ruegg PL, Goodger WJ, Holmberg LD, et al. Relation among body condition score, serum urea nitrogen and cholesterol concentrations, and reproductive performance in high-producing Holstein dairy cows in early lactation. Am J Vet Res 1992;53:10–4.
121. Moss N. The epidemiology of subfertility in Australian dairy cows. PhD thesis. Sydney: University of Sydney; 2001.
122. Burke JM, Carroll DJ, Rowe KE, et al. Intravascular infusion of lipid into ewes stimulates production of progesterone and prostaglandin. Biol Reprod 1996; 55:169–75.
123. Carroll DJ, Hossain FR, Keller MR. Effect of supplemental fish meal on the lactation and reproductive performance of dairy cows. J Dairy Sci 1994;77:3058–72.
124. Ferguson JD, Sklan D, Chalupa WV, et al. Effects of hard fats on in vitro and in vivo rumen fermentation, milk production, and reproduction in dairy cows. J Dairy Sci 1990;73:2864–79.
125. Sklan D, Moallem U, Folman Y. Effect of feeding calcium soaps of fatty acids on production and reproductive responses in high producing lactating cows. J Dairy Sci 1991;74:510–7.
126. Son J, Grant RJ, Larson LL. Effects of tallow and escape protein on lactational and reproductive performance of dairy cows. J Dairy Sci 1996;79:822–30.
127. Sklan D, Kaim M, Moallem U, et al. Effect of dietary calcium soaps on milk yield, body weight, reproductive hormones, and fertility in first parity and older cows. J Dairy Sci 1994;77:1652–60.
128. Lucy MC, Staples CR, Thatcher WW, et al. Influence of diet composition, dry-matter intake, milk production and energy balance on time of post-partum ovulation and fertility in dairy cows. Anim Prod 1992;54:323–31.
129. Thatcher WW, Santos JE, Staples CR, et al. The science of Omega-3 fatty acids on dairy cows reproduction. In: J Dairy Sci ADSA Series. Quebec (Canada): 2002.
130. von Soosten D, Meyer U, Piechotta M, et al. Effect of conjugated linoleic acid supplementation on body composition, body fat mobilization, protein accretion, and energy utilization in early lactation dairy cows. J Dairy Sci 2012;95:1222–39.
131. Palmquist DL, Jenkins TC. Fat in lactation rations: review. J Dairy Sci 1980;63: 1–14.
132. Kay JK, Mackle TR, Auldist MJ, et al. Endogenous synthesis of cis-9, trans-11 conjugated linoleic acid in dairy cows fed fresh pasture. J Dairy Sci 2004;87: 369–78.
133. Hutchinson I, de Veth MJ, Stanton C, et al. Effects of lipid-encapsulated conjugated linoleic acid supplementation on milk production, bioenergetic status and indicators of reproductive performance in lactating dairy cows. J Dairy Res 2011;78:308–17.
134. Bines JA, Hart IC, Morant SV. Endocrine control of energy metabolism in the cow: the effect on milk yield and levels of some blood constituents of injecting growth hormone and growth hormone fragments. Br J Nutr 1980;43:179–88.

135. Pocius PA, Herbein JH. Effects of in vivo administration of growth hormone on milk production and in vitro hepatic metabolism in dairy cattle. J Dairy Sci 1986;69:713–20.
136. Gulay MS, Garcia AN, Hayen MJ, et al. Responses of Holstein cows to different bovine somatotropin (bST) treatments during the transition period and early lactation. Asian-Australian Journal of Animal Sciences 2004;17:784–93.
137. Gulay MS, Hayen MJ, Liboni M, et al. Low doses of bovine somatotropin during the transition period and early lactation improves milk yield, efficiency of production, and other physiological responses of Holstein cows. J Dairy Sci 2004;87:948–60.
138. Lean IJ, Troutt HF, Bruss ML, et al. Postparturient metabolic and production responses in cows previously exposed to long-term treatment with somatotropin. J Dairy Sci 1991;74:3429–45.
139. Bobe G, Young YW, Beitz DC. Pathology, etiology, prevention, and treatment of fatty liver in dairy cows. J Dairy Sci 2004;87:3105–24.
140. Ametaj BN. A new understanding of the causes of fatty liver in dairy cows. Adv Dairy Tech 2005;17:97–112.
141. Durand D, Chilliard Y, Bauchart D. Effects of lysine and methionine on in vivo hepatic secretion of VLDL in the high yielding dairy cow [abstract]. J Dairy Sci 1992;75(Suppl 1):279.
142. Gruffat D, Durand D, Graulet B, et al. Regulation of VLDL synthesis and secretion in the liver. Reprod Nutr Dev 1996;36:375–89.
143. Emmanuel B, Kennelley JJ. Kinetics of methionine and choline and their incorporation into plasma lipids and milk components in lactating goats. J Dairy Sci 1984;67:1912–8.
144. Pinotti L, Baldi A, Dell'Orto V. Comparative mammalian choline metabolism with emphasis on the high-yielding dairy cow. Nutr Res Rev 2002;15:315–31.
145. Davidson B, Hopkins BA, Odle J, et al. Supplementing limited methionine diets with rumen-protected methionine, betaine, and choline in early lactation Holstein cows. J Dairy Sci 2008;91:1552–9.
146. Oikawa S, Katoh N, Kawawa F, et al. Decreased serum apolipoprotein B-100 and A-1 concentrations in cows with ketosis and left displacement of the abomasum. Am J Vet Res 1997;58:121–5.
147. Atkins KB, Erdman RA, Vandersall JH. Dietary choline effects on milk yield and duodenal choline flow in dairy cattle. J Dairy Sci 1988;71:109–16.
148. Hartwell JR, Cecava MJ, Donkin SS. Impact of dietary rumen undegradable protein and rumen-protected choline on intake, peripartum liver triacylglyceride, plasma metabolites and milk production in transition dairy cows. J Dairy Sci 2000;83:2907–17.
149. Piepenbrink MS, Overton TR. Liver metabolism and production of cows fed increasing amounts of rumen-protected choline during the periparturient period. J Dairy Sci 2003;86:1722–33.
150. Cooke RR, Silva del Rio N, Caraviello DZ, et al. Supplemental choline for prevention and alleviation of fatty liver in dairy cattle. J Dairy Sci 2007;90:2413–8.
151. Pinotti L, Baldi A, Politis I, et al. Rumen-protected choline administration to transition cows: effects on milk production and vitamin E status. J Vet Med A Physiol Pathol Clin Med 2003;50:18–21.
152. Zom RL, van Baal J, Goselink RM, et al. Effect of rumen-protected choline on performance, blood metabolites, and hepatic triacylglycerols of periparturient dairy cattle. J Dairy Sci 2001;94:4016–27.

153. Lima FS, Sa Filho MF, Greco LF, et al. Effects of feeding rumen-protected choline on incidence of diseases and reproduction of dairy cows. Vet J 2012; 193:140–5.
154. Elek P, Newbold JR, Gaal T, et al. Effects of rumen-protected choline supplementation on milk production and choline supply of periparturient dairy cows. Animal 2008;1:1595–601.
155. Oelrichs WA, Lucy MC, Kerley MS, et al. Feeding soybeans and rumen-protected choline to dairy cows during the parturient period and early lactation: effects on plasma lipid balance [abstract]. J Dairy Sci 2004;87(Suppl):441.
156. Janovick-Guretzky NA, Carlson DB, Garrett JE, et al. Lipid metabolite profiles and milk production for Holstein and Jersey cows fed rumen-protected choline during the periparturient period. J Dairy Sci 2006;89:188–200.
157. Grummer RC. Choline: a limiting nutrient for transition dairy cows. In: Proceedings of the Cornell Nutrition Conference for Feed Manufacturers. Syracuse (NY): 2012. p. 16–8.
158. Sales J, Homolka P, KoukolovÃ¡ V. Effect of dietary rumen-protected choline on milk production of dairy cows: a meta-analysis. J Dairy Sci 2010;93:3746–54.
159. Bergen WG, Bates DB. Ionophores: their effect on production efficiency and mode of action. J Anim Sci 1984;58:1465–83.
160. Richardson LF, Raun AP, Potter EL, et al. Effect of monensin on rumen fermentation in vitro and in vivo. J Anim Sci 1976;43:657–64.
161. Russell JB, Strobel HJ. Effect of ionophores on ruminal fermentation. Appl Environ Microbiol 1989;55:1–6.
162. Van Nevel CJ, Demeyer DI. Effect of monensin on rumen metabolism in vitro. Appl Environ Microbiol 1977;34:251–7.
163. Duffield TF, Rabiee AR, Lean IJ. A meta-analysis of the impact of monensin in lactating dairy cattle. Part 3. Health and reproduction. J Dairy Sci 2008;91: 2328–41.
164. Duffield TF, Rabiee AR, Lean IJ. A meta-analysis of the impact of monensin in lactating dairy cattle. Part 2. Production effects. J Dairy Sci 2008;91:1347–60.
165. Duffield TF, Rabiee AR, Lean IJ. A meta-analysis of the impact of monensin in lactating dairy cattle. Part 1. Metabolic effects. J Dairy Sci 2008;91:1334–46.
166. Osweiler GD. Mycotoxins - Contemporary issues of food animal health and productivity. Vet Clin North Am Food Anim Pract 2000;16:511–30.
167. Oswald IP, Marin DE, Bouhet S, et al. Immunotoxicological risk of myoctoxins for domestic animals. Food Addit Contam 2005;22:354–60.
168. Fink-Gremmels J. The role of mycotoxins in the health and performance of dairy cows. Vet J 2008;176:84–92.
169. Kiessling KH, Pettersson H, Sandholm K, et al. Metabolism of aflatoxin, ochratoxin, zearalenone and three trichothecenes by intact rumen fluid, rumen protozoa and rumen bacteria. Appl Environ Microbiol 1984;47:1070–3.
170. Caloni F, Spotti M, Auerbach H, et al. In vitro metabolism of fumonisin B1 by rumen microflora. Vet Res Commun 2000;24:379–87.
171. Escoula L. Patulin production by *Pencillium granulatum* and inhibition of rumen flora. J Environ Pathol Toxicol Oncol 1992;11:45–8.
172. Morgavi D, Boudra H, Jouany J, et al. Prevention of patulin toxicity on rumen microbial fermentation by SH-containing reducing agents. J Agric Food Chem 2003;51:6906–10.
173. Logrieco A, Moretti A, Castella G, et al. Beavuericin production by *Fusarium* species. Appl Environ Microbiol 1998;64:3084–8.

174. Xiao H, Marquardt RR, Frohlich AA, et al. Effect of a hay and grain diet on the rate of hydrolysis of ochratoxin A in the rumen of sheep. J Anim Sci 1991;69:3706–14.
175. Bolsen KK, Huck GL, Siefers MK, et al. Silage management: five key factors. Manhattan (KS): Kansas State University; 1999. Available at: http://www.ksre.ksu.edu/pr_silage/bunker_silo_mgmt.htm. Accessed January 12, 2013.
176. Buening GM, Mann DD, Hook B, et al. The effect of T-2 toxin on the immune bovine system: cellular factors. Vet Immunol Immunopathol 1982;3:411–7.
177. Pier AC. Major biological consequences of aflatoxicosis in animal production. J Anim Sci 1992;70:3964–7.
178. Morris CA, Towers NR, Tempero HJ. Breeding for resistance to facial eczema in dairy cattle. In: Proceedings of the New Zealand Grassland Association. 1991. p. 221–4.
179. Lean IJ. Perennial ryegrass endophytes - effects on dairy cattle. In: Reed KF, Page SW, Lean IJ, editors. Perennial ryegrass toxicosis in Australia. Attwood (Australia): Meat & Livestock Australia; 2005. p. 29–36.
180. Reed KF. Perennial rye grass toxins in Australian pasture. In: Reed KF, Page SW, Lean IJ, editors. Perennial ryegrass toxicosis in Australia. Attwood (Australia): Meat & Livestock Australia; 2005. p. 11–9.

Mineral and Antioxidant Management of Transition Dairy Cows

Ian J. Lean, BVSc, DVSc, PhD, MANZCVS[a,*],
Robert Van Saun, DVM, MS, PhD[b], Peter J. DeGaris, BVSc (Hons), PhD[c]

KEYWORDS

• Transition • Calcium • Skeleton • Antioxidant • Vitamins

KEY POINTS

- Effective transition management requires an integrated approach to nutritional and environmental management to provide cows with freedom from rumen disruption, mineral deficiencies, immunosuppression, disorders of lipid metabolism, and other forms of stress (eg, toxic feeds, social disruption).
- The skeleton is an important regulator of energy and protein metabolism.
- Although calcium is pivotal in the pathogenesis of milk fever, the most significant factor influencing risk of milk fever is the magnesium content of the diet.
- Vitamin and mineral status of cattle should not be considered in isolation from other antioxidants or from the level of oxidative challenge. Adequacy is a function of these interactions, not just a single vitamin or mineral, and increased concentrations of 1 of these may also not be better.

INTRODUCTION

Although controlling disorders of macromineral metabolism, and in particular milk fever, forms a small part of the overall management of the transition cow, it is often the focus at a producer level. As a result, it is critical to ensure that any transition cow program is effective in controlling macromineral disorders. Further, recent developments in understanding of the role of calcium in metabolism and bone as an integrator of metabolism reinforce the need to ensure that there is careful attention to calcium metabolism. The concept of milk fever and hypocalcemia being central to the interactions of other diseases has been well understood since the pivotal studies of Curtis and colleagues.[1] Recent understandings of the role of bone in integrated

[a] SBScibus, PO Box 660, Camden, New South Wales 2570, Australia; [b] Department of Veterinary & Biomedical Sciences, Pennsylvania State University, University Park, PA 16802, USA; [c] Tarwin Veterinary Group, 32 Anderson St, Leongatha, Victoria 3953, Australia
* Corresponding author.
E-mail address: ianl@sbscibus.com.au

Vet Clin Food Anim 29 (2013) 367–386
http://dx.doi.org/10.1016/j.cvfa.2013.03.004 vetfood.theclinics.com

metabolism (reviewed later) provide a basis on which to understand the gateway role of milk fever in other disorders and reproduction.

The pathophysiology of hypocalcemia and dietary manipulations to control the risk of milk fever have been extensively reviewed,[2–5] and insights from these reviews are incorporated in this article. Further, the understanding that transition management needs to be fully integrated to be effective[6] is discussed in the context of review of a study that integrated these priniciples.[7–9] Micronutrient needs are addressed in the context of vulnerability of cattle to oxidative stress and inflammatory disorders. This article concludes with a series of practical approaches to improving transition diets.

Approach to transition management: correcting 1 area of challenge is not enough. Effective solutions are derived from ensuring freedom from rumen disruption, mineral deficiencies, immunosuppression, and disorders of lipid metabolism and that further other forms of stress (eg, toxic feeds, social disruption) are reduced and cows are comfortable.

Milk Fever Control

The following recommendations for the dietary control of hypocalcemia are based on 4 meta-analyses examining factors influencing the risk of milk fever.[10–13] These meta-analyses showed that the risk of milk fever can be predicted from dietary levels of calcium, magnesium, phosphorus, dietary cation-anion difference (DCAD) (as calculated by $[Na^+ + K^+] - [Cl^- + S^{2-}]$), breed of cattle, and duration of exposure to the diet. To effectively prevent these disorders, careful attention is needed to concentrations of calcium, magnesium, and phosphorus as well as the DCAD of the prepartum diet (**Table 1**).

What is meta-analysis?: a form of study design that uses previous studies to provide a pooled estimate of effect of an observation or intervention. Well-conducted meta-analyses are the gold standard for assessing these effects and provide more precise estimates of the effect of interventions. Ideally, these studies are based on randomized controlled studies.

DCAD

The DCAD theory of milk fever prevention has its basis in the strong ion model of acid: base balance,[14] modified in the 1980s[15] and simplified in the late 1990s.[16] Some contention still exists regarding the most appropriate equation for predicting DCAD. Charbonneau and colleagues[13] preferred the equation $(Na^+ + K^+) - (Cl^- + 0.6\ S^{2-})$ on the basis that it was the best equation at predicting blood pH, whereas DeGaris and Lean[3] preferred the equation $(Na^+ + K^+) - (Cl^- + S^{2-})$, because the equations were equivalent for predicting the risk of milk fever. Given that the equations are equivalent for predicting milk fever, we recommend use of the latter and more simple equation.

The simplified strong ion model[17] to predict plasma pH is:

$$pH = pK_1' + \log \frac{[SID^+] - K_a[A_{TOT}]/(K_a + 10^{-pH})}{S * p_{co2}}$$

where pK'_1 is the ion product of water, K_a is the effective equilibrium disassociation constant for plasma nonvolatile weak acids, $[SID^+]$ is the strong ion difference,

Table 1
Logistic meta-regression analysis of the dietary components and variables that predict the incidence of milk fever (random effects model)

Predictor Variable	Coefficient	Standard Error	*P* Value	Odds Ratio	95% Confidence Interval
Constant	−5.76	1.028	0.001	0.003	0.001–0.024
Breed 1[a]	0.86	0.382	0.024	2.374	1.122–5.023
Breed 2[b]	1.49	0.824	0.071	4.424	0.880–22.235
Ca[c]	5.48	1.729	0.013	239.362	8.082–7089.244
Mg[c]	−5.05	1.618	0.002	0.006	0.001–0.152
P[c]	1.85	0.716	0.010	6.376	1.566–25.958
DCAD 1[d]	0.02	0.007	0.040	1.015	1.001–1.030
Ca * Ca	−2.03	0.819	0.013	0.131	0.026–0.654
Exposure[e]	0.03	0.014	0.030	1.030	1.003–1.058
Trial	−0.01	0.001	0.369	—	—
Variance (σ)	1.33	0.357	—	—	—

[a] Breed 1, Jerseys (Holstein Friesian used as the reference breed).
[b] Breed 2, Norwegian Red and White (Holstein Friesian used as the reference breed).
[c] Ca, Mg, and P expressed as % of DM.
[d] DCAD 1 = (Na + K) − (Cl + S) in mEq/100 g DM.
[e] Exposure is the mean time in days that the cows in a study were exposed to the precalving transition diet.

From Lean IJ, DeGaris PJ, McNeil DM, et al. Hypocalcemia in dairy cows: meta analysis and dietary cation anion difference theory revisited. J Dairy Sci 2006;89:673.

$[A_{TOT}]$ is the plasma nonvolatile weak acid concentration, S is the solubility of CO_2 in plasma, and p_{co2} is the partial pressure of CO_2 in plasma. The implication of this equation is that the major variable factor that can be readily influenced is the strong ion difference and prevention of milk fever involves, in part, the appropriate application of DCAD theory to reduce the strong ion difference ($[SID^+]$) by lowering plasma pH and producing strong ion metabolic acidosis. This goal can be achieved by feeding salts of the strong cations ($CaCl_2$, $CaSO_4$, $MgCl_2$, $MgSO_4$, NH_4Cl, and $(NH_4)_2SO_4$) or acids of the anions (HCl and H_2SO_4). The strong cations Ca^{2+}, Mg^{2+}, and NH_4^+ are absorbed to a lesser extent from the gastrointestinal tract (GIT) than are the strong anions Cl^- and SO_4^{2-}. The differential absorption results in a relative excess of absorbed anions compared with absorbed cations lowering the $[SID^+]$ and subsequently plasma pH. Because Na^+ and K^+ are absorbed with near 100% efficiency in the intestine, NaCl and KCl have a net effect of zero on the $[SID^+]$.

Inducing a mild metabolic acidosis in the prepartum cow reduces milk fever risk through changes in calcium metabolism. Numerous effects of decreasing or increasing the DCAD of precalving diets have been reported. Among the effects reported are:

- Metabolic acidosis in goats[18,19] and cattle[20]
- Decreased renal sensitivity to parathyroid hormone (PTH) in cows fed a strongly positive DCAD precalving diet[20,21]
- Enhanced renal production of 1,25(OH) vitamin D_3 in response to a low-DCAD precalving diet[20,21]
- Increased responsiveness of target tissues to 1,25(OH) vitamin D_3 associated with increased calcium absorption from the intestinal tract[22]

- Increased resorption of calcium from bone stores[23–25]
- Calciuria[20,26–28]
- Increased plasma ionized calcium concentrations[26,28]

Critically, the overall effect is to increase calcium turnover through increased GIT absorption and increased sensitivity of target tissues to homeostatic signals, rather than an improvement in overall calcium balance. The meta-analyses of milk fever risk factors[10–13] have identified that the effect of DCAD on the risk of milk fever is linear and independent of the important effects of dietary Ca, Mg, and P concentrations. Consequently, any reduction in the DCAD decreases the risk of milk fever. This linear relationship should not be confused with the curvilinear relationship between DCAD and urine pH, with DCAD having little impact on urine pH until it reaches approximately 20 mEq/100 g dry matter (DM) (**Fig. 1**). This curvilinear relationship is caused by renal buffering systems that maintain an alkaline urinary pH until overwhelmed. Although recommendations exist for target urine pH to ensure adequate acidification, these assess only effectiveness of DCAD management of the diet and not the risk of milk fever.

> **Urinary pH:** monitors efficacy of the DCAD; does not monitor milk fever risk. Good transition diets prevent milk fever; urinary acidification is only part of this, and urinary pH is not a good predictor of milk fever risk. We recommend sampling and testing feeds for mineral concentrations and assessing quality in preference to (but not exclusive of) testing urine.

Our recommendations for the balancing of the macromineral component of transition diets are listed in a series of recommendations at the end of this article.

Calcium

The optimum concentration of dietary Ca intake for the control of milk fever is also contentious, with Lean and colleagues[6] and Thilsing-Hansen and colleagues[5] suggesting that the precalving intake of calcium be limited to 60 on a negative DCAD diet and 20 g per day, respectively. McNeill and colleagues[2] also concluded that excessive calcium intake was an important risk factor for milk fever, but less so than potassium. However, Goff[4] concluded that calcium concentration in precalving diets had little influence on the incidence of milk fever when fed at levels higher

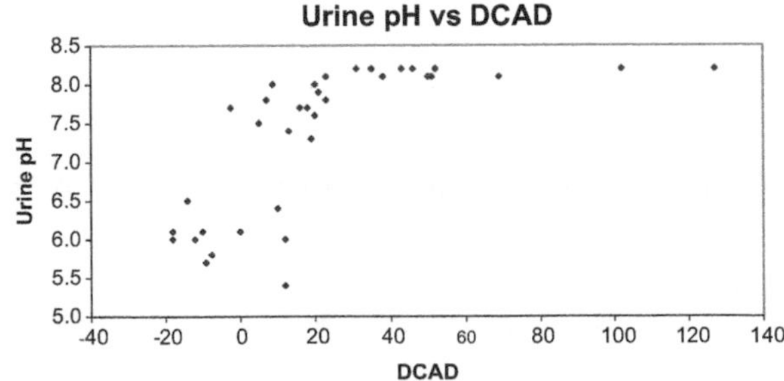

Fig. 1. Curvilinear relationship between urine pH and DCAD $[(Na^+ + K^+) - (Cl^- + S^{2-})]$. (*From* DeGaris PJ, Moss N, Lean IJ, et al. The transition period–preventing milk fever and more. In: Proceedings of the Australian Cattle Vets 2005 - Gold Coast AVA Conference. Gold Coast: Australian Association of Cattle Veterinarians. 2005. p. 66.)

than the daily requirements of the cow (approximately 30 g/d). Oetzel[29] recommended a daily intake in the precalving diet of 150 g/d, a calcium concentration of between 1.1% and 1.5% of DM, in conjunction with a dietary DCAD of approximately −15 mEq/100 g DM. However, the meta-analyses of Oetzel[10] and Lean and colleagues[12] found that a calcium concentration of 1.1% to 1.5% of DM provided near-maximal risk of milk fever (**Fig. 2**). When the effects of length of time cattle were exposed to a transition ration before calving were investigated, a quadratic interaction with calcium was found.[12] This relationship suggests that short exposures to high concentrations of calcium markedly increase milk fever risk, whereas a prolonged exposure to the same concentrations produces only a moderate risk (**Fig. 3**). These observations may explain the differences in recommended calcium concentrations of different workers.

The total exchangeable body calcium mass is only 1.5% of total body calcium in mature cows.[30] Goff and colleagues[21] estimated an even smaller pool of readily labile calcium bone stores, 6 to 10 g, based on responses of cattle to ammonium chloride-induced acidosis.[31] We have observed mild milk fever cases arising before calving with low-DCAD and low-calcium diets, possibly reflecting calciuria stimulated by the low-DCAD diets, and find that diets containing 0.4% to 0.6% calcium overcome this problem.

Magnesium

The most significant factor influencing risk of milk fever is the magnesium content of the diet.[12] Magnesium may prevent milk fever through roles in

- The release of PTH and in the synthesis of 1,25-dihydroxycholecalciferol
- In hypomagnesemic states, kidney and bone are less responsive to PTH[4,32]
- Reducing renal calcium excretion. Wang and Beede[33] found that nonpregnant, nonlactating cows fed a diet high in Mg had lower renal calclum excretion than those fed a diet low in Mg

Contreras and colleagues[34] and van de Braak and colleagues[35] reported poor calcium mobilization in hypomagnesemic cattle. Although clinical hypomagesemia is rare in dairy cattle, very low dietary Na or high dietary K concentrations may interfere with

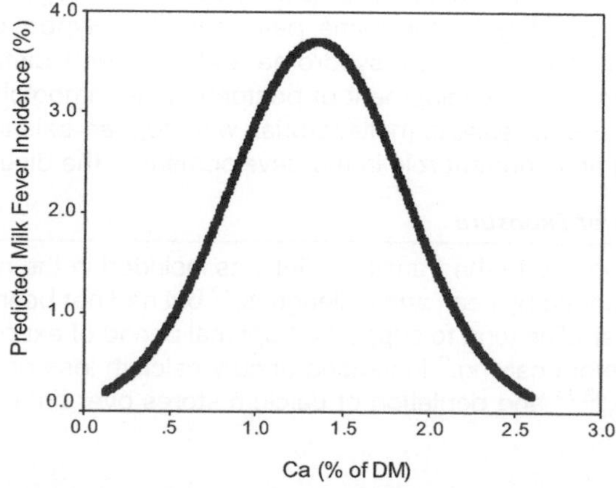

Fig. 2. Milk fever incidence in response to varying dietary Ca concentrations. (*From* Lean IJ, DeGaris PJ, McNeil DM, et al. Hypocalcemia in dairy cows: meta analysis and dietary cation anion difference theory revisited. J Dairy Sci 2006;89:674.)

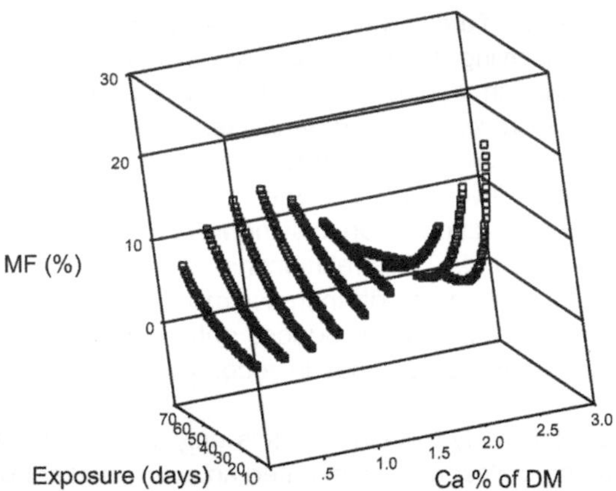

Fig. 3. Relationship between calcium %, days exposure to the transition diet, and milk fever incidence (MF %). (*Adapted from* DeGaris PJ, Lean IJ. Milk fever in dairy cows - A review of pathophysiology and control principles. Vet J 2008;176:64; with permission.)

Mg transport across the rumen wall and result in clinical disease. Magnesium is best supplied as magnesium sulfate, magnesium chloride, and magnesium oxide; caution needs to be applied to supply in the chloride form, because this is unpalatable (we have observed successful application in water). As with any other mineral, it should not be assumed that more is better; we have observed problems associated with supply of 0.8% magnesium in diets.

Phosphorus

Phosphorus also plays an important role in milk fever, with increasing phosphorus concentrations increasing milk fever risk. Although phosphorus concentrations are not as tightly regulated as calcium, both are closely related, with plasma PO_4 concentrations regulated directly by 1,25(OH) vitamin D_3 and indirectly by the PTH/calcium negative feedback loop.[36] However, in rats, hyperphosphatemia can inhibit the renal production of 1,25(OH) D_3 sufficiently to cause hypocalcemia.[37–39] In cattle, there is evidence that a prepartum diet high in phosphorus can have a negative impact on calcium homeostasis, possibly by the same pathways.[40–42] Hypophosphatemia may contribute to the alert downer cow syndrome and long-term dietary P deficiency has been implicated in the development of postparturient hemoglobinuria; however, it is likely that the latter disease is multifactorial, with copper, selenium, and antioxidant status playing an important role in the development of the disease.

Optimum Duration of Exposure

The duration of exposure to the transition diet was included in the models to predict milk fever risk developed by Lean and colleagues,[12] but had not been validated in trial work. Subsequent studies tend to support an optimal period of exposure to transition diets of 25 days before calving.[9] Increased urinary calcium loss on low-DCAD diets has been reported,[43,44] and depletion of calcium stores over time may explain part of this effect.

Age and Protein

There is good evidence that increasing age increases the risk of milk fever as a result of decreased intestinal calcium absorption and responsiveness to hypocalcemia,[45–47] reduced bone turnover,[48] and decreased bone responsiveness to PTH and vitamin D.[21] We found that the risk of milk fever increased by 9% per lactation in the subpopulation of studies used for a meta-analysis[12] that reported age (unpublished data).

Increased protein concentration in the diet increased the risk of milk fever in some models and approached significance in many models tested by Lean and colleagues[12] (unpublished data). This effect was not large compared with magnesium and calcium concentrations. However, too few studies provided data on this finding to include in final published meta-analytical models.

Importance of Bone in Energy Metabolism

Important homeostatic links between bone and energy metabolism have been established. This relationship was first postulated when obesity was discovered to reduce the risk of osteoporosis in humans.[49] Ducy and colleagues[50] then proposed that the bone and energy metabolism may be regulated by the same hormones. Mouse models show that osteocalcin, produced by mature osteoblasts, completes the negative feedback loop between bone and energy metabolism, which is the hallmark of homeostatic regulation.[51] The uncarboxylated form of osteocalcin promotes

- β-cell proliferation
- Insulin secretion
- Independently increases peripheral tissue insulin sensitivity
- Adiponectin secretion by adipose cells

Although there is no specific research in cattle linking bone and energy metabolism, there are findings that support the hypothesis that these may be linked, and this interaction seems to be a vital aspect of the homeorhetic adaptations to lactation. Many studies support this conceptual framework at the physiologic level, and clinically, Heuer and colleagues[52] found that obese cows (body condition scoring [BCS] >4.5/5) were at greater risk of milk fever. Binger and colleagues[53] found an increase in insulin resistance in cows fed low-DCAD rations before calving. DeGaris and colleagues[8] found a positive relationship between BCS and area under the curve of blood Ca after calving, and reanalysis of the data used in that study using time series techniques found significant, positive correlations between blood calcium and glucose both before and after calving (DeGaris, and Lean, unpublished data). Associations between ketosis and hypocalcemia are well recognized and have been recently reconfirmed in prospective, randomized trials with anionic diets[54] and cohort studies examining the effects of hypocalcemia.[55]

Critically, links between calcium metabolism and health and reproduction are also evident. Hypocalcemia is a risk factor for many of the important diseases of lactation, including mastitis, ketosis, retained placenta, displaced abomasums, and uterine prolapse. Hypocalcaemia is also a risk factor for reproductive disorders and is an indirect risk factor for increased culling.[25,56,57] Curtis and colleagues[58] observed an increased odds of mastitis of 8-fold for cows with milk fever. Although such increases have been ascribed to recumbency and failure of teat sphincter closure, these mechanisms are speculative. Cows with subclinical hypocalcemia (defined as <8.59 mg/dL) were at greater risk of developing fever, metritis, and puerperal metritis compared with normocalcemic cows.[55] There are differences in peripheral mononuclear cells function, which indicate impaired function in hypocalcemic cows.[59] Borsberry and Dobson[60] in the United Kingdom found that cows with clinical milk fever had 13 more days from calving to conception, a finding supported by Martinez and colleagues[55] in hypocalcemic cows. These investigators also found lower conception rates in hypocalcemic cows and that 66.6% of metritis and 91.3% of puerperal metritis in this population was attributable to hypocalcemia. New Zealand studies[61,62] found a tendency to improved interval to conception in cows treated with calcium-containing products after calving. Although further targeted research is needed to explore this potentially important aspect of energy and bone metabolism in dairy cattle, those evaluating or formulating diets should work on the premise that these links between bone health and energy metabolism are substantial.

Specific Interventions

Vitamin D and calcium

One of the emerging areas of understanding is the important role of vitamin D in immune function.[63] Vitamin D has roles in both innate and adaptive immune responses. Although cattle exposed to sunlight may obtain sufficient vitamin D, it is clear that housed cattle do not unless supplemented. The target levels for optimal performance are being identified, as are the optimal forms of supplementation. Supplying 40,000 IU of vitamin D_3 may be appropriate; however, there should be careful consideration of the optimal timing of such supplementation before calving.

The potential benefits of the use of vitamin D metabolites have been recognized for many years. Problems in finding satisfactory therapies have been encountered as a result of needs to predict calving dates, variation in responses associated with different prepartum calcium intakes,[22,64] and the potential for toxic reactions to arise from the administration of the vitamin D metabolites as a result of persistent hypercalcemia, such as the deposition of calcium in tissues, particularly the cardiovascular system.[65,66] Notwithstanding these limitations, several studies have reported positive responses to 25-OH cholecalciferol on milk fever risk and metabolism. As better understandings of vitamin D, calcium, and energy metabolism emerge, more detailed recommendations on vitamin D use can be anticipated.

Acidifying feeds

Lowering the DCAD of the prepartum diet using mineral salts has produced a significant increase or a trend toward increased milk production in lactation.[23,67–70] These responses are approximately 1 to 2 L per cow per day. The most researched of the interventions is the acidifying protein meal BioChlor (Church and Dwight, NJ), produced using sulfuric and hydrochloric acids. Soychlor (West Central Soy, IA) is another acidifying protein meal that is based on hydrochloric acid and soya-proteins. Corbett[71] retrospectively examined 13,000 DairyComp 305 records and found an increase in daily milk yields of between 2.0 and 3.0 L for cows exposed to a transition diet containing BioChlor for 15 to 21 days compared with 0 to 7 days' exposure. DeGroot[72] in a randomized controlled trial found an average 2.0 L/d production response in cows exposed to a prepartum diet containing BioChlor for 21 days over cows fed control diet with a similar DCAD.

After calving

Recommendations for the target DCAD for lactating cows range from +35 to +40 mEq/100 g DM and are based on the meta-analysis of Hu and Murphy.[73] Increasing the lactating diet DCAD to these levels has been shown to increase DM intake (DMI), milk components, and milk yield and possibly improve amino acid balance.[73–77]

Zeolites and calcium binding

Thilsing-Hansen and colleagues[5] concluded that limiting the precalving calcium intake to 20 g/d or less is 100% effective at preventing milk fever, but may be too low to incorporate with a negative DCAD diet. However, it is often difficult to limit daily calcium intake to these levels. Calcium-binding agents (eg, zeolite A) have been shown to bind calcium and reduce Ca availability in precalving diets. However, some binders have been associated with reduced DMI before calving and because they are nonspecific, the potential exists for reduced availability of other divalent cations such as magnesium, an action that would increase the risk of milk fever.[5,78,79]

Calcium drenches

Calcium drenches and gels are available and have been widely used to prevent and treat hypocalcemia. Preventive gels are given as an oral drench during the 24-hour period around calving. Most calcium gels are based on calcium chloride, which supplies a soluble form of calcium and acidifies. Goff and Horst[80] compared the effectiveness of various calcium salts, including calcium propionate, calcium chloride, and calcium carbonate. Although calcium chloride increased plasma calcium concentrations higher than those of the other products, it could cause a severe acidosis[80] and may irritate the oral and ruminal mucosa. Calcium propionate has the advantage of being glucogenic and may reduce the risk of ketosis.[81]

Micromineral metabolism: free radicals and antioxidants in transition The homeorhetic and homeostatic responses to lactation can be exaggerated or perturbed by release of inflammatory mediators from lipid mobilization, environmental stressors, or subclinical disease conditions that increase postparturient disease risks[82–87] (see also the article by Sordillo and colleagues elsewhere in this issue). The magnitude of effects of these responses are most clearly shown by studies in which the antiinflammatory agent acetylsalicylate (aspirin), either fed or injected, markedly reduced the risks of disorder after calving, increased milk production, and improved reproduction.[88]

Clinical situations in which inflammation is increased and free radicals may be generated include:

- Challenge from infectious agents (novel agents, highly pathogenic, substantial exposure)
- Deficiency states of antioxidants, either single antioxidants or several antioxidants
- Parturition when cows are exposed to bacterial contamination of the reproductive tract, increased metabolic demands, and depletion of antioxidants associated with lactation and production of colostrum
- Higher-producing animals have higher metabolic activity rates and greater loss of antioxidants in the milk
- Excessive intakes of prooxidants (eg, polyunsaturated fatty acids or catalysts such as iron, copper or zinc)
- Estrus activity; there is a considerable capacity for free radical generation and challenge during steroidogenesis and in the period of growth and atresia of ovarian structures[89]; reproduction is not a sterile process, and consequently, there is considerable potential for bacteria to create free radical challenge during conception and early embryonic development

The processes of calving and lactation are proinflammatory. Inflammation is a critical part of innate immune responses and is an adverse response only when uncontrolled. Control of inflammation is exerted by ensuring that there is a good balance between exposure to pathogens and that cows are able to mount effective innate and humoral immune responses. When inflammatory effects are uncontrolled, these effects are often mediated through propagating reactions that involve the generation of free radicals.

Free radicals are generated as a normal part of metabolism in cellular respiration, electron transport via cytochrome P450, enzymatic reactions, and significantly in the killing systems used by macrophages, neutrophils, and other phagocytic leucocytes. This controlled release of free radicals is part of the immune response through the respiratory burst of phagocytic leucocytes. Granulocytes, mononuclear macrophages, and lymphocytes use free radicals such as H_2O_2, myeloperoxides, and superoxides as a means of destroying invading organisms and damaged tissue. The oxidative agents released extracellularly or within phagosomes are a controlled response to defined activated pathways.[90] This process involves the production of high levels of superoxide, which can cause significant damage to biological molecules in an iron catalyzed reaction, in which $OH^{\cdot}$ is an intermediate. This reaction is called the Fenton reaction and allows the formation of free radicals that are destructive to tissues.[91] Free radicals are unstable, react with the environment, and create toxic lipids, reactive proteins, and other free radicals and further damaging tissues, DNA and RNA.[92] Damage from free radicals is more severe when systems that quench propagating reactions are impaired, often through deficiencies in the antioxidant vitamins and minerals.

The balance of radical generation and antioxidant control is complex, because the processes involved are highly interrelated, and excesses of trace elements can be as damaging as deficiencies. Iron and copper are needed in key protective enzymes such as transferrin, catalase (Fe), and Cu/Zn superoxide dismutase (Cu) that bind these; however, excessive supplementation with copper or iron saturates potential binding sites and increases the level of these metals in their free states. Free iron and copper may catalyze oxidative reactions, as shown in the spectacular sudden death syndromes associated with acute and chronic copper toxicity.

Serum concentrations of the fat-soluble vitamins retinol (vitamins A) and α-tocopherol (vitamin E) decline around the time of calving,[93] a decline that cannot be completely accounted for by losses through the mammary gland.[94] Curtis[83] serially sampled Holstein cows from 1 month before calving until 1 month after calving and identified the likely transfer of many antioxidants to the calf, in utero and through colostrum, a finding supported by many other studies. Plasma retinol, α-tocopherol and β-carotene concentrations were depleted to nadirs at a mean of 4.5 days after calving. Subsequently, plasma retinol and α-tocopherol concentrations increased.[83] At the time that plasma retinol, α-tocopherol, and β-carotene concentrations were lowest, plasma ceruloplasmin activities were highest, but these decreased at the end of the sampling period. Whole blood glutathione peroxidase activities increased and peaked 3.6 days before calving. Plasma ascorbate concentrations and erythrocyte Cu/Zn superoxide dismutase activities did not display consistent patterns of change over the sampling period. There were significant correlations between the changes in plasma retinol, α-tocopherol, and β-carotene concentrations and also between plasma ceruloplasmin and whole blood glutathione peroxidase activities. Initial increases in malondialdehyde (an indicator of free radical damage) concentrations were associated with decreases in concentrations of the fat soluble vitamins and the decrease in malondialdehyde over calving was associated with increases in plasma ceruloplasmin and whole blood glutathione. The findings of Curtis[83] show strong interactions among antioxidants.

At calving, cows with plasma α-tocopherol concentrations less than 3.0 μg/mL were at 9.4 times greater risk of having mastitis within the first 7 days of lactation compared with cows with higher concentrations.[95] LeBlanc and colleagues[96] did not find a protective effect of prepartum serum α-tocopherol concentration on mastitis, but for every 1 μg/mL increase, retained placenta incidence was reduced 21%. Because serum retinol concentration increased 100 ng/mL during the last week of gestation, risk of clinical mastitis in early lactation was decreased 60%.[96] Serum vitamin concentrations can be augmented with appropriate dietary supplementation.[97–100] However, caution should be exercised in use of transition metal and vitamins antioxidants, because these can have adverse or no effects when fed greater than requirements. Responses to additional vitamin E in dairy cattle have been variable, and a meta-analysis of use of vitamin E and selenium in beef feedlot cattle indicated that feeding vitamin E at concentrations greater than the National Research Council (NRC) recommendation, or the administration of vitamin E as an injection, did not improve average daily gain, efficiency of gain, or morbidity in feedlot cattle.[101]

Although trace mineral nutrition of dairy cattle is of great importance and many trace minerals improve immune function,[102] the capacity for interactions with other dietary inputs and variation in individual animal requirements means that despite extensive study, there are still many areas that require clarification. Although the inflammatory pathways that influence health, productivity, and reproduction are complex, the clinician need not understand all of the pathways to be aware and enact preventive strategies. Ensuring that mineral and vitamin intakes meet or moderately exceed NRC requirements is essential. The source of such minerals may be important because responses have been noted in both production and reproduction to organic sources of minerals.[103]

Table 2 highlights the dietary sources, active forms, sites of action, and types of action of antioxidants in cattle.

> **Free radical management and controlling inflammation:** the major implication of Curtis' work is that vitamin and mineral status of cattle should not be considered in isolation of other antioxidants, nor of the level of oxidative challenge; adequacy is a function of these interactions, not just a single vitamin or mineral; increased concentrations of 1 of these may also not be better.

Putting it all Together: a Cohort Study of Integrated Interventions

In a large, prospective observational study examining the effect of increasing days exposure to a BioChlor-based transition diet that was formulated to deliver on a DM basis, 16.0% CP (crude protein), 4.2% rumen undegradable protein, and 6.9 MJ/kg (0.65 Mcal/#) NE_L.[7–9] The diets provided an average metabolizable protein balance of 286 g/d based on the Cornell Net Protein and Carbohydrate Model and a dietary cation anion difference of −15.0 mEq/100 g, provided micronutrients to meet or exceed NRC requirements, and rumen modification to control risk of acidosis. Increasing exposure to the prepartum transition diet had positive effects on milk and milk protein yield. The increase in production reported between minimal exposure (3 days or less) and optimal exposure (22 days for milk yield and 25 days for milk protein yield) was approximately 3.75 L of 4.0% fat and 3.2% protein corrected milk per day and 100 g of milk protein per day (**Figs. 4** and **5**). DeGaris and colleagues[7] also found that exposure to the transition diet increased risk of conception by 1.2% per day on the transition diet. This effect is large and is shown in **Fig. 6**, showing the cumulative pregnancy rate for cows exposed to the diet for less than 10 days, those exposed for 10 to 20 days, and those cows exposed for more than 20 days. Numerically, more cows were in calf at the end of the mating periods for cows with greater exposure to the transition diet.

Putting it all Together: Troubleshooting/Formulating: a Checklist

The following guidelines are useful when formulating or troubleshooting transition diets and management. Given the multivariable nature of the disorder and other benefits

Table 2
Dietary sources, active forms, sites of action and type of action of antioxidants in cattle

Dietary Input[a]	Biologically Active Antioxidant	Site of Action	Type of Action
Selenium	GSHPx	IC/membrane	ROOH, H_2O_2
Copper	Cu/Zn superoxide dismutase	IC	O_2^-
	Caeruloplasmin	EC	Binds Cu/oxidizes Fe, weak O_2^- scavenger
	EC superoxide dismutase	EC	O_2^-
Zinc	Cu/Zn superoxide dismutase	IC	O_2^-
	EC superoxide dismutase	EC	O_2^-
	Metallothionine	EC	Binds metal ions
Manganese	Mn superoxide dismutase	IC	O_2^-
Iron	Catalase	IC	H_2O_2
	Transferrin	EC	Binds Fe
	Lactoferrin	EC-milk/sweat	Binds Fe
Cobalt	Vitamin B_{12}		
Vitamin E	α-Tocopherol	Membrane	Blocks peroxidation in lipids especially
Vitamin A	Retinol	EC	Maintains cell integrity
β-Carotene	β-Carotene	Membrane	Scavenges singlet O_2
	Retinol	EC	Cell integrity
Glucose	Ascorbate	EC	Vitamin E, GSSG reduction, radical scavenger
Sulfur amino acids	GSSG	IC	Replenishes GSHPx
Protein	Albumin	EC	Binds Fe and Cu
	Hemopexin	EC	Binds Fe
	Haptopexin	EC	Binds Fe
	Histidine-rich glycoproteins	EC	Binds other metal ions
	Erythrocytes	EC	Transport radicals IC
	Mucins	EC	$OH^\cdot$ Scavenging

Abbreviations: EC, extracellular; GSHPx, glutathione peroxidase; GSSG, glutathione; H_2O_2, controls hydrogen peroxide; IC, intracellular; NIR, near infrared spectroscopy; O_2^-, controls superoxides; $OH^\cdot$, controls hydroxyl radicals; ROOH, controls lipid peroxides.

[a] Limiting dietary component.

Data from Lean IJ, Westwood CT, Rabiee AR, et al. Recent advances in nutrition and reproduction in temperate dairy management. In: Webber W, ed. Proceedings of the Society of Dairy Cattle Veterinarians of the NZVA Annual Conference. Palmerston North, New Zealand: VetLearn Foundation, 1998. p. 87–118.

of correct transition diets, care should be taken not to crudely apply rules of thumb, but to evaluate the diets in total.

1. Analyze available feeds for macromineral content using wet chemistry methods. NIR can be unreliable for determination of mineral composition of forages in particular. Analyze feeds to allow macronutrient balancing. Comprehensive and cost-effective feed testing can be performed (eg, using an accredited laboratory from http://www.foragetesting.org [National Forage Testing Association]).
2. Select feed ingredients that have a low DCAD (<20 mEq/100 g DM). Of particular importance are forages that are low in K (<2.0%) and possibly Ca Select forages, which allow adaptation of the cow's rumen to the early lactation diet. Forages (hays/silages) or paddocks may need to be specifically grown or prepared for transition cows and receive minimal potassium-based fertilizers or manure applications.

e. As many as possible of the postcalving feed ingredients are included in the precalving diet
f. Avoid feeding transition diets through dairy parlors; this can result in unsatisfactory intake in some cows and increases risk of mastitis in some herds by stimulating mammary letdown; cows fed in dairies should have teat spray applied.

16. Monitor the effectiveness of the DCAD aspects of the transition diet by measuring urine pH targets should be 6.2 to 6.8 for Holsteins and 5.8 to 6.3 for Jerseys. Urine pHs less than 5.8 suggest excessive metabolic acidosis that compromise cow health. The aim is to prevent milk fever and not necessarily reduce urine pH. Measure and analyze feeds in preference to testing urine (if you can choose to do only one or the other, getting the diet correct is more critical).
17. Aim to have cows on a transition diet for 21 days.

REFERENCES

1. Curtis CR, Erb EH, Sniffen CJ, et al. Path analysis of dry period nutrition, postpartum metabolic and reproductive disorders, and mastitis in Holstein cows. J Dairy Sci 1985;68:2347–60.
2. McNeill DM, Roche JR, McLachlan BP, et al. Nutritional strategies for the prevention of hypocalcaemia at calving for dairy cows in pasture-based systems. Aust J Agr Res 2002;53:755–70.
3. DeGaris PJ, Lean IJ. Milk fever in dairy cows–a review of pathophysiology and control principles. Vet J 2007;176:58–69.
4. Goff JP. Pathophisiology of calcium and phosphorus disorders. Vet Clin North Am Food Anim Pract 2000;16:319–37.
5. Thilsing-Hansen T, Jorgensen RJ, Ostergaard S. Milk fever control principles: a review. Acta Vet Scand 2002;43:1–19.
6. Lean IJ, DeGaris PJ, Wade LK, et al. Transition management of dairy cows: 2003. In: Parkinson TJ, editor. Taupo (New Zealand): Proceedings of the Australian and New Zealand Combined Dairy Cattle Veterinarians Conference—incorporating the 20th Annual Seminar of the Society of Dairy Cattle Veterinarians of the New Zealand Veterinary Association. New Zealand, Veterinary Association; 2003.
7. DeGaris PJ, Lean IJ, Rabiee AR, et al. Effects of increasing days of exposure to pre-partum diets on reproduction and health in dairy cows. Aust Vet J 2010;88:84–92.
8. DeGaris PJ, Lean IJ, Rabiee AR, et al. Effects of increasing days of exposure to a pre-partum diet on the concentration of certain blood metabolites in dairy cows. Aust Vet J 2010;88:137–45.
9. DeGaris PJ, Lean IJ, Rabiee AR, et al. Effects of increasing days of exposure to pre-partum transition diets on milk production and milk composition in dairy cows. Aust Vet J 2008;86:341–51.
10. Oetzel GR. Meta-analysis of nutritional risk factors for milk fever in dairy cattle. J Dairy Sci 1991;74:3900–12.
11. Enevoldsen C. Nutritional risk factors for milk fever in dairy cattle: meta-analysis revisited. Acta Vet Scand 1993;89:131–4.
12. Lean IJ, DeGaris PJ, McNeil DM, et al. Hypocalcemia in dairy cows: meta analysis and dietary cation anion difference theory revisited. J Dairy Sci 2006;89:669–84.
13. Charbonneau E, Pellerin D, Oetzel GR. Impact of lowering dietary cation-anion difference in nonlactating dairy cows: a meta-analysis. J Dairy Sci 2006;89:537–48.

14. Singer RB, Hastings AB. An improved clinical method for the estimation of disturbances of the acid-base balance of human blood. Medicine 1948;27:223–42.
15. Stewart PA. Strong ions, plus carbon dioxide, plus weak acid, isolated blood plasma and isolated intracellular fluid. How to understand acid-base. New York: Elsevier; 1981. p. 110–44.
16. Constable PD. A simplified strong ion model for acid-base equilibria: application to horse plasma. J Appl Physiol 1997;83:297–311.
17. Constable PD. Clinical assessment of acid-base status: strong ion difference theory. Vet Clin North Am Food Anim Pract 1999;15:447–71.
18. Fredeen AH, DePeeters EJ, Baldwin RL. Characterisation of acid-base disturbances on calcium and phosphorus balances of dietary fixed ions in pregnant or lactating does. J Anim Sci 1988;66:157–73.
19. Fredeen AH, DePeeters EJ, Baldwin RL. Effects of acid-base disturbances caused by differences in dietary fixed ion balance on kinetics of calcium metabolism in ruminants with high calcium demand. J Anim Sci 1988;66:174–84.
20. Gaynor PJ, Mueller FJ, Miller JK, et al. Parturient hypocalcemia in Jersey cows fed alfalfa haylage-based diets with different cation to anion ratios. J Dairy Sci 1989;72:2525–31.
21. Goff JP, Horst RL, Mueller FJ, et al. Addition of chloride to a prepartal diet high in cations increases 1,25-dihydroxyvitamin D response to hypocalcemia preventing milk fever. J Dairy Sci 1991;74:3863–71.
22. Allsop TF, Pauli JV. Failure of 25-hydroxycholecalciferol to prevent milk fever in dairy cows. N Z Vet J 1985;13:19–22.
23. Block E. Manipulating dietary anions and cations for prepartum dairy cows to reduce incidence of milk fever. J Dairy Sci 1984;67:2939–48.
24. Goff JP, Horst RL. Effects of the addition of potassium or sodium but not calcium to prepartum rations on milk fever in dairy cows. J Dairy Sci 1997;80:176–86.
25. Leclerc H, Block E. Effects of reducing dietary cation-anion balance for prepartum dairy cows with specific reference to hypocalcemic parturient paresis. Can J Anim Sci 1989;69:411–23.
26. Phillipo M, Reid GW, Nevison IM. Parturient hypocalcaemia in dairy cows: effects of dietary acidity on plasma mineral and calciotropic hormones. Res Vet Sci 1994;56:303–9.
27. Lomba F, Chauvaux G, Teller E, et al. Calcium digestibility in cows as influenced by the excess of alkaline ions over stable acid ions in their diets. Br J Nutr 1978;39:425–9.
28. Oetzel GR, Fettemn MJ, Hamar DW. Screening of anionic salts for palatability, effects on acid-base status, and urinary calcium excretion in dairy cows. J Dairy Sci 1991;74:965–71.
29. Oetzel GR. Management of dry cows for the prevention of milk fever and other mineral disorders. Vet Clin North Am Food Anim Pract 2000;16:369–86.
30. Ramberg CF, Ferguson JD, Galligan DT. Feeding and managing the transition cow: metabolic basis of the cation anion difference concept. 1996. Available at http://cahpwww.vet.upenn.edu/node/15.
31. Vagg MJ, Payne JM. The effect of ammonium chloride induced acidosis on calcium metabolism in ruminants. Br Vet J 1970;126:531–7.
32. Sampson BF, Manston R, Vagg MJ. Magnesium and milk fever. Vet Rec 1983;112:447–9.
33. Wang C, Beede DK. Effects of diet magnesium on acid-base status and calcium metabolism of dry cows fed acidogenic salts. J Dairy Sci 1992;75:829–36.

34. Contreras PA, Manston R, Samson BF. Calcium homeostasis in hypomagnesaemic cattle. Res Vet Sci 1982;33:10–6.
35. van de Braak AE, Van't Klooster AT, Malestein A. Influence of a deficient supply of magnesium during the dry period on the rate of calcium mobilization by dairy cows at parturition. Res Vet Sci 1987;42:101–8.
36. Goff JP. Treatment of calcium, phosphorus and magnesium balance disorders. Vet Clin North Am Food Anim Pract 1999;15:619–39.
37. Masuyama R, Kajita Y, Odachi J, et al. Chronic phosphorus supplementation decreases the expression of renal PTH/PTHrP receptor mRNA in rats. J Nutr 2000; 112:480–7.
38. Silver J, Yalcindag C, Sela-Brown A, et al. Regulation of the parathyroid hormone gene by vitamin D, calcium and phosphate. Kidney Int Suppl 1999;56:2–7.
39. Tallon S, Berdud I, Hernandez A, et al. Relative effects of PTH and dietary phosphorus on calcitriol production in normal and azotemic rats. Kidney Int 1996;49: 1441–6.
40. Barton BA, Jorgensen NA, DeLuca HF. Impact of prepartum dietary phosphorus intake on calcium homeostasis at parturition. J Dairy Sci 1987;70: 1186–91.
41. Julien WE, Conrad HR, Hibbs JW, et al. Milk fever in dairy cows. VIII. Effect of injected vitamin D3 and calcium and phosphorus intake on incidence. J Dairy Sci 1977;60:431–6.
42. Kichura TS, Horst RL, Beitz DC, et al. Relationships between prepartal dietary calcium and phosphorus, vitamin D metabolism, and parturient paresis in dairy cows. J Nutr 1982;112:480–7.
43. Vagnoni DB, Oetzel GR. Effects of dietary cation-anion difference on the acid-base status of dry cows. J Dairy Sci 1998;81:1643–52.
44. van Mosel M, Van't Klooster AT, van Mosel F, et al. Effects of reducing dietary $[(Na^+ + K^+) - (Cl^- + SO_4^=)]$ on the rate of calcium mobilisation by dairy cows at parturition. Res Vet Sci 1993;54:1–9.
45. Hansard SL, Comar CL, Plumlee MP. The effects of age upon calcium utilization and maintenance requirements in the bovine. J Anim Sci 1954;13:25.
46. Horst RL, DeLuca HF, Jorgensen NA. The effect of age on calcium absorption and accumulation of 1,25-dihydroxyvitamin D_3 in intestinal mucosa of rats. Metab Bone Dis Relat Res 1978;1:29–33.
47. Horst RL, Goff JP, Reinhardt TA. Advancing age results in reduction of intestinal and bone 1,25-dihydroxyvitamin D receptor. J Endocrinol 1990;126:1053–7.
48. Parfitt AM. The cellular basis of bone remodelling: the quantum concept re-examined in the light of recent advances in the cell biology of bone. Calcif Tissue Int 1984;36(Suppl 1):37–45.
49. Felson DT, Zhang Y, Hannan MT, et al. Effects of weight and body mass index on bone mineral density in men and women: the Framington study. J Bone Miner Res 1993;8:567–73.
50. Ducy P, Amling M, Takeda S, et al. Leptin inhibits bone formation through a hypothalamic relay: a central control of bone mass. Cell 2000;100:197–207.
51. Lee NK, Sowa H, Hinoi E, et al. Endocrine regulation of energy metabolism by the skeleton. Cell 2007;132:456–69.
52. Heuer C, Schukken YH, Dobbleaar P. Postpartum body condition score and results from the first test day milk as predictors of disease, fertility, yield and culling in commercial dairy herds. J Dairy Sci 1999;82:295–304.
53. Bigner DR, Goff JP, Faust MA, et al. Acidosis effects on insulin response during glucose tolerance tests in Jersey cows. J Dairy Sci 1996;79:2182–8.

54. DeGroot MA, Block E, French PD. Effect of prepartum anionic supplementation on periparturient feed intake, health and milk production. J Dairy Sci 2010;93: 5268–79.
55. Martinez N, Risco CA, Lima FS, et al. Evaluation of peripartal calcium status, energetic profile and neutrophil function in dairy cows at low or high risk of developing uterine disease. J Dairy Sci 2012;95:7158–72.
56. Erb HN, Smith RD, Oltenacu PA, et al. Path model of reproductive disorders and performance, milk fever, mastitis, milk yield and culling in Holstein cows. J Dairy Sci 1985;68:3337–49.
57. Stevenson JS, Call EP. Reproductive disorders in the periparturient dairy cow. J Dairy Sci 1985;71:2572–83.
58. Curtis CR, Erb EH, Sniffen CJ. Association of parturient hypocalcemia with eight periparturient disorders in Holstein cows. J Am Vet Med Assoc 1983; 183:559.
59. Kimura K, Reinhardt TA, Goff JP. Parturition and hypocalcemia blunts calcium signals in immune cells of dairy cows. J Dairy Sci 2006;89:2588–95.
60. Borsberry S, Dobson H. Periparturient diseases and their effect on reproductive performance in five dairy herds. Vet Rec 1989;124:217–9.
61. McKay B. Subclinical hypocalcaemia: a possible affect on fertility. In: Proceedings of the 11th seminar for the Society of Dairy Cattle Veterinarians of the New Zealand Veterinary Association. Queenstown (New Zealand): New Zealand Veterinary Association. 1994.
62. Stevenson MA, Williamson NB, Hanlon DW. The effects of calcium supplementation of dairy cattle after calving on milk, milk fat and protein production, and fertility. N Z Vet J 1999;47:53–60.
63. Nelson CD, Reinhardt TA, Lippolis JD, et al. Vitamin D signalling in the bovine immune system: a model for understanding human vitamin D requirements. Nutrients 2012;4:181–96.
64. Goff JP, Horst RL, Beitz DC, et al. Use of 24-F-1, 25-dihydroxyvitamin D3 to prevent parturient paresis in dairy cows. J Dairy Sci 1988;71:1211–9.
65. Petrie L, Breeze RG. Hypervitaminosis D and metastatic pulmonary calcification in a cow. Vet Rec 1977;101:480–2.
66. Littledike ET, Horst RL. Vitamin D3 toxicity in dairy cows. J Dairy Sci 1982;65: 749–59.
67. Walker RG, Carter RR, McGuigan KR, et al. The effect of altering the cation-anion balance of the pre-calving diet of dairy cows on post-calving milk production and health. Proc Aust Soc Anim Prod 1998;22:372.
68. Joyce PW, Sanchez WK, Goff JP. Effect of anionic salts in prepartum diets based on alfalfa. J Dairy Sci 1997;80:2866–75.
69. McLachlan BP, Watson P, Ternouth J, et al. Effect of prepartum diet on subclinical hypocalcaemia and milk production in dairy cows. Asian Australas J Anim Sci 2002;13(Suppl A):264.
70. Beede DK, Sanchez WK, Wang C. Macrominerals. In: Van Horn HH, Wilcox CJ, editors. Large dairy herd management. Gainesville (FL): University of Florida; 1992. p. 272–86.
71. Corbett RB. Influence of days fed a close-up dry cow ration and heat stress on subsequent milk production in western dairy herds [abstract]. J Dairy Sci 2002; 85(Suppl 1):191.
72. DeGroot MA. The effect of prepartum anionic supplementation on periparturient feed intake and behavior, health and milk production. PhD. Oregon State University; 2004. http://ir.library.oregonstate.edu/xmlui/handle/1957/22408.

73. Hu W, Murphy MR. Dietary cation-anion difference effects on performance and acid-base status of lactating dairy cows: a meta-analysis. J Dairy Sci 2004;87: 2222–9.
74. Hu W, Murphy MR, Constable PD, et al. Dietary cation-anion difference effects on performance and acid-base status of dairy cows postpartum. J Dairy Sci 2007;90:3367–75.
75. Hu W, Murphy MR, Constable PD, et al. Dietary cation-anion difference and dietary protein effects on performance and acid-base status of dairy cows in early lactation. J Dairy Sci 2007;90:3355–66.
76. Wildman CD, West JW, Bernard JK. Effect of dietary cation-anion difference and dietary crude protein on milk yield, acid-base chemistry and rumen fermentation. J Dairy Sci 2007;90:4693–700.
77. Wildman CD, West JW, Bernard JK. Effect of dietary cation-anion difference and dietary crude protein on performance of lactating dairy cows during hot weather. J Dairy Sci 2007;90:1842–50.
78. Wilson GF. A novel nutritional strategy to prevent milk fever and stimulate milk production in dairy cows. N Z Vet J 2001;49:78–80.
79. Wilson GF. Stimulation of calcium absorption and reduction in susceptibility to fasting-induced hypocalcaemia in pregnant ewes fed vegetable oil. N Z Vet J 2001;49:115–8.
80. Goff JP, Horst RL. Oral administration of calcium salts for treatment of hypocalcemia in cattle. J Dairy Sci 1993;76:101–8.
81. Goff JP, Horst RL, Jardon PW, et al. Field trials of an oral calcium propionate paste as an aid to prevent milk fever in periparturient dairy cows. J Dairy Sci 1996;79:378–83.
82. Trevisi E, Amadori M, Cogrossi S, et al. Metabolic stress and inflammatory response in high-yielding periparturient dairy cows. Res Vet Sci 2012;93: 695–704.
83. Curtis MA. Epidemiology of uterine infections in dairy cows. Antioxidant and metabolic investigations. PhD. Sydney: University of Sydney; 1997.
84. Bernabucci U, Ronchi B, Lacetera N, et al. Influence of body condition score on relationships between metabolic status and oxidative stress in periparturient dairy cows. J Dairy Sci 2005;88:2017–26.
85. Bertoni G, Trevisi E, Han X, et al. Effects of inflammatory conditions on liver activity in puerperium period and consequences for performance in dairy cows. J Dairy Sci 2008;91:3300–10.
86. Zebeli Q, Sivaraman S, Dunn SM, et al. Intermittent parenteral administration of endotoxin triggers metabolic and immunological alterations typically associated with displaced abomasum and retained placenta in periparturient dairy cows. J Dairy Sci 2011;94:4968–83.
87. Bradford BJ, Mamedova LK, Minton E, et al. Daily injection of tumor necrosis factor-alpha increases hepatic triglycerides and alters transcript abundance of metabolic genes in lactating dairy cattle. J Nutr 2009;139:1451–6.
88. Trevisi E, Bertoni G. Attenuation with acetylsalicylate treatments of inflammatory condition in periparturient dairy cows. In: Quinn PI, editor. Aspirin and health research progress. Hauppauge (NY): Nova Science Publishers; 2008. p. 22–37.
89. Riley JC, Behrman HR. Oxygen radicals and reactive oxygen species in reproduction. Proc Soc Exp Biol Med 1991;198:781–91.
90. Dean R, Simpson J. Free radical damage to proteins and its role in the immune response. Mol Aspects Med 1991;12:121–8.
91. Draper HH. Advances in nutritional research. Plenum Press; 1990.

92. Mead JF, Stein RA, Guey-Shuang W. Metabolic fate of lipid peroxidation products. In: Chow CK, editor. Cellular antioxidant defense mechanisms. Boca Raton: CRC Press; 1988.
93. Goff JP, Stabel JR. Decreased plasma retinol, alpha tocopherol and zinc concentration during the periparturient period: effect of milk fever. J Dairy Sci 1990;73:3195–9.
94. Goff JP, Kimura K, Horst RL. Effect of mastectomy on milk fever, energy and vitamins A, E, and beta-carotene status at parturition. J Dairy Sci 2002;85:1427–36.
95. Weiss WP, Hogan JS, Todhunter DA, et al. Effect of vitamin E supplementation in diets with low concentration of selenium on mammary gland health of dairy cows. J Dairy Sci 1997;80:1728–37.
96. LeBlanc SJ, Herdt TH, Seymour WM, et al. Peripartum serum vitamin E, retinol and beta-carotene in dairy cattle and their associations with disease. J Dairy Sci 2004;87:609–19.
97. Chawla R, Kaur H. Plasma antioxidant vitamin status of periparturient cows supplemented with alpha-tocopherol and alpha-carotene. Anim Feed Sci Technol 2004;114:279–85.
98. Weiss WP, Hogan JS, Smith KL, et al. Effect of supplementing periparturient cows with vitamin E on distribution of alpha-tocopherol in blood. J Dairy Sci 1992;75:3479–85.
99. Weiss WP, Hogan JS, Smith KL, et al. Effect of dietary fat and vitamin E on alpha-tocopherol and beta-carotene in blood of peripartum cows. J Dairy Sci 1994;77:1422–9.
100. Weiss WP, Todhunter DA, Smith KL. Effect and duration of supplementation of selenium and vitamin E on periparturient cows. J Dairy Sci 1990;1990:3187–94.
101. Cusack PM, McMeniman NP, Rabiee AR, et al. Assessment of the effects of supplementation with vitamin E on health and production of feedlot cattle using meta-analysis. Prev Vet Med 2009;88:229–46.
102. Gaylean ML, Perino LJ, Duff GC. Interaction of cattle health/immunity and nutrition. J Anim Sci 1999;77:1120–34.
103. Rabiee AR, Lean IJ, Stevenson MA, et al. Effects of feeding organic trace minerals on milk production and reproductive performance in lactating dairy cows: a meta-analysis. J Dairy Sci 2010;93:4239–51.

Using Nonesterified Fatty Acids and β-Hydroxybutyrate Concentrations During the Transition Period for Herd-Level Monitoring of Increased Risk of Disease and Decreased Reproductive and Milking Performance

Paula A. Ospina, DVM, MPH, PhD[a], Jessica A. McArt, DVM, PhD[b], Thomas R. Overton, PhD[a], Tracy Stokol, BVSc, PhD[c], Daryl V. Nydam, DVM, PhD[d,*]

KEYWORDS

- Dairy cows • Negative energy balance • Nonesterified fatty acids
- β-Hydroxybutyrate • Herd-level tests

KEY POINTS

- Nonesterified fatty acids (NEFA) and β-hydroxybutyrate (BHB) are energy metabolites that can be used as markers of excessive negative energy balance in dairy cows during the transition period.
- When sampled in the appropriate time frame, prepartum and postpartum NEFA and BHB concentrations above certain thresholds are associated with negative downstream outcomes such as increased risk of disease, and decreased milking and reproductive performance at the level of the individual cow.
- BHB concentrations can be measured qualitatively or quantitatively with several tests of varying sensitivities and specificities both cow-side and in laboratories. At present, NEFA concentrations can be measured only quantitatively in laboratories.

Continued

Disclosures: Nil.

[a] Department of Animal Science, Cornell University, 272 Morrison Hall, Ithaca, NY 14850, USA; [b] Department of Clinical Sciences, Colorado State University, B217 VTH, 300 West Drake, Fort Collins, Colorado 80523-1601, USA; [c] Department of Population Medicine and Diagnostic Sciences, Cornell University, S3 110 Schurman Hall, Ithaca NY 14853, USA; [d] Department of Population Medicine and Diagnostic Sciences, Veterinary Medical Center, Cornell University, Room C2 562, Ithaca, NY 14850, USA
* Corresponding author.
E-mail address: dvn2@cornell.edu

Vet Clin Food Anim 29 (2013) 387–412
http://dx.doi.org/10.1016/j.cvfa.2013.04.003

Continued

- At the cow level, the following metabolite concentrations are associated with negative downstream outcomes: prepartum BHB 0.6 to 0.8 mmol/L and greater; prepartum NEFA 0.3 to 0.5 mEq/L and greater; postpartum NEFA 0.7 to 1 mEq/L and greater; and postpartum BHB 1.0 to 1.4 mmol/L and greater.
- At the herd level, negative downstream outcomes can be seen when more than 15% to 25% of the individual cows sampled (given the appropriate sample size) are higher than the aforementioned metabolite concentrations. Herd-level sensitivity is adversely affected by low cow-level test sensitivity, especially at lower prevalences and smaller sample sizes.
- Rational metabolite-testing protocols can lead to appropriate identification of herd-level risk for transition problems in cows, based on which preventive and corrective management strategies can be used, including treating individual cows with propylene glycol.

INTRODUCTION

All dairy cows visit a state of negative energy balance (NEB) as they transition from late gestation to early lactation. This imbalance in energy is the result of both an increase in energy requirements (more than twice as high when compared with prepartum levels[1]) and a decrease in dry matter intake (DMI[2]). The increase in energy demand is due to lactogenesis, which depends on available glucose concentrations[3] from gluconeogenesis in the liver.[4]

At the individual animal level there are several metabolic adaptations to manage NEB, including mobilization of nonesterified fatty acids (NEFA) from body fat reserves and glucose sparing for lactogenesis. However, some animals will experience excessive NEB, and it is this excess that is associated with negative downstream outcomes, such as increased risk of disease development and a decrease in both milk production and reproductive performance.

Several groups that have evaluated elevated NEFA and BHB concentrations as markers of excessive NEB report an increased risk of disease development[5–10] and a decrease in both milk production and reproductive performance.[11–14] As some degree of NEB postpartum is physiologically normal, it is the depth, duration, and timing of it that influences the cow's health and performance.

Based on current pen-level feeding and management practices, strategies to minimize excessive NEB in both the individual and the herd should focus on herd-level testing and management. This article reviews strategies for the testing and monitoring of excessive NEB at the herd level through individual-level testing of 2 energy markers: NEFA and BHB.

PHYSIOLOGY

The metabolites NEFA and BHB can be used as markers of NEB because of the relationship between energy demands, energy reserves, and the metabolic association between NEFA and BHB. **Fig. 1** is a graphic representation of the association between these factors.

Adipose Tissue

Glycerol and NEFA are released from adipose tissue in response to hormonal cues such as glucagon, corticosteroids, corticotropin, and catecholamines. Insulin is the

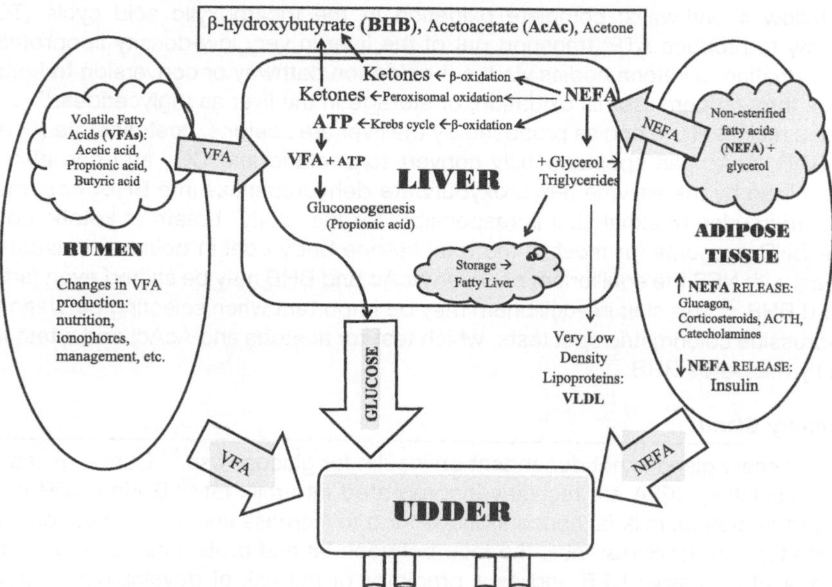

Fig. 1. The relationship between energy demands, energy reserves, and the metabolic association between nonesterified fatty acids (NEFA) and β-hydroxybutyrate (BHB). *Abbreviations:* ACTH, corticotropin; ATP, adenosine triphosphate.

only hormone that will act to inhibit lipolysis and therefore decrease the amount of NEFA released from adipose tissue.

Early in the postpartum period, there is both a decrease in insulin production[15] and a transient state of insulin resistance.[1] These 2 mechanisms allow glucose sparing for lactogenesis by decreasing glucose use by insulin-sensitive tissues, and allowing continued lipolysis even when insulin concentrations increase.[16]

The continual release of NEFA into circulation is not always detrimental: NEFA is a good source of energy for several tissues in the body, and can be used to synthesize milk fat. However, elevated levels of NEFA can result in excessive accumulation of triglycerides in the liver, resulting in hepatic lipidosis. In addition to the overtly detrimental effects of hepatic lipidosis,[17] more recent research has demonstrated that elevated NEFA concentrations can also adversely affect immune function[18,19] (see also the article by Sordillo and colleagues[20] elsewhere in this issue), and an excessive amount of circulating fatty acids may promote inflammation, which is an important factor in common diseases such as metritis and mastitis.

Rumen

Several factors (eg, nutrition, ionophore use, and DMI) determine the amount and proportion of the 3 major volatile fatty acids (VFA; acetic acid, propionic acid, and butyric acid) produced by microbes in the rumen. Acetic acid is used mainly in the liver as a major source of acetyl coenzyme A to generate adenosine triphosphate (ATP). Butyric acid is absorbed from the rumen as a ketone body, BHB. Propionic acid is taken up by the liver via portal circulation and serves as the major substrate for gluconeogenesis.[4]

Liver

The liver receives approximately one-third of cardiac output and removes approximately 15% to 20% of the NEFA in circulation.[21,22] Once inside the liver, fatty acids can follow 4 pathways: complete oxidation in the tricarboxylic acid cycle (TCA) pathway to produce ATP; transport out of the liver in very low-density lipoproteins; transformation to ketone bodies via the β-oxidation pathway or conversion to ketone bodies through peroxisomal oxidation; or storage in the liver as triglycerides.[15]

The 3 major ketone bodies produced by the liver are acetone, acetoacetate (AcAc), and BHB. AcAc can spontaneously convert to acetone and CO_2 and can also be metabolized by the enzyme β-hydroxybutyrate dehydrogenase into BHB. Acetone is excreted in urine or exhaled; it is responsible for the "fruity" breath of ketotic cows. While BHB accounts for most of the total ketone body pool in bovines, in lactating animals with NEB the equilibrium between AcAc and BHB may be shifted even farther toward BHB.[23] This shift in equilibrium may be important when selecting between the nitroprusside colorimetric spot tests, which test for acetone and AcAc, and a test that directly measures BHB.

Mammary Gland

The mammary gland is not dependent on insulin for glucose use.[24] During excessive NEB, circulating NEFA are regularly incorporated into milk fat.[25] During NEB in the postpartum period, milk fat concentrations tend to increase and milk protein concentrations tend to decrease; thus, the ratio between fat and protein can be used as an indicator of excessive NEB and as a predictor of the risk of developing metabolic diseases.[26–28] To use milk fat and protein information as a predictor of metabolic diseases that commonly occurs within 30 days in milk (DIM), samples should be evaluated within 9 days postpartum.[28]

DIAGNOSTIC TEST ACCURACY: INDIVIDUAL ANIMAL TESTS

Sensitivity and Specificity

In epidemiology, sensitivity is defined as the ability of a test to correctly identify those who have the disease (true positive risk), and specificity is defined as the ability of a test to correctly identify those who do not have the disease. In this context, the sensitivity and specificity of a test are routinely evaluated against a gold standard whereby the true status of the individual is known. The ideal test would have both high sensitivity and high specificity, but commonly there is a trade-off between the two.

To illustrate the trade-off between sensitivity and specificity when selecting a cut-point from a continuous distribution, data from a previous study[9] are used here. In this study the postpartum NEFA concentration was measured in animals 3 to 14 DIM, the objective being to determine a cut-point above which an animal was at higher risk of developing a displaced abomasum (DA), for example. **Fig. 2** is a frequency distribution of NEFA concentrations in the sampled animals.

Three major factors should be apparent from this example: (1) NEFA concentrations do not follow a normal distribution; (2) relatively few animals developed a DA; and (3) there is an overlap in NEFA concentrations between those animals that developed a DA and those that did not. It is this overlap between the 2 groups that forces the trade-off between sensitivity and specificity. Animals with postpartum NEFA concentration of 0.7 mEq/L or more were 10 times more likely to develop a DA than those with NEFA concentrations of less than 0.7 mEq/L.[9] In this example, if the NEFA cut-point is increased (eg, 1.0 mEq/L), the sensitivity of this test goes down and specificity goes up; that is, animals whose NEFA concentration is below the new higher cut-point but that develop a DA will result in a false negative, but there will simultaneously be fewer false positives. The converse is also true if the cut-point is chosen to be lower than 0.7 mEq/L.

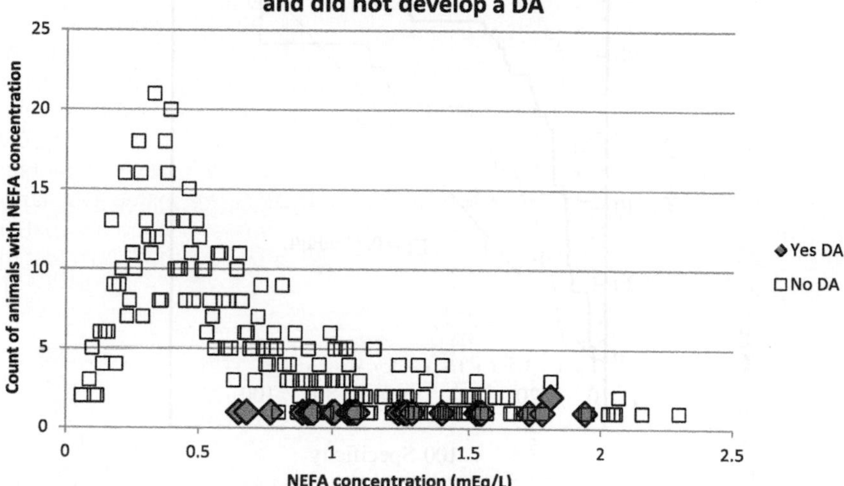

Fig. 2. Frequency distribution of NEFA postpartum in animals that developed a displaced abomasum (Yes DA; n = 26) versus those that did not (No DA; n = 800).

Because there is usually an overlap between the 2 populations of interest (ie, those with and without the outcome of interest), the cut-point chosen at the individual animal level could provide either the highest sensitivity if the consequence of false negatives are a concern, or the highest specificity if the consequence of false positives are a concern. However, in most cases it is ideal to use a test with both high sensitivity and high specificity. To identify this threshold, a receiver-operator characteristic (ROC) curve can be used to compare continuous predictors with a single dichotomous outcome. An example of the ROC curve evaluating NEFA in cows sampled postpartum versus DA as the outcome is shown in **Fig. 3**.

The area under the ROC curve can be interpreted as the probability that a randomly selected diseased individual has a greater test value than an individual without the disease.[29] When evaluating the association between elevated NEFA and BHB and the development of disease, both metabolites were treated as tests with continuous concentrations and were evaluated against the development of disease. The diseases under evaluation were DA, metritis (MET) and/or retained placenta (RP), and clinical ketosis (CK), or any of the three.[9]

The ROC curves were used to estimate sensitivity and specificity for various cut-points and diseases (**Table 1**). The study evaluated these cut-points at the individual animal level and determined the risk ratio associated with having elevated NEFA or BHB.[9] **Table 2** is a summary of the risk ratios of developing any disease (DA, CK, MET, or RP) based on the cut-points with the highest combined sensitivity and specificity.

Likelihood Ratios and Predictive Values

Table 1 also reports the likelihood ratio positive (LR+) and negative (LR−). In general, the LR measures how much a test result will change the odds that the animal has the disease, and incorporates both the sensitivity and specificity of the test. The LR+ indicates how much the odds of the disease increase when a test is positive. Similarly,

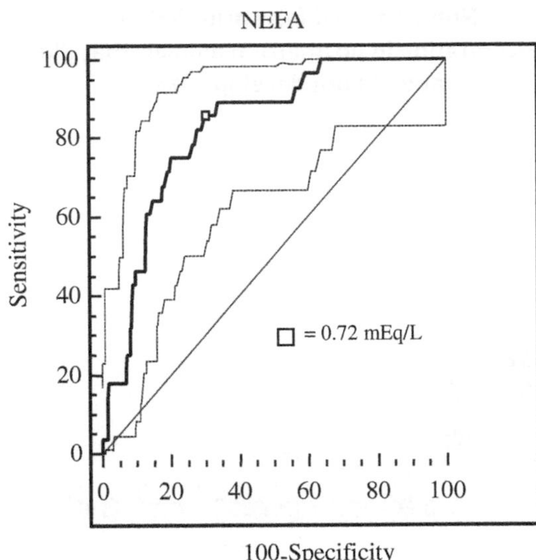

Fig. 3. Receiver-operator characteristic curve (*solid line*) that determines the critical threshold (*open square* in upper left corner) for NEFA concentrations (≥0.72 mEq/L) predicting displaced abomasa in animals sampled postpartum. The dotted curves represent the 95% confidence interval for the ROC curve. The diagonal line represents the sensitivity and specificity level at which the test is noninformative.

the LR– indicates how much the odds of the disease decrease when a test is negative.[29]

Because odds are difficult to interpret but LRs are commonly reported, a simpler approach is proposed for evaluation of LRs.[30] This approach estimates the change in probability associated with different LRs, and is based on the pretest probability. A pretest probability refers to the probability of an animal having the target disorder before the results of the diagnostic test is known. For example, an LR+ of 2 can be interpreted as a 15% increase in the probability of disease above the current pretest probability; LR+ of 3 is 20%, LR+ of 4 is 25%, and so forth. An LR– of 0.1 reduces the probability of a disease given the test result by 45%, LR– of 0.2 by 30%, LR– of 0.3 by 25 and so forth, below the current pretest probability.[30] In **Table 1**, for example, an LR+ of 1.9 when postpartum NEFA is at least 0.6 mEq/L means that an animal with NEFA of 0.6 mEq/L or greater has a 15% increased probability (above the pretest probability) of having any of the diseases (DA, CK, MET, or RP).

Although the predictive value positive (PV+) and negative (PV–) are not reported in **Table 1**, these values are a useful tool for interpreting test results. The PV+ is the probability that, given a positive test, the animal actually has the disease; PV– is the probability that, given a negative test, the animal does not have the disease.[29] The same test will have different PV+ and PV– in different populations because it is driven by the underlying true population prevalence.

Available Tests

Ketone bodies

Recently, the Precision Xtra meter (Abbott Laboratories, Abbott Park, IL), a handheld device for measuring blood BHB concentrations, was validated for use in ruminants.[31,32] The sensitivity and specificity are 88% and 96%, respectively, when using a cutoff value of 1.2 mmol/L; and 96% and 97% when using a cutoff value of

Table 1
Receiver-operator characteristic curve determination of critical NEFA (mEq/L) and BHB (mmol/L) thresholds as predictors of disease in transition dairy cows

Disease	Critical Threshold[a]	Sen	95% CI for Sen	Spec	95% CI for Spec	LR+[b]	LR−[c]	AUC	*P* Value
Animals sampled prepartum (n = 1440); thresholds for NEFA prepartum									
DA	0.3	57	42–72	62	60–65	1.5	0.7	0.6	.01
CK	0.3	53	43–64	61	58–64	1.4	0.8	0.6	.001
MET and/or RP	0.4	37	30–45	80	78–83	1.9	0.8	0.6	.0001
Any 3	0.3	48	42–54	69	67–72	1.6	0.8	0.6	<.001
Animals sampled postpartum (n = 1318); thresholds for NEFA postpartum									
DA	0.7	80	65–91	73	70–75	3.0	0.3	0.8	<.001
CK	0.6	74	61–84	59	57–62	1.8	0.4	0.7	<.001
MET	0.4	97	86–100	30	28–33	1.4	0.1	0.6	.009
Any 3	0.6	75	66–82	61	58–64	1.9	0.4	0.7	<.001
Animals sampled postpartum (n = 1318); thresholds for BHB postpartum									
DA	1.0	71	55–84	80	77–82	3.5	0.4	0.78	<.001
CK	1.0	57	44–70	80	78–82	2.8	0.5	0.74	<.001
MET	0.7	63	46–78	59	56–61	1.5	0.6	0.61	.03
Any 3	1.0	57	47–66	82	79–84	3.1	0.5	0.74	<.001

Abbreviations: AUC, area under the curve; CI, confidence interval; CK, clinical ketosis; DA, displaced abomasum; MET, metritis; RP, retained placenta; Sen, epidemiologic sensitivity; Spec, epidemiologic specificity.

[a] Highest combined specificity and sensitivity.

[b] Likelihood ratio positive.

[c] Likelihood ratio negative.

Data from Ospina PA, Nydam DV, Stokol T, et al. Evaluation of nonesterified fatty acids and beta-hydroxybutyrate in transition dairy cattle in the northeastern United States: critical thresholds for prediction of clinical diseases. J Dairy Sci 2010;93(2):546–54.

Table 2
The risk ratios for developing any disease[a] based on NEFA concentrations sampled prepartum and postpartum and BHB sampled postpartum

Critical Threshold	Risk Ratio	95% CI	*P* Value
0.3 mEq/L prepartum NEFA	1.8	1.4–2.2	<.001
0.6 mEq/L postpartum NEFA	4.4	2.6–7.3	<.001
1.0 mmol/L postpartum BHB	4.4	3.1–6.3	<.001

[a] Any disease indicates displaced abomasum, clinical ketosis, metritis, or retained placenta.

1.4 mmol/L.[31,32] The cost of this test is approximately US$1.30 per strip and the meter costs approximately US$30.00.

There are other ketone body tests on the market with varying degrees of sensitivity and specificity. The Ketostix strip (Bayer Corp, Elkhart, IN) evaluates AcAc in urine. Relative to serum BHB concentrations of 1.4 mmol/L and higher, the strip had 90% sensitivity and 86% specificity when read as a "trace," and when read as "small" it had 78% sensitivity and 96% specificity.[33] A limitation of the test is that only 50% of the cows could be induced to urinate while sampling. The cost of this test is $0.20 per strip.

The Ketotest (Sanwa Kagaku Co Ltd, Nagoya, Japan) for BHB in milk when read at 0.1 mmol/L or greater had 73% sensitivity and 96% specificity; at greater than 0.2 mmol/L it had 27% and 99% sensitivity and specificity, respectively, when compared with serum BHB 1.4 mmol/L or greater.[33] The cost is $1.70.

The KetoCheck powder for milk AcAc (Great States Animal Health, St. Joseph, MO), had a very low sensitivity, ranging from 41% to 2% when reading the test from trace to large, respectively; but the specificity was high, ranging from 99% to 100%, when compared with BHB 1.4 mmol/L or greater in serum.[33] The cost of this test ranges from $0.50 to $1.00 per test.

The accuracy of PortaBHB (PortaCheck, Moorestown, NJ), a newer cow-side milk test, has been reported to have sensitivity and specificity of 89% and 80% when using a threshold of 100 μmol/L, and 40% and 100% when using a threshold of 2 mmol/L, compared with a serum BHB concentration of 1.4 mmol/L or greater.[34] It costs approximately $2.05 per strip.

NEFA

At present, NEFA testing is limited to processing blood or serum samples at a diagnostic laboratory. The recommended procedure for sample collection and processing is: collect with ethylenediaminetetraacetic acid or non-anticoagulant tubes, immediately cool to 4°C, and separate serum within 24 hours.[35] Although NEFA values can be more stable throughout the day in comparison with BHB,[36] NEFA values may be affected by stress at sampling and sample handling, given that in vitro hemolysis can increase or decrease the NEFA concentration depending on reagents used.[37,38] The current cost at the New York State Animal Health Diagnostic Center is $11.00 per sample. However, it is important that when both NEFA and BHB were evaluated in the same model, NEFA had a stronger association than BHB with the outcomes of interest.[9]

Incidence versus prevalence testing

There are 2 measures that can be used to evaluate the amount of NEB in a herd: incidence and prevalence. By definition, incidence is the number of new cases in a given time, whereas prevalence is the number of existing cases (both new and ongoing) at any point in time. Incidence is more difficult to estimate because it requires testing animals frequently enough to detect all new cases. Prevalence is simpler to measure because a simple cross-sectional sample can be taken to estimate it. Understanding the difference between incidence and prevalence is essential for comparison of on-farm results with the published literature data, some of which report associations based on incidence and others on prevalence.

When evaluating NEB, for example, the incidence can be estimated by identifying new instances of cows with high NEFA or high BHB divided by the number of cows that have gone through the time period at risk. It is important to stress that to estimate incidence only cows at risk, that is, those that were not previously positive, should be tested, and the test must be done frequently enough to identify new cases. The prevalence can be estimated by identifying the cows with existing high NEFA or BHB and dividing this number by the number of animals that were tested. Prevalence can be estimated by cross-sectional sampling.

When evaluating NEB, the distinction between incidence and prevalence tests is important because they can yield different results based on the frequency of sampling. This difference is based on the average duration of disease; for example, the prevalence of a disease that has a short duration may be low, whereas the incidence may be high. In the case of NEB the average duration of subclinical ketosis (SCK; BHB concentrations ≥1.2 mmol/L on Abbott BHB meter) was 5 days.[39] In this case, a minimum of biweekly sampling (of all animals at risk) will be needed to estimate incidence. If less frequent prevalence testing is done, the prevalence estimate may be half of the incidence, a large underestimate.[39,40]

COW-LEVEL ASSOCIATION OF EXCESSIVE NEB AND NEGATIVE DOWNSTREAM OUTCOMES

When measured approximately 2 weeks prepartum to 2 weeks postpartum, the metabolites NEFA and BHB can be used as markers of excessive NEB; however, of importance is that some amount of NEB is normal in the transition period. In addition, although the physiology of NEB may be similar between cows, the transition period is dynamic and individual variation may be amplified. Lastly, because both NEFA and BHB are not normally distributed, calculations of standard deviation are inadequate for the definition of objective thresholds for excessive NEB.

Several research groups have evaluated the association between excessive NEB and negative downstream outcomes at the individual animal level, and have reported NEFA and BHB cut-points associated with these outcomes of interest.[5,8–14,41] Some of these cut-points were reported earlier (see **Table 1**).[9,13]

Diseases and Culling

The association between elevated NEFA and disease and culling was done in a study of 67 high-producing herds comprising 1170 multiparous Holstein cows in Michigan.[5] This study concluded that cows with prepartum NEFA concentrations greater than 0.3 mEq/L had a higher risk of developing a DA. This study was also one of the first to report several herd-level risk factors for increased risk of a DA, including summer and winter season, high-energy forage in the dry period, poor bunk management, and increased body condition score.

A study involving 25 dairy farms and approximately 1000 cows near Guelph (Ontario, Canada) also explored the association between excessive NEB and negative downstream outcomes.[10,11,41] ROC curves were used to determine the cut-point for prepartum NEFA and postpartum BHB above which cows had higher odds of developing a DA.[41] When prepartum NEFA concentrations were measured 4 to 10 days prepartum, cows with concentrations greater than 0.5 mEq/L had 4.1 greater odds of developing a DA. The sensitivity, specificity, and LR of this cut-point were 46%, 82%, and 2.6, respectively. The odds of developing a DA in cows with serum postpartum BHB concentration greater than 1.2 mmol/L measured 1 to 7 DIM were 8 times greater than that of cows below this threshold. The sensitivity, specificity, and LR of this cut-point were 62%, 82%, and 3.5, respectively. Cows with BHB concentrations in milk (Ketotest, Elanco) greater than 0.2 mmol/L had 3.4 greater odds of developing a DA; this cut-point had 47% sensitivity, 79% specificity, and LR 2.4. In this study, BHB measured in the postpartum period was a better predictor of the risk of developing a DA than was NEFA sampled prepartum; however, NEFA in the postpartum period was not evaluated.[41]

The effect of elevated BHB concentrations postpartum on both health and milk production was evaluated.[11] Two-by-two tables for cut-points between 6 and 20 mmol/L in 2-mmol/L increments were evaluated, and the cut-point with the highest sensitivity, highest specificity, largest impact, and smallest chance of committing a type I error was reported. The impact was evaluated through the odds ratio (OR). The ORs for the development of a DA were 2.6 and 6.2; the BHB concentration cut-points were 1.2 mmol/L and 1.8 mmol/L for week 1 and week 2, respectively. The sensitivity, specificity, and LR for these cut-points were 44%, 77%, and 1.9 for week 1 and 45%, 88%, and 3.9 for week 2, respectively. When clinical ketosis (CK) was evaluated as the outcome, the cut-points were 1.4 mmol/L for both week 1 and week 2. The ORs were 4.2 and 5.9, and the sensitivity, specificity, and LR were 46%, 83%, and 2.8 for week 1 and 57%, 82%, and 3.1 for week 2, respectively. Only week-1 BHB was associated with metritis, the cut-point being 1.2 mmol/L; sensitivity was 52%, specificity 76%, and LR 2.1.

Ospina and colleagues[9] studied more than 2700 cows in 100 free-stall dairies in New York, Pennsylvania, and Vermont. Approximately half the animals were sampled 14 to 3 days prepartum and the other half sampled 3 to 14 days postpartum in a cross-sectional sample. This study established critical thresholds above which cows were more likely to develop disease (DA, CK, or RP/MET). The ROC curves were used to identify the cut-point with the highest sensitivity and specificity, with the presence or absence of the disease as the outcome (see **Table 1**).

The prevalence of SCK (BHB concentrations ≥1.2 mmol/L) was 18%; prevalence of excessive NEB (defined as having postpartum NEFA ≥0.7 mEq/L) was 32%. In the 1439 animals sampled prepartum, the prevalence of excessive NEB defined as having prepartum NEFA of at least 0.3 mEq/L was 34%. Animals with excessive NEB were twice as likely to be culled within 30 DIM.

In addition to sensitivity and specificity, LR were also reported (see **Table 1**). The thresholds with the largest combined sensitivity and specificity associated with the development of any of the diseases of interest were: prepartum NEFA 0.3 mEq/L or greater; postpartum NEFA 0.6 mEq/L; postpartum BHB 1.0 mmol/L. The LRs ranged from 1.2 to 4.9 across different NEFA and BHB cut-points. In the original article[9] several different cut-points are reported, including those with higher sensitivity or higher specificity, so that the reader can select the appropriate cut-point based on the desired criteria.

In a study including more than 2300 cows in 55 free-stall Holstein dairies across the United States and parts of Canada, the association between elevated NEFA and BHB and the development of diseases was studied.[10] This study is the first to evaluate on a large scale the association between prepartum BHB and disease outcomes. The investigators reported that cows with prepartum NEFA concentrations of 0.3 mEq/L or greater had higher odds of developing RP (OR 1.8; 95% confidence interval [CI] 1.3–2.6; sensitivity 67%, specificity 46%) and metritis (OR 1.8; 95% CI 1.5–2.9; sensitivity 75%, specificity 40%), than cows with prepartum NEFA below this cut-point. However, there were some regional differences for metritis. The odds of developing a DA in animals sampled prepartum with NEFA concentrations of 0.5 mEq/L or greater was 2.9; the sensitivity and specificity of this cut-point were 49% and 75%, respectively. In animals sampled postpartum, those with NEFA concentrations greater than or equal to 1.0 mEq/L had higher odds of developing a DA (OR 4.3; sensitivity 51%, specificity 80%). Although this study found a univariable association between elevated prepartum BHB 0.8 mmol/L or greater and increased risk of DA, the sensitivity was low (22%) and the number of animals at risk was also low, so these findings should be interpreted with caution.

Most recently, the epidemiology of hyperketonemia (BHB $\geq$1.2 mmol/L) was intensively studied in 4 herds (2 in New York and 2 in Wisconsin).[39] Cows with elevated BHB concentrations were 19.3 times more likely than nonketotic cows to develop a DA ($P<.001$), and ketotic cows were also 3 times more likely to be culled or die within the first 30 DIM ($P<.001$).[42]

Reproduction and Milk Production

The effect of SCK on the probability of becoming pregnant after the first artificial insemination was studied in 2007.[11] It was reported that cows with elevated BHB concentrations in the first or second week postpartum were 20% less likely to get pregnant after the first insemination; the cut-points were 1.0 mmol/L and 1.4 mmol/L, respectively. Cows that had concentrations higher than the cut-points during both weeks were 50% less likely to conceive.

In the first and second week postpartum, the effect of elevated BHB in 25 herds in Ontario, Canada that did not feed a total mixed ration were evaluated.[10] The greatest impact on milk yield, measured at the first Dairy Herd Improvement Association (DHIA) test, was seen at 1.4 mmol/L in the first week (milk yield decreased by 1.88 kg/d) and 2.0 mmol/L in the second week (milk yield decreased by 3.3 kg/d).

Milk production was estimated with mature equivalent milk 305 (ME305) from at least 4 DHIA test days (at approximately 120 DIM) in a study done in 2007.[12] Multiparous animals with elevated BHB and NEFA concentrations produced less milk. However, in this study primiparous animals with elevated BHB in the postpartum period produced more milk. Although the biological basis of this finding is not clearly understood, it is hypothesized that first-lactation animals may mobilize energy resources such as lipid more readily than multiparous cows because they have to balance maintenance, growth, and milk production. The concept of homeorhesis, the orchestrated or coordinated changes in metabolism of body tissues necessary to support a physiologic state,[43] may help explain these findings. The effect of elevated NEFA peripartum and BHB postpartum on reproduction was similar between parity groups. Animals with prepartum NEFA 0.3 mEq/L or more had a 19% decreased risk of pregnancy, postpartum cows with NEFA 0.7 mEq/L or more had a 16% decreased risk of pregnancy, and those with elevated postpartum BHB 1.0 mmol/L or more had a 13% decreased risk.

A multicenter study examined the effect of peripartum NEFA and BHB on both milk production and reproduction.[14] In this study, elevated NEFA ($\geq$0.5 mEq/L), and elevated BHB ($\geq$0.6 mmol/L) prepartum were associated with reduced milk production across the first 4 DHIA tests. Elevated NEFA (week 1 at 0.7 and week 2 at 1.0 mEq/L) and BHB (week 1 at 1.4 and week 2 at 1.2 mmol/L) also resulted in decreased milk at first DHIA test. There was no association between these metabolites and pregnancy at first artificial insemination.

Most recently, the effect of elevated BHB (≥1.2 mmol/L) on reproduction parameters and milk yield was studied.[44] There was no difference between ketotic and nonketotic cows regarding conception to first service ($P = .55$) and time to conception in 3 farms ($P = .4$). However, nonketotic cows produced 0.4 kg more milk per milking than SCK-positive cows in the first 30 DIM, for a total difference of approximately 1.2 kg/cow/d ($P = .006$).

HERD-LEVEL ASSOCIATION OF EXCESSIVE NEB AND NEGATIVE DOWNSTREAM OUTCOMES

As already reviewed, objective cow-level thresholds have been determined for elevated BHB and NEFA concentrations that are associated with disease or a decline in reproduction and milk production.[5,8–14,41] This information allows the identification of individual cows at risk for these downstream outcomes based on their NEB status during the transition period. However, despite all of the NEB information available at the cow level and its association with negative downstream outcomes, individual strategies for prevention and treatment of NEB in cows are still a challenge.[6] Efforts to improve NEB are better implemented at the herd level, where decisions about nutritional and herd management are routinely addressed.

Unfortunately, parameters to identify herds at increased risk of negative downstream outcomes as a result of excessive NEB at the individual cow level have not been well defined.[45] In the last 5 years, only 2 large studies have examined the herd-level associations of serum NEFA and BHB with negative downstream outcomes.[46,47] Both of these studies empirically report a critical herd-level threshold, based on individual animal testing, above which there was an association with negative downstream outcomes.

Herd Alarm Levels

Tables 3 and **4** summarize the herd alarm levels reported from these studies.[46,47] Both report a herd alarm level based on a proportion of animals above a predetermined cut-point for the NEFA or BHB concentration. The individual cut-points were determined from prior studies that investigated the association of elevated NEFA or BHB on individual animal outcomes.[9–14] The second part of the herd alarm level, the proportion of animals above the predetermined cut-point, was selected based on the largest change in the herd-level outcome and lowest chance of committing a type I error (stating that there is a difference when there really is no difference). The herd-level outcomes of interest were increased probability of disease, decreased milk production, and decreased reproduction.

Fig. 4 is a graphic representation of the change in herd-level prevalence of disease with increasing proportion of animals that were above the cut-point.[47] It shows a dose-response effect; that is, as the proportion of animals that test positive increases, the disease incidence also increases. In this study, the prevalence of herds with more than 15% of sampled animals above the metabolite threshold was 75% with prepartum NEFA 0.30 mEq/L or greater, 40% with BHB 1.2 mmol/L or greater, and 65% with postpartum NEFA 0.70 mEq/L or greater.

To correctly evaluate excessive NEB at the herd level, appropriate sample collection is critical, and it is important to decide when to sample cows, how many cows to sample, how often to sample, and how to evaluate the samples, including whether

Table 3
Herd-level associations of increased metabolite concentrations within 1 week before or after calving with displaced abomasum (DA), milk production (kg/d at first DHIA test), and pregnancy at first AI

Proportion of Animals Above Cut-Point (%)	Metabolite Concentration (Cut-Point)	Sampling Time (Reference to Calving) (wk)	Odds Ratio (95% CI; ± Standard Error)	*P* Value	Outcome of Interest
≥25	BHB ≥1.4 mmol/L	+1	2.1 (1–4.2)	.04	Odds of developing DA
≥25[a]	BHB ≥1.4 mmol/L	+1	1.9 (1.0–3.3)	.04	Odds of developing DA
≥15	BHB ≥8 mmol/L	−1	−4.4 (±1.7) kg/d/cow	.01	Milk Production
≥30[a]	NEFA ≥0.5 mEq/L	−1	−3 (±1.5) kg/d/cow	.04	Milk Production
≥20[a]	BHB ≥8	−1	−5.5 (±1.5) kg/d/cow	.01	Milk Production
≥30	NEFA ≥1.0 mEq/L	+1	0.6 (0.4–0.9)	.02	Odds of pregnancy by first AI
≥50[a]	NEFA ≥0.5 mEq/L	−1	0.5 (0.2–0.9)	.03	Odds of pregnancy by first AI
≥30[a]	NEFA ≥1.0 mEq/L	+1	0.6 (0.4–1.0)	.04	Odds of pregnancy by first AI

Abbreviations: AI, artificial insemination; DHIA, Dairy Herd Improvement Association.
[a] Only multiparous animals were included in the analysis.
Data from Chapinal N, LeBlanc SJ, Carson ME, et al. Herd-level association of serum metabolites in the transition period with disease, milk production, and early lactation reproductive performance. J Dairy Sci 2012;95(10):5676–82.

it is possible to pool the samples. These questions are of particular importance because the test results will influence management decisions at the herd level.

Sample Size for a Herd-Based Test

Determining sample size is an important first step in herd evaluation. There is no single sample size that is appropriate in all contexts; the number of animals to be sampled must be based on the reason for sampling. Herds can be sampled to estimate the true or apparent prevalence of a disease or condition. Considerations for sampling and evaluating data are discussed here, using NEFA and BHB as indicators of NEB.

Estimating population proportion from a sample

The following parameters will determine the sample size needed to estimate the prevalence of animals with excessive NEB at the herd level, assuming a near perfect test:

1. Precision, which refers to the reproducibility of the measure and has the greatest impact on sample size. An estimate with high precision, that is, a small acceptable bound above and below the estimate, will require a large sample size.
2. Confidence, which refers to the level of certainty with which one wants to estimate the answer. The more confidence one wants to have in the estimate, the larger is the sample size required.

Table 4
Herd-level associations of increased metabolite concentrations from animals sampled 3 to 14 days prepartum and 3 to 14 DIM relative to increased risk of displaced abomasum or clinical ketosis; mature equivalent (ME) 305 milk measured at 120 DIM; and change in pregnancy rate at the herd level measured at 70 days after voluntary waiting period

Proportion of Animals Above Cut-Point (%)	Metabolite Concentration (Cut-Point)	Sampling Time (Reference to Calving)	Change in Outcome (Standard Error)	*P* Value	Outcome of Interest
>15	NEFA ≥0.27 mEq/L	Prepartum	3.6 (±1.3)	.006	Change in disease
>15	NEFA ≥0.70 mEq/L	Postpartum	1.7 (±0.8)	.04	Change in disease
>15	BHB ≥1.2 mmol/L	Postpartum	1.8 (±0.8)	.03	Change in disease
>15	NEFA ≥0.27 mEq/L	Prepartum	−282 kg (±91)	.002	Difference in ME305 milk
>15[a]	NEFA ≥0.60 mEq/L	Postpartum	−288 kg (±159)	.07	Difference in ME305 milk
>15[b]	NEFA ≥0.70 mEq/L	Postpartum	−593 kg (±107)	<.0001	Difference in ME305 milk
>20[a]	BHB ≥1.2 mmol/L	Postpartum	−534 kg (±141)	.0002	Difference in ME305 milk
>15[b]	BHB ≥1.0 mmol/L	Postpartum	−368 (±99)	.0004	Difference in ME305 milk
>15	NEFA ≥0.27 mEq/L	Prepartum	−1.2 (±0.4)	.006	Change in pregnancy rate
>15	NEFA ≥0.70 mEq/L	Postpartum	−0.9 (±0.5)	.05	Change in pregnancy rate
>15	BHB ≥1.2 mmol/L	Postpartum	0.8 (±0.4)	.03	Change in pregnancy rate

[a] Only multiparous animals included in the analysis.
[b] Only primiparous animals included in the analysis.
Data from Ospina PA, Nydam DV, Stokol T, et al. Association between the proportion of sampled transition cows with increased nonesterified fatty acids and β-hydroxybutyrate and disease incidence, pregnancy rate, and milk production at the herd level. J Dairy Sci 2010;93(4):3595–601.

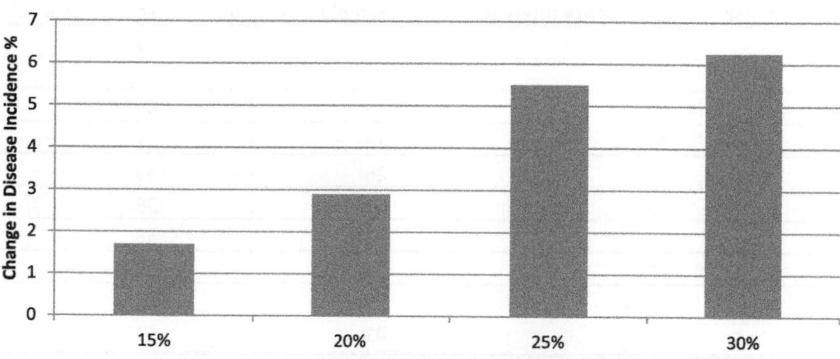

Fig. 4. Change in disease incidence at the herd level based on the proportion of animals 3 to 14 DIM with NEFA concentrations 0.7 mEq/L or greater (n = 805) from herd-level samples (60 herds). Disease is defined as displaced abomasum and/or clinical ketosis.

3. Expected prevalence: Few research groups have reported the prevalence or incidence of SCK and elevated NEFA, albeit at different concentration cut-points for NEFA and BHB and slightly different sampling windows.
   a. For prevalence of SCK a range of 20%,[41] 31%,[48] 18%,[9] and, most recently, 12%.[10]
   b. The prevalence of elevated NEFA was 37% in the first week and 34% the second week postpartum,[48] and 32% in.[9]
4. Number of animals at risk: Not all animals on the farm will be at risk for transition cow NEB disorders on any given day. Research groups have focused on the period between 14 to 3 days prepartum and 3 to 14 DIM, and some have narrowed it even more.
   a. Considering a 3 to 14 DIM sampling window, a herd that milks 1000 cows and has average reproductive performance (thus having approximately 3–4 calvings per day) will have approximately 35 postpartum animals in the at-risk period.

Table 5 lists the sample sizes necessary in a 1000-cow dairy with 35 animals at risk or a 2000-cow dairy with 75 cows at risk, with the CI ranging from 75% to 99%, the desired precision at ±10 and ±5, and the expected prevalence set at 20%.

Evaluating Individual Animal Tests at the Herd Level

Herd-level sensitivity, specificity, and predictive value positive and negative

The herd alarm levels were identified as having more than 15% of sampled transition animals with BHB concentrations of 1.2 mmol/L or greater.[47] Herds above this alarm level empirically had higher incidence of DA and CK, as well as decreased pregnancy rate (PR) and milk production. The accuracy of this herd-based test depends primarily on the underlying true prevalence of the disease being monitored, individual test sensitivity, and individual test specificity; however, herd-level parameters such as herd-level sensitivity (HSe), herd-level specificity (HSp), herd-level predictive value positive (HPV+), and herd-level predictive value negative (HPV−) should also be evaluated.

Table 5
Sample size necessary to estimate the prevalence of animals with elevated energy metabolites with various numbers of animals at risk, confidence intervals, and desired precision around the estimate

Animals at Risk	Confidence Interval (%)	Sample Size (±10)[a]	Sample Size (±5)[a]
35	75	14	25
35	85	18	28
35	90	20	30
35	95	22	31
35	99	26	33
70	75	17	39
70	85	23	46
70	90	27	50
70	95	33	55
70	99	43	61

[a] Precision around the confidence interval.

The HSe is the probability of a herd being correctly identified as positive when it truly has excessive NEB, whereas the HSp is the probability of a herd being correctly identified as negative. The HPV+ estimates the probability that a positive test came from a positive herd; conversely, the HPV− determines the probability that a negative test came from a negative herd.

Herd-level diagnostic test accuracy

Although the sensitivity and specificity of tests at the individual animal level are well understood, the impact of the underlying true prevalence on herd-level sensitivity and herd-level specificity is more difficult to understand and may deviate from what is expected.[49] At present there is a Microsoft Windows–based program, Herdacc,[50] that will estimate the herd-level sensitivity, specificity, and PVs based on individual test sensitivity, specificity, herd size, sample size, prevalence, and cut-point used to determine whether a herd is classified as positive or negative. Herdacc uses an approximation based on the expected number of test-positive animals in the population; the cutoff is the minimum number of animals that test positive before the herd is considered positive.[51,52]

Based on the previously reported prevalence of elevated BHB concentrations, most farms will fall into the category of less than 40% prevalence.[9,10,41,48] In this category, the characteristics of the test at the individual animal level may affect the herd-level sensitivity and specificity differently than what is expected. This difference is most apparent when the test is considered positive based on a proportion of positive animals rather than an absolute number, which is how the herd alarm level is defined above.

Table 6 shows the results of using the Herdacc software to estimate the HSe for a herd with the true prevalence ranging from 0.2 to 0.6 in increments of 0.1; the sample size ranging from 20 to 35; and the cut-point ranging from 3 to 5 (~15% of 20–35, respectively).[47] In this example, the HSe (ie, the probability of correctly identifying the herd as positive) decreases when a test with low sensitivity (eg, Ketocheck powder, sensitivity 41%) is used and sample size increases, which results in an increase in the number of positive animals required to identify the herd as positive.

Because the test sensitivity is low, false negatives are increased. In some cases, a test with a lower specificity may result in a higher HSe, despite a low test sensitivity resulting from false positives. However, the marginal increase in HSe does not warrant

Table 6
Estimation of herd-level sensitivity (HSe) using Herdacc software (with Herdacc option[50]) for tests with different individual animal-level sensitivity and specificity in a herd with 1000 animals

	Herd Level Prevalence				
	0.2	0.3	0.4	0.5	0.6
HSe based on individual animal test sensitivity = 41%, specificity = 99%[31] (Ketocheck powder; Great States Animal Health, St. Joseph, MO)					
20[a] animals sampled	0.27	0.49	0.69	0.83	0.91
35[b] animals sampled	0.2	0.49	0.74	0.89	0.96
HSe based on individual animal test sensitivity = 78%, specificity = 96%[29] (Ketostix; Bayer Corp, Elkhart, IN)					
20[a] animals sampled	0.76	0.93	0.98	1	1
35[b] animals sampled	0.82	0.97	1	1	1
HSe based on individual animal test sensitivity = 96%, specificity = 97%[29] (Precision Xtra meter; Abbott Laboratories, Abbott Park, IL)					
20[a] animals sampled	0.84	0.97	1	1	1
35[b] animals sampled	0.91	0.99	1	1	1

[a] Three or more (~15%) animals sampled would need to test positive to call the herd positive.[47]
[b] Five or more (~15%) animals sampled would need to test positive to call the herd positive.[47]

selecting a test with lower specificity. A test with high sensitivity and high specificity (eg, Precision Xtra BHB meter, sensitivity 96%, specificity 97%) results in almost perfect HSe at higher levels of underlying prevalence.

When evaluating herds, a high HSe is desirable because it increases the chance that a herd at risk for negative downstream outcomes, such as increased disease and decreased milking and reproductive performance, will be identified. Misclassifying herds at this level would result in missed opportunities for improvement. When selecting individual animal tests to use at the herd level, one must keep in mind that in addition to the test sensitivity and specificity previously defined, there is another level of test sensitivity and specificity. This second level refers to the estimated metabolite concentration cut-point and proportion of animals above that cut-point that defines a herd as positive or negative. Additional methods, including Bayesian approaches, are necessary to more precisely define this herd alarm level sensitivity and specificity, but this requires a very large herd-level sample size. However, a safe assumption is that the sensitivity and specificity are not 100%. In an effort to minimize the effect of the uncertainty in this measure, it is recommended that the individual animal test with the highest combined sensitivity and specificity be used to correctly identify herds at risk for negative downstream outcomes.

Sources of Error in Herd Testing

Nonrepresentative sample and other confounders

When evaluating herd status based on individual tests, there is an additional potential bias: not sampling the animals that are at risk and, therefore, not having a representative sample. It is important that the NEFA and BHB tests used to determine the risk both at the individual and herd level are based on sampling animals that are subjectively healthy.

In addition, it is important to focus the sampling time frame. Samples obtained within a few days of calving will be elevated[41] and may not indicate a true excess of

NEB. For this reason, studies have focused on sampling 14 to 3 days prepartum and 3 to 14 days postpartum.

The current parity of the animal may be a confounder. Both the herd-level studies reported a difference in the effects of elevated NEFA and BHB between primiparous and multiparous cows.[46,47] It is recommended that primiparous animals be evaluated separately from multiparous animals, if they are housed and managed separately.

Pooling versus individual animal tests

A data set that evaluated both NEFA and BHB at the individual animal level was used to estimate the sensitivity and specificity of a pooled testing approach versus using individual samples to classify a herd as positive or negative for excessive NEB.[9] Twelve herds with a minimum of 12 samples were rerun in the laboratory as pooled and individual samples. Herds were defined as having excessive NEB if the proportion of individual samples with a metabolite concentration above the threshold was more than 15% (≥2 animals from 12).[47] The metabolite threshold for BHB was 1.2 mmol/L or greater. Herds with pooled sample BHB concentrations 1.2 mmol/L or more were considered to have excessive NEB. A similar evaluation was performed for NEFAs, the cut-points for NEFA concentration being 0.3 mEq/L prepartum and 0.7 mEq/L postpartum. Herds with more than 15% of animals with elevated NEFA concentrations were considered positive, and herds with a pooled concentration of greater than 0.3 mEq/L or greater than 0.7 mEq/L were considered positive.

The results were similar to those of a previous report[53]; pooled samples were well correlated with the arithmetical means of individual samples. McNemar's *P* value, κ, sensitivity, and specificity were evaluated to compare individual and pooled tests. Sensitivity and specificity analyses compared the pooled test with the individual tests (**Table 7**). When compared with the individual test, the pooled test had a low sensitivity for correctly identifying herds above the herd alarm level.

The McNemar *P* value evaluates bias between the 2 tests[29]; however, in this example a low McNemar *P* value is most likely consistent with true differences in the tests. The McNemar *P* values were: prepartum NEFA $P = .03$, postpartum NEFA $P = .03$, and BHB $P = .008$.

The κ statistic evaluates the agreement beyond chance between tests.[29] The κ statistics for the individual versus pooled tests were low, indicating low agreement between the tests. The κ statistics were: 0.17 (95% CI −0.14 to 0.48) for prepartum NEFA, 0.25 (95% CI −0.08 to 0.58) for postpartum NEFA, and 0.13 (95% CI −0.08

Table 7
Sensitivity and specificity of pooled samples compared with the proportion of individual samples

Category	Sensitivity (%)	95% CI for Sensitivity	Specificity (%)	95% CI for Specificity
Prepartum NEFA[a]	55	24–83	100	16–100
Postpartum NEFA[b]	50	19–81	100	19–100
BHB[c]	30	7–65	100	19–100

[a] Prepartum NEFA: cutoff concentration 0.3 mEq/L.
[b] Postpartum NEFA: cutoff concentration 0.7 mEq/L.
[c] BHB: cutoff concentration 1.2 mmol/L.

Data from Ospina PA, Nydam DV, Stokol T, et al. Association between the proportion of sampled transition cows with increased nonesterified fatty acids and β-hydroxybutyrate and disease incidence, pregnancy rate, and milk production at the herd level. J Dairy Sci 2010;93(4):3595–601.

to 0.33) for BHB. In addition, the proportion of herds categorized as having excessive NEB based on individual tests was different from the proportion of herds with excessive NEB based on pooled samples, which was 0.5, 0.4, and 0.3 for prepartum NEFA, postpartum NEFA, and BHB, respectively.

The sensitivity of the individual versus pooled test for prepartum NEFA, postpartum NEFA, and BHB was low; however, the specificity was high (see **Table 7**). Low test sensitivity can lead to a large number of false negatives, which means that herds at risk will not be identified and opportunities for improvement may be lost. The wide CIs for specificity of the pooled test indicate uncertainty about the estimate; additional herds would need to be tested to improve the accuracy of this estimate.

Pooled samples are good estimates of the arithmetical means of individual samples, but may be misleading when evaluating herd NEB status. All animals have a normal baseline concentration for NEFA and BHB; disease is associated with metabolite levels above a certain biological threshold.[45] At the herd level there is an association between a certain proportion of animals above that biological threshold and negative downstream outcomes.[47] Although pooled samples to determine herd NEB status may seem desirable owing to lower laboratory costs, the low sensitivity and lack of agreement between pooled samples and the proportion of affected individuals can lead to an increased number of false negatives. An increased number of false negatives may result in missed opportunities for improving the health and productivity of transition cows.

NEFA versus BHB testing

Although NEFA can be metabolized to BHB in the liver, this is only 1 of several pathways for NEFA in the cow (see **Fig. 1**). When animals were sampled simultaneously 3 to 14 DIM for both NEFA and BHB measurement,[9] the correlation between NEFA and BHB was 0.18 (**Fig. 5**). This finding means that only 18% of the variability in BHB concentration was explained by NEFA concentration. The lack of correlation may be related to the fact that not all NEFA is metabolized to BHB in all cows in the same way. There could also be a temporal delay between elevation of NEFA and metabolism to BHB. However,

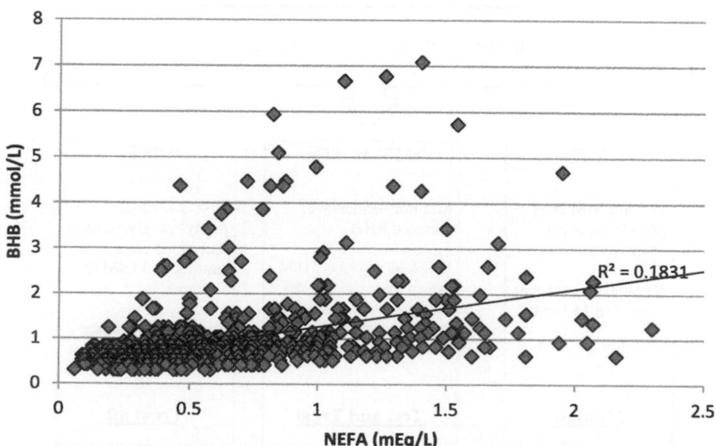

Fig. 5. Correlation between simultaneous evaluation of BHB (mmol/L) and NEFA (mEq/L) in animals sampled 3 to 14 (n = 783) days postpartum. $R^2 = 0.1831$.

further evaluation of the relationship between these 2 metabolites may prove useful in understanding the biological mechanisms of adaptation or maladaptation to NEB.

At present, the recommendations for testing depend on the purpose of testing and the current herd situation. Most herds will monitor NEB in transition cows by checking BHB concentrations with the Precision Xtra meter between 3 and 14 DIM at a frequency ranging from biweekly to every other week. This strategy is a good one because the meter is accurate and timely, and the test is inexpensive. Of course another test with similar test sensitivity and specificity, cow-side friendliness, and cost-effectiveness could also be used. However, although BHB is a good predictor of negative downstream outcomes, NEFA was a better predictor in some studies. Therefore, in herds where transition cow diseases are higher than expected and BHB test results do not indicate that the herd is experiencing excessive NEB, evaluation of the prevalence of elevated NEFA, either postpartum or both prepartum and postpartum, may be warranted.

Sample Frequency

The minimum recommended sampling frequency is before and after a significant change in management or nutrition is being made. The purpose of this sampling scheme is 2-fold: first, to evaluate management changes, and second, to allow prompt action to correct increased NEB at both herd and individual levels. Based on previous studies, any animal that has an elevated BHB test (BHB ≥1.2 mmol/L) should be treated with propylene glycol (300 mL by mouth once daily for 5 days[42,44]).

In cases where more aggressive monitoring is necessary, additional testing strategies are necessary. To determine whether more aggressive monitoring and, perhaps,

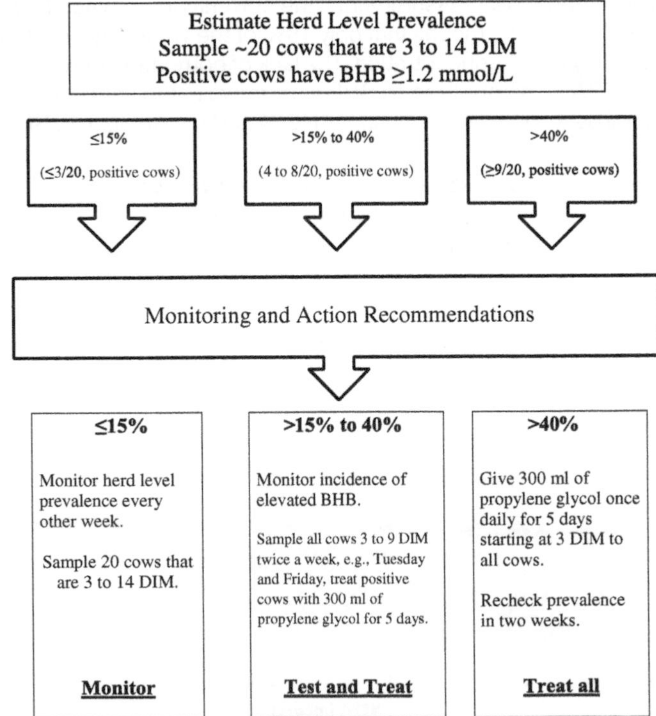

Fig. 6. Monitoring recommendations for BHB testing based on herd-level prevalence of elevated BHB.

treatment is necessary, an initial sample of the at-risk population is necessary. It is recommended to sample at least 20 animals at risk, that is, animals 3 to 14 DIM. A more specific sample size could be based on the parameters in **Table 3**. Based on the initial prevalence determined, 3 different testing frequencies are suggested (**Fig. 6**).

The recommendations for the 3 testing frequencies are based on evaluation of a stochastic Monte Carlo partial budget model using @ Risk, version 6.1.1 (Palisade Corporation, Ithaca, NY). The model estimates the cost-benefit of various testing and treating protocols at many different herd-level incidences of SCK using 10,000 iterations. Included in the model are the costs associated with labor to test cows, BHB test strips, labor to treat cows with propylene glycol, propylene glycol, and feed cost. Also modeled are the associated gain in milk production, decrease in DA, and early removal risks of animals treated with propylene glycol.

The estimates used to quantify changes in milk production, decrease in DA, and early removal risks were based on previous reports.[39,42,44] This study was a randomized trial that evaluated the effect of propylene glycol on cows with BHB level of 1.2 mmol/L or greater. The cows in this study were sampled 3 times per week to identify new cases (ie, incidence sampling).

Tables 8 and **9** demonstrate the economic returns based on this stochastic model per 100 fresh cows, and include: the percentage of the time that the outcome was positive (ie, >$0 return); the percentage of the time that the return was more than $500; and the average increase in cash flow. In addition to the economic returns, the sample prevalence of SCK and estimated incidence are included in these tables. **Table 8** shows the monetary return for testing all animals at risk twice weekly at various prevalences because the model indicated it was more cost-effective to test and treat at lower prevalences. **Table 9** shows the monetary return for treating all cows that are 3 DIM at higher prevalences because the model indicated that it becomes more cost-effective to simply treat all cows rather than spend time and resources on testing.

The relationship between incidence and prevalence was evaluated by randomly sampling 20 cows from the control group once a week and then comparing this

Table 8
Stochastic simulation results for testing all cows 3 to 9 DIM 2 times per week and treating those cows with BHB ≥1.2 mmol/L with 300 mL of propylene glycol orally for 5 days

Sample Prevalence	Estimated Incidence[a]	Percentage of Time that Outcome is Positive (%)	Percentage of Time that Outcome is >$500 per 100 Cows (%)	Mean of Distribution ($)
15	20	90	18	289
20	30	98	59	618
25	35	99	73	780
30	45	99	88	1108
35	50	99.9	92	1271
40	60	99.9	96.2	1598
45	65	99.9	97.4	1765
50	75	100	98.8	2092
60	90	100	99.5	2582

The expected monetary return is per 100 fresh cows at various incidence levels of BHB ≥1.2 mmol/L.
[a] Conservative approximation of incidence (1.5 times prevalence): for ease of interpretation, the number was rounded down to the nearest 5th or 10th.

Table 9
Stochastic simulation results for treating all cows with 300 mL of propylene glycol orally for 5 days starting at 3 DIM

Sample Prevalence	Estimated Incidence[a]	Percentage of Time that Outcome is Positive (%)	Percentage of Time that Outcome is >$500 (%)	Mean of Distribution ($)
45	65	100	98.1	1860
50	75	100	98.6	2088
60	90	100	99.5	2578

The expected monetary return is per 100 fresh cows at various incidence levels of BHB ≥1.2 mmol/L.
[a] Conservative approximation of incidence (1.5 times prevalence): for ease of interpretation, the number was rounded down to the nearest 5th or 10th.

number with the incidence.[39,42,44] Although there was some week-to-week variability, on average the incidence was approximately 1.8 times the prevalence. This association is consistent with that shown by other reports.[40]

Testing strategies

An initial sample for prevalence estimation should be performed following the sample size guidelines described; for example, test at least 20 at-risk animals who are subjectively healthy and 3 to 14 DIM (see **Fig. 6**). Any animal with a BHB concentration of at least 1.2 mmol/L should receive 300 mL propylene glycol for 5 days.[42,44]

1. If 15% or fewer of the animals sampled (3–14 DIM) have a BHB concentration 1.2 mmol/L or greater, the recommendation is to sample again every other week to monitor herd-level prevalence of elevated BHB. More frequent sampling may be indicated when there are significant changes in diet formulation, management, or environment.
2. If greater than 15% to 40% of the animals sampled (3–14 DIM) have a BHB concentration greater than or equal to 1.2 mmol/L, the recommendation is to test all animals that are 3 to 9 DIM twice weekly (eg, Tuesday and Friday) and treat all positive cows. This more frequent testing scheme is warranted to identify and treat most of the cows with elevated BHB, thus reducing their risk of negative downstream outcomes. If at least 2 consecutive prevalence tests independently result in fewer than 15% of the animals testing positive, one could consider stopping this testing and treating protocol and monitor the prevalence every 2 weeks as described earlier.
3. If more than 40% of the animals sampled (3–14 DIM) have a BHB concentration of 1.2 mmol/L or greater, the recommendation is to start treating all fresh cows with propylene glycol at 3 DIM for 5 days. This treatment scheme will help reduce the negative effects of elevated BHB concentrations in herds with a very high prevalence. Recheck the prevalence in 2 weeks to determine the next course of action; for example one may stop treating all cows and move to the test-and-treat positive cow scheme, or remain in the treat-all-cows protocol. This monitoring scheme should continue until at least 2 consecutive prevalence tests independently result in fewer than 40% of the animals testing positive.

RECOMMENDATIONS

As summarized earlier, several studies have reported that there is an association between elevated NEFA and BHB and negative downstream outcomes. There are also several concentration thresholds above which negative outcomes are more likely; the chosen NEFA and BHB cut-point used will depend on the level of sensitivity and specificity that is most important in the situation.

At present, there are only 2 studies that have reported herd alarm levels.[46,47] These herd-level cut-points should be applied in the same way as individual cut-points: if false negatives are more important, the cut-point with the highest sensitivity (ie, lower herd alarm level) should be used for evaluation; conversely, if false positives are more important, the cut-point with the highest specificity (ie, higher alarm level) should be chosen (see **Tables 3** and **4**).

Metabolite Testing

NEFA versus BHB

Concentrations of BHB and NEFA are not well correlated when sampled on the same day; that is, they are not both elevated in the same animal at the same time. In addition, reports that evaluated both NEFA and BHB more often than not found an association between NEFA and negative downstream outcomes when the association was not present with BHB (see **Fig. 5**).

In general, NEFA was found to be a better predictor of negative downstream outcomes; however, BHB is easy and inexpensive to measure accurately cow-side if the appropriate test is chosen. Therefore, BHB should be used as the primary monitoring tool, but when there is evidence that the herd is experiencing issues with transition cows without significant elevation in BHB, NEFA should be evaluated.

Sample Size

When evaluating prevalence, it is recommended to sample at least 20 cows at risk; a larger sample size will result in a more precise estimate (see **Table 5**).

Sampling Time Frame

The first time cows are sampled on a farm, the sampling window should include cows between 3 and 14 DIM. However, when twice-weekly sampling is warranted, this window is decreased to cows between 3 and 9 DIM.

Sample Frequency, Testing, and Treatment Strategies

Fig. 6 provides an overview of the sampling guidelines based on initial prevalence of elevated BHB concentrations. **Tables 8** and **9** show the expected monetary return based on the sampling schemes.

Take-Home Message

In conjunction with BHB or NEFA monitoring, it is necessary to continuously evaluate other herd-level factors that increase the risk of excessive NEB, such as overcrowding, lack of heat abatement, excessive pen moves, excessive energy in dry cow diets, and unbalanced dietary protein. The goal is to prevent excessive NEB and to use these testing and monitoring guidelines to evaluate the effectiveness of the program, or make changes based on objective measures of the success of the dairy.

The metabolites NEFA and BHB can be used as markers of NEB, owing to the relationship between energy demands, energy reserves, and the metabolic association between NEFA and BHB.

REFERENCES

1. Bell AW. Regulation of organic nutrient metabolism during transition from late pregnancy to early lactation. J Anim Sci 1995;73(9):2804–19.

2. Hayirli A, Grummer RR, Nordheim EV, et al. Animal and dietary factors affecting feed intake during the prefresh transition period in Holsteins. J Dairy Sci 2002; 85(12):3430–43.
3. Mepham TB. The development of ideas on the role of glucose in regulating milk secretion. Aust J Agric Res 1993;44:509–22.
4. Reynolds CK, Huntington GB, Tyrrell HF, et al. Net portal-drained visceral and hepatic metabolism of glucose, L-lactate, and nitrogenous compounds in lactating Holstein cows. J Dairy Sci 1988;71(7):1803–12.
5. Cameron RE, Dyk PB, Herdt TH, et al. Dry cow diet, management, and energy balance as risk factors for displaced abomasum in high producing dairy herds. J Dairy Sci 1998;81(1):132–9.
6. Duffield T. Subclinical ketosis in lactating dairy cattle. Vet Clin North Am Food Anim Pract 2000;16(2):231–53, v.
7. Dohoo IR, Martin SW. Subclinical ketosis: prevalence and associations with production and disease. Can J Comp Med 1984;48(1):1–5.
8. Andersson L. Subclinical ketosis in dairy cows. Vet Clin North Am Food Anim Pract 1988;4(2):233–51.
9. Ospina PA, Nydam DV, Stokol T, et al. Evaluation of nonesterified fatty acids and beta-hydroxybutyrate in transition dairy cattle in the northeastern United States: critical thresholds for prediction of clinical diseases. J Dairy Sci 2010;93(2): 546–54.
10. Chapinal N, Carson M, Duffield TF, et al. The association of serum metabolites with clinical disease during the transition period. J Dairy Sci 2011;94(10):4897–903.
11. Duffield TF, Lissemore KD, McBride BW, et al. Impact of hyperketonemia in early lactation dairy cows on health and production. J Dairy Sci 2009;92(2):571–80.
12. Walsh RB, Walton JS, Kelton DF, et al. The effect of subclinical ketosis in early lactation on reproductive performance of postpartum dairy cows. J Dairy Sci 2007;90(6):2788–96.
13. Ospina PA, Nydam DV, Stokol T, et al. Associations of elevated nonesterified fatty acids and beta-hydroxybutyrate concentrations with early lactation reproductive performance and milk production in transition dairy cattle in the northeastern United States. J Dairy Sci 2010;93(4):1596–603.
14. Chapinal N, Carson ME, LeBlanc SJ, et al. The association of serum metabolites in the transition period with milk production and early-lactation reproductive performance. J Dairy Sci 2012;95(3):1301–9.
15. Drackley JK, Overton TR, Douglas NG. Adaptations of glucose and long chain fatty acid metabolism in liver of dairy cows during the periparturient period. J Dairy Sci 2001;84(Suppl E):E100–12.
16. Vernon RG, Finley E. Roles of insulin and growth hormone in the adaptations of fatty acid synthesis in white adipose tissue during the lactation cycle in sheep. Biochem J 1988;256(3):873–8.
17. Herdt TH. Fatty liver in dairy cows. Vet Clin North Am Food Anim Pract 1988; 4(2):269–87.
18. Contreras GA, O'Boyle NJ, Herdt TH, et al. Lipomobilization in periparturient dairy cows influences the composition of plasma nonesterified fatty acids and leukocyte phospholipid fatty acids. J Dairy Sci 2010;93(6):2508–16.
19. Ster C, Loiselle MC, Lacasse P. Effect of postcalving serum nonesterified fatty acids concentration on the functionality of bovine immune cells. J Dairy Sci 2012;95(2):708–17.
20. Sordillo LM, Contreras GA, Aitken SL. Metabolic factors affecting the inflammatory response of periparturient dairy cows. Anim Health Res Rev 2009;10(1):53–63.

21. Huntington GB, Eisemann JH, Whitt JM. Portal blood flow in beef steers: comparison of techniques and relation to hepatic blood flow, cardiac output and oxygen uptake. J Anim Sci 1990;68(6):1666–73.
22. Drackley JK, Andersen JB. Splanchnic metabolism of long-chain fatty acids in ruminants. In: Sejrsen K, Hvelplund T, Nielsen MO, editors. Wageningen (The Netherlands): Wageningen Academic Publishers; 2006. p. 199–224.
23. Mills SE, Beitz DC, Young JW. Characterization of metabolic changes during a protocol for inducing lactation ketosis in dairy cows. J Dairy Sci 1986;69(2): 352–61.
24. Komatsu T, Itoh F, Kushibiki S, et al. Changes in gene expression of glucose transporters in lactating and nonlactating cows. J Anim Sci 2005;83(3):557–64.
25. Bauman DE, Griinari JM. Regulation and nutritional manipulation of milk fat: low-fat milk syndrome. Livest Prod Sci 2001;70:15–29.
26. Duffield TF, Kelton DF, Leslie KE, et al. Use of test day milk fat and milk protein to detect subclinical ketosis in dairy cattle in Ontario. Can Vet J 1997;38(11): 713–8.
27. Heuer C, Schukken YH, Dobbelaar P. Postpartum body condition score and results from the first test day milk as predictors of disease, fertility, yield, and culling in commercial dairy herds. J Dairy Sci 1999;82(2):295–304.
28. Toni F, Vincenti L, Grigoletto L, et al. Early lactation ratio of fat and protein percentage in milk is associated with health, milk production, and survival. J Dairy Sci 2011;94(4):1772–83.
29. Dohoo IR, Wayne M, Stryhn H. Veterinary epidemiological research. Charlottetown (Canada): AVC Inc, University of Prince Edward Island; 2003.
30. McGee S. Simplifying likelihood ratios. J Gen Intern Med 2002;17(8):646–9.
31. Iwersen M, Falkenberg U, Voigtsberger R, et al. Evaluation of an electronic cowside test to detect subclinical ketosis in dairy cows. J Dairy Sci 2009; 92(6):2618–24.
32. Konkol K, Godden P, Rapnicki P, et al. Validation of a rapid cow-side test for the measurement of blood beta-hydroxybutyrate in fresh cows. Proceedings 42nd Annual Conference. American Association of Bovine Practitioners; 2009. p. 190.
33. Carrier J, Stewart S, Godden S, et al. Evaluation and use of three cowside tests for detection of subclinical ketosis in early postpartum cows. J Dairy Sci 2004; 87(11):3725–35.
34. Denis-Robichaud J, DesCôteaux L, Dubuc J. Accuracy of a new milk strip cow-side test for diagnosis of hyperketonemia. Bov Pract 2011;45(2):100.
35. Stokol T, Nydam DV. Effect of anticoagulant and storage conditions on bovine nonesterified fatty acid and beta-hydroxybutyrate concentrations in blood. J Dairy Sci 2005;88(9):3139–44.
36. Eicher R, Liesegang A, Bouchard E, et al. Effect of cow-specific factors and feeding frequency of concentrate on diurnal variations of blood metabolites in dairy cows. Am J Vet Res 1999;60(12):1493–9.
37. Leroy JL, Bossaert P, Opsomer G, et al. The effect of animal handling procedures on the blood non-esterified fatty acid and glucose concentrations of lactating dairy cows. Vet J 2011;187(1):81–4.
38. Stokol T, Nydam DV. Effect of hemolysis on nonesterified fatty acid and beta-hydroxybutyrate concentrations in bovine blood. J Vet Diagn Invest 2006; 18(5):466–9.
39. McArt JA, Nydam DV, Oetzel GR. Epidemiology of subclinical ketosis in early lactation dairy cattle. J Dairy Sci 2012;95(9):5056–66.

40. Duffield TF, Sandals D, Leslie KE, et al. Efficacy of monensin for the prevention of subclinical ketosis in lactating dairy cows. J Dairy Sci 1998;81(11):2866–73.
41. LeBlanc SJ, Leslie KE, Duffield TF. Metabolic predictors of displaced abomasum in dairy cattle. J Dairy Sci 2005;88(1):159–70.
42. McArt JA, Nydam DV, Oetzel GR. A field trial on the effect of propylene glycol on displaced abomasum, removal from herd, and reproduction in fresh cows diagnosed with subclinical ketosis. J Dairy Sci 2012;95(5):2505–12.
43. Bauman DE, Currie WB. Partitioning of nutrients during pregnancy and lactation: a review of mechanisms involving homeostasis and homeorhesis. J Dairy Sci 1980;63(9):1514–29.
44. McArt JA, Nydam DV, Ospina PA, et al. A field trial on the effect of propylene glycol on milk yield and resolution of ketosis in fresh cows diagnosed with subclinical ketosis. J Dairy Sci 2011;94(12):6011–20.
45. Oetzel GR. Monitoring and testing dairy herds for metabolic disease. Vet Clin North Am Food Anim Pract 2004;20(3):651–74.
46. Chapinal N, LeBlanc SJ, Carson ME, et al. Herd-level association of serum metabolites in the transition period with disease, milk production, and early lactation reproductive performance. J Dairy Sci 2012;95(10):5676–82.
47. Ospina PA, Nydam DV, Stokol T, et al. Association between the proportion of sampled transition cows with increased nonesterified fatty acids and β-hydroxybutyrate and disease incidence, pregnancy rate, and milk production at the herd level. J Dairy Sci 2010;93(4):3595–601.
48. Seifi HA, LeBlanc SJ, Leslie K, et al. Metabolic predictors of post-partum disease and culling risk in dairy cattle. Vet J 2011;188:216–20.
49. Carpenter TE, Gardner IA. Simulation modeling to determine herd-level predictive values and sensitivity based on individual-animal test sensitivity and specificity and sample size. Prev Vet Med 1996;27:57–66.
50. AusVet Animal Health Services. Calculate SeH and SpH for range of sample sizes and cut-points for given herd size and imperfect tests. Available at: http://epitools.ausvet.com.au/content.php?page=HerdSens4. Accessed January 24, 2013.
51. Jordan D, McEwen SA. Herd-level test performance based on uncertain estimates of individual test performance, individual true prevalence and herd true prevalence. Prev Vet Med 1998;36(3):187–209.
52. Martin SW, Shoukri M, Thorburn MA. Evaluating the health status of herds based on tests applied to individuals. Prev Vet Med 1992;14:33–43.
53. Borchardt S, Staufendbiel H. Evaluation of the use of nonesterified fatty acids and β-hydroxybutyrate concentrations in pooled serum samples for herd-based detection of subclinical ketosis in dairy cows during the first week after parturition. J Am Vet Med Assoc 2012;240(8):1003–11.

Use of the Liver Activity Index and Other Metabolic Variables in the Assessment of Metabolic Health in Dairy Herds

Giuseppe Bertoni*, Erminio Trevisi, PhD

KEYWORDS

• Metabolic profile • Inflammation • Sampling standardization • Liver functionality
• Transition period • Dairy cows

KEY POINTS

- Metabolic profiling as a tool to diagnose the nutritional-management causes of health problems in dairy farms is of limited use except as part of an integrated diagnostic system (first-step evaluation of the whole farm and animal conditions followed, if needed, by the second step, metabolic profiling).
- Rather than general profiling of animals across several lactation stages, targeting animals in the transition period appears to have more promise as a valuable tool in the management of dairy cow health.
- The development of metabolic indices for application during the transition period is challenging because of the tremendous physiologic changes taking place during this time.
- Reference ranges need to be developed in a way that take into careful account the interval between calving and blood sampling.
- Composite indices based on multiple variables, including variables associated with inflammation, have promise for use as an aid in the diagnosis and correction of management and nutritional problems on dairy farms.

INTRODUCTION

Most metabolic diseases (milk fever, ketosis, retained placenta, and displacement of abomasum) of dairy cows occur within the first 2 weeks of lactation.[1] In the same period the majority of infectious diseases (eg, mastitis, metritis) also occur. Furthermore, some other metabolic diseases that manifest clinically later in the lactation (eg, laminitis) can be traced back to metabolic insults that occurred during early

Institute of Zootechnic, Faculty of Agriculture, Università Cattolica del Sacro Cuore, Via Emilia Parmense, 84, Piacenza 29122, Italy
* Corresponding author.
E-mail address: giuseppe.bertoni@unicatt.it

Vet Clin Food Anim 29 (2013) 413–431
http://dx.doi.org/10.1016/j.cvfa.2013.04.004 vetfood.theclinics.com
0749-0720/13/$ – see front matter

lactation (ie, rumen acidosis as suggested by Nocek[2]). One of the reasons, particularly of the higher frequency of infectious disease, is the immune depression typical of this period.[3] This depression is often attributed to energy deficiency, and is related to higher serum concentrations of nonesterified fatty acids (NEFA) and β-hydroxybutyric acid (BHBA).[4] There is therefore a close relationship between metabolic and infectious diseases; both of these types of disease may lead to inflammation, which can be responsible for lower milk production and impaired fertility.[5,6] Poor reproductive performance, like poor health and production, may also be traced back to problems occurring in the transition stage.

The ever increasing milk yields of modern dairy cows are generally considered as an important risk factor in the development of metabolic disease. However, this is only partly true because nutritional (inadequate feed intake) and environmental stressors are also of relevant importance.[7] This issue has been recently discussed with respect to the apparent antagonistic association between milk production and fertility.[8] The investigators suggest that in the case of multifactorial associations, such as those between milk yield and fertility, it is essential to understand the complexities of the variables affecting fertility (i.e. the relationships between milk production, nutrition, and metabolic diseases). Then, it is of paramount importance, particularly for high-yield cows, to exercise great care in feeding[9,10] and management so as to minimize multiple stressors.[11]

Consequently, there is intense interest in nutrition and management during the transition phase[4,12] and perhaps some time before (eg, at the end of previous lactation to avoid overfattening). Attention to feeding details and adherence to recognized nutritional guidelines[13,14] is the first step in managing metabolic disease. However, additional strategic tools may be useful in reducing the overwhelming risks during the transition period, one of which is appropriate application of blood analysis. There are 2 main aims in such analyses:

- Herd-level evaluation to assess overall feeding and management adequacy in dry and early lactation periods
- Cow-level evaluation to assess the status of individual animals relative to clinical or subclinical disease, the objective being to monitor herd incidences of disease and to provide an opportunity for early treatment of prophylaxis

HERD-LEVEL METABOLIC EVALUATION

Historically the use of blood analysis to evaluate the metabolic health of cows can be traced back to Payne and colleagues[15] and their metabolic profile, which can be considered a presymptomatic diagnostic tool to prevent metabolic disorders and diseases in dairy farms. This approach was later almost abandoned, owing to cost and insensitivity relative to nutritional inadequacies.[16] Today it seems counterintuitive to view metabolic profiles as a means of ration evaluation because precise means of ration formulation and evaluation are otherwise available.[17] By contrast, there is opportunity to use blood analysis as the last step in an Integrated Diagnostic System (IDS) to solve nutrition-management problems at the farm level. The first step is the collection of available data concerning the herd, namely feeding, management, performance, environment, body condition score (BCS), disease frequency, or any other problem,[18] thus avoiding new analysis. This approach obviously implies that blood profiling (second step) is recommended for the diagnosis and evaluation of problems not identified in the first step. Blood profiling would be used only when other more simple and less expensive diagnostic tools have failed. To properly interpret metabolic profiles, Bertoni and colleagues[18] suggest well-standardized techniques for sample collection and analysis, as well as an appropriate approach to the evaluation of blood changes based on their biochemical meaning and on specific reference values. For this purpose, namely to evaluate the metabolic status in cows without clear clinical signs of disease, the variation in blood analyte concentrations associated with subclinical abnormalities will not be as extreme as in the case of clinical disease. Thus, meticulous attention should be given to the avoidance of extraneous causes of variation in blood variables in the use of reference ranges specifically established for this purpose.

Minimizing Extraneous Sources of Variation in Blood Analyte Concentrations

Animal selection and sampling

Sources of variation other than those expected in response to metabolic or nutritional challenges, that is, the response variables of interest, may be minimized by proper animal selection, proper timing of sample collection, and proper sample handling after collection. Animals showing signs of clinical disease should not be selected when sampling for herd-level evaluation. Clinical disease frequently causes secondary changes in blood variables that can interfere with herd-level interpretation. Furthermore, timing of sampling relative to feeding is important, as there is prandial variation among several metabolites of interest including glucose, NEFA, and BHBA as well as among some hormones such as insulin, thyroid hormones, and growth hormone.[19,20] Prandial effects may be reduced when totally mixed rations (TMR) diets are available continually throughout the day,[21] but even in these types of feed delivery systems it is most desirable to sample just before daily delivery of fresh feed. During restraint and sample collection animals should remain as calm as possible to avoid stress-related changes in blood variables. For some variables, sampling site (jugular, mammary, or coccygeal vein) is also a potential cause of extraneous variation. Selection of sampling site may also affect the risk of sample hemolysis (higher in tail samples), which should be avoided.[22] **Box 1** lists specific instructions for animal selection and sampling.

Sample analysis Analytical techniques are often beyond the control of the clinician, but it is advisable to understand the control procedures used by the laboratory. The use of bovine-origin control samples is recommended, as is the use of 1 or 2 commercial standards for the calibration of equipment.[23]

Interpretation

For interpretation of analytical results it is important to have a clear understanding of the physiologic influences affecting the concentration of blood analytes, and how these influences are affected by nutritional status and physiologic state. In addition, it is critical to have appropriately constructed reference intervals available.

To illustrate that the relationship between blood metabolite concentrations and nutrition is not always simple or direct, the following examples are offered:

- Blood urea is not an index of rumen ammonia concentration only, as is often supposed.[24,25] Amino acid oxidation is also an important factor.[26,27] Thus, a high intake of any protein source tends to increase blood urea concentration (**Fig. 1**).
- The sudden and marked decrease in serum zinc concentration, and partly of serum calcium concentration, is generally due to inflammatory phenomena,[28,29] almost never due to deficiency.
- Reduced serum concentrations of albumin, cholesterol, and vitamin A can at least partly be a consequence of a reduced liver synthesis of usual proteins; lower lipoprotein concentrations result in lower serum cholesterol, and lower serum retinol-binding protein concentrations result in lower vitamin A. This situation can occur during an acute-phase reaction that diverts the activity of the liver

Box 1
Instructions to collect blood samples from dairy cows for a proper assessment of the metabolic profile

1. Select 6 to 8 cows between 25 and 80 days in milk, when the health problems of farm concern mainly fertility, lameness, mastitis. Select 6 to 8 cows during the dry period (between 30 and 10 days before the expected date of the calving), when the health problems of farm concern the puerperium (milk fever, retained placenta, metritis, ketosis, displaced abomasum)
2. Exclude from bleeding the sick cows (affected by lameness, mastitis, diarrhea, and so forth) or the cows with an irregular feed intake
3. Withdraw the blood samples immediately before the main morning meal: before the Total Mixed Ration distribution or before the administration of forages (in case the feeds are administered separately)
4. Maintain unchanged feeding habits in the days before the blood sampling (including the day of sampling)
5. Avoid any physical effort, fear, or anxiety in cows during their capture. Any stress should be transient and limited to a few seconds during the blood sampling.
6. Collect about 10 mL of whole blood from each cow, preferably from the jugular vein and in a vacuum tube, containing lithium heparin as anticoagulant (gently mix after the sampling). Alternatively, sampling from the caudal vein is permitted, but should be done with caution to avoid hemolysis or mixing with the arterial blood (as much as possible).
7. Cool down the sample very quickly in iced water and centrifuge the samples as soon as possible (at least within 2 hours from the collection).

Courtesy of Institute of Zootechnics, Università Cattolica S. Cuore, Piacenza, Italy.

to the synthesis of other proteins such as haptoglobin, fibrinogen, C-reactive protein, ceruloplasmin, or metallothionein, instead of the aforementioned more normal hepatic protein products.[16,30]

- Glucose, NEFA, and BHBA are useful as energy indicators, but mainly at the end of pregnancy and in the first weeks of lactation, or in the case of great and prolonged energy deficiencies, the latter being an infrequent occurrence in dairy cows.

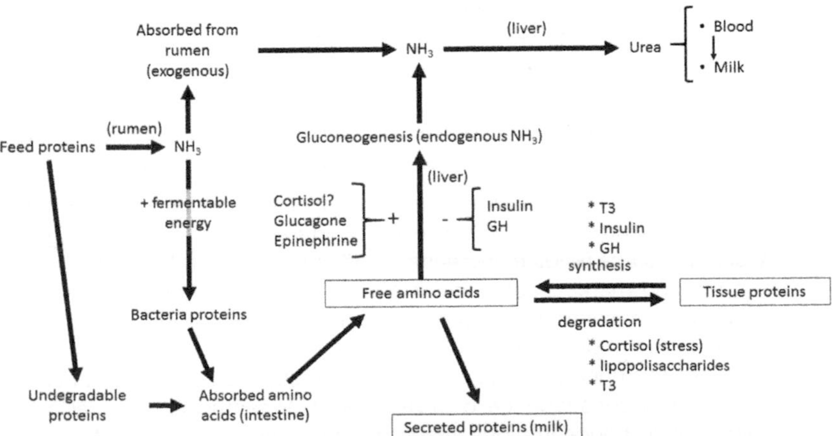

Fig. 1. Sources of the ammonia nitrogen in the liver of ruminants and regulatory mechanisms of the protein metabolism. GH, growth hormone; T3, Thyroid hormone.

- Among minerals, only P (inorganic), Mg, Se, and I can be monitored in blood to establish their dietary availability.

The use of reference values specific to the metabolic profile application is a critical point. In fact, given the aims, which are to detect herd-level deviation of blood values in clinically normal cows, one cannot use the usual clinical biochemistry reference values, which are designed to identify animals with clinical illness. For many years[31] our Institute has maintained that reference values for the interpretation of dairy herd metabolic profiles must be obtained with proper trials, performed on clinically healthy animals, correctly fed and managed, and also (we can add today) without important inflammatory events. The same concepts have been substantially expressed by the International Federation of Clinical Chemistry (IFCC) for humans, through many contributions to the theory of reference values (1987–1991). In particular, IFCC rules suggest that "reference values from an individual or a group of individuals are only meaningful when the individual(s) and method of production of values are adequately described." Consequently, to obtain these appropriate reference values for herd-level metabolic profile interpretation, a population of reference herds must be established. These herds should be well managed, appropriately fed, and with a low frequency of clinical diseases. Furthermore, the selection of animals, method of sample collection and handling, and methods of sample analysis should all be standardized, as already discussed. Using these criteria, the reference values obtained for dairy cows are shown in **Table 1**.[32] These values may vary depending on the physiologic stage (dry vs fresh) or age (primiparous vs multiparous) of animals.

To conclude this section it must be emphasized that, despite the several cautions suggested to minimize extraneous variation of blood values and to increase the validity of data interpretation, the usefulness of this type of metabolic profile in the farm context is doubtful. The main reason is inherent in the relationship between dietary errors and blood variables. If the errors are small, as happens in modern dairy farms and particularly in dry and lactation periods, excluding the transition period, the related blood variations are often ambiguous. By contrast, if the errors are considerable, blood changes can be better appreciated, but such nutritional errors might be more easily identified through animal performance and diet evaluation.

Nevertheless, the metabolic profile (blood analysis) could be included in an IDS aimed to solve any kind of farm problems.[18] The first step is to create a precise clinical evaluation of the farm (management conditions for animals, health problems, feeds and diets, animal characteristics [eg, BCS, cleanliness, teat score], digestive function [rumination, fecal characteristics], milk yield and quality [eg, fat, protein, somatic cells number], animal behavior, and so forth. The metabolic profile, as a second step, could be a useful complement for the better understanding of more difficult situations such as subclinical inflammations (see the following sections of this article and the article by Sordillo and colleagues elsewhere in this issue), which can be the consequence of nutritional errors (eg, excess of energy, deficiency of specific nutrients), digestive disorders, and infections. Inflammation, as may be present at a low grade, represents a metabolic disease risk per se and may interfere with nutrition balance.

Special Laboratory Procedures for Evaluation of Health in Transition Cows

In dairy cows, the first phase of lactation is characterized by a high incidence of diseases such as mastitis and endometritis,[33] and also metabolic disorders, particularly in high-producing dairy cows.[34] These metabolic disorders can have their root cause in the last weeks of pregnancy. The several diseases are related to each other, and the

Table 1
Plasma reference values of some blood parameters in dairy cows categorized in accordance to the parity and the lactation stage

					Lactating Cows (25–80 d in milk)				
	Units of	Dry Cows			Multiparous			Primiparous[a]	
Plasma Parameter	**Measurement**	**68%**		**95%**	**68%**		**95%**	**68%**	**95%**
Hematocrit	L/L	0.29–0.34		0.27–0.36	0.27–0.31		0.25–0.33	0.28–0.32	0.26–0.34
Glucose	mmol/L	3.64–4.06		3.43–4.26	3.67–4.08		3.46–4.28	3.76–4.22	3.55–4.41
NEFA	mmol/L	0.13–0.37	@	0.03–0.46	0.12–0.38	@	0.01–0.52	—	—
BHBA	mmol/L	0.19–0.33		0.12–0.40	0.23–0.45	@	0.16–0.65	—	—
Total cholesterol[b]	mmol/L	2.19–3.06	@	1.82–3.77	3.84–5.81		2.90–6.76	—	—
Total cholesterol[c]	mmol/L	—		—	4.78–6.73		3.85–7.66	—	—
Triglycerides	mmol/L	0.17–0.28		0.12–0.34	0.08–0.12		0.07–0.13	—	—
Creatinine	μmol/L	101.4–128.9		88.1–142.1	82.8–98.5		75.3–106.0	—	—
Urea	mmol/L	2.74–4.31		1.99–5.07	4.41–5.97		3.67–6.71	—	—
Calcium	mmol/L	2.42–2.61		2.33–2.71	2.38–2.59		2.28–2.69	—	—
Inorganic phosphorous	mmol/L	1.72–2.20		1.60–2.83	1.57–2.17		1.28–2.46	—	—
Magnesium	mmol/L	0.88–0.96		0.84–1.00	0.91–1.03		0.85–1.08	—	—
Sodium	mmol/L	142.1–147.9		139.4–150.7	141.1–145.5	@	139.0–147.7	142.4–146.0	140.7–147.7
Potassium	mmol/L	3.86–4.62		3.50–4.99	3.67–4.64		3.21–5.11	—	—

Chlorine	mmol/L	105.1–110.0		102.7–112.3	100.2–106.6	@	94.7–109.0	102.3–107.4		99.8–109.8
Zinc	μmol/L	13.7–18.5		11.5–20.7	11.5–16.3		9.2–18.6	—		—
Ceruloplasmin	μmol/L	2.18–3.11		1.74–3.55	2.19–3.15		1.73–3.62	—		—
Total protein	g/L	73.9–82.2	@	68.8–85.0	77.0–84.9		73.3–88.6	74.8–82.7		71.0–86.5
Globulin	g/L	38.5–48.9		33.6–53.8	41.5–51.2	@	38.3–57.6	37.7–49.3	@	37.6–54.7
Albumin	g/L	34.6–36.2	@	33.8–37.0	33.3–35.0	@	32.3–35.9	—		—
GOT/AST	IU/L (at 37°C)	50.6–72.1	@	46.5–82.6	67.1–89.6	@	61.1–103.0	—		—
GGT	IU/L (at 37°C)	21.0–30.9	@	17.8–38.0	25.3–34.5	@	20.8–45.1	23.4–31.5	@	20.8–37.3
Alkaline phosphatase	IU/L (at 37°C)	34.1–57.3	@	27.3–72.9	34.5–55.8		27.3–70.0	50.9–74.1		39.8–85.2
LDH	IU/L (at 37°C)	1307–1779		1081–2005	1469–1987		1220–2236	1640–2195		1374–2461
GSH-Px	mU/mg Hb	27.7–68.3		8.2–87.8	26.5–66.3		7.4–85.4	—		—

The reference values are calculated in 68% and 95% of the population, respectively. @: normalized parameter.

Abbreviations: AST, aspartate aminotransferase; BHBA, β-hydroxybutyric acid; GGT, γ-glutamyltransferase; GOT, glutamate oxaloacetate transaminase; GSH-Px, glutathione peroxidase; LDH, lactate dehydrogenase; NEFA, nonesterified fatty acids.

[a] For the primiparous cows, only shown are the reference values statistically different in comparison with multiparous cows.

[b] Diets without fat supplementation.

[c] Diets with fat supplementation.

Data from Bertoni G, Calamari L, Trevisi E. Nuovi criteri per l'individuazione dei valori di riferimento di taluni parametri ematici in bovine da latte. La Selezione Veterinaria 2000;Suppl:S261–8.

existence of one disease can increase the risk for others and vice versa. This relationship explains the typical syndromes of multiple diseases occurring during the peripartum period. It also illustrates the challenge in properly separating the root sources of each problem, which is essential in diagnosing the fundamental causes of disease. This complexity leads to the observation of Chapinal and colleagues[35] that "maintaining health and productivity in the transition period is one of the most difficult challenges that dairy herds face." Moreover, the importance of meeting this challenge becomes even more critical because the occurrence of metabolic diseases in early lactation is strongly and negatively associated with subsequent fertility.[6,36] Again this suggests the diagnostic utility of metabolic indicators that could be "… associated with herd-level incidence of retained placenta, metritis and displaced abomasum, milk production, and probability of pregnancy at the first artificial insemination."[35]

Blood variables as metabolic indicators could be useful as monitors of metabolic health, but the situation is very complex because the causes and effects of transition-cow diseases occur within the framework of the tremendous physiologic changes (endocrine and metabolic) characteristic of the transition period. These physiologic changes are part of some complex mechanisms needed, first to prepare the cow for parturition and lactogenesis, and then to achieve the homeorhetic changes[37] required to sustain milk synthesis despite negative nutrient balance.

In this context, the better known blood changes concern those of glucose, NEFA, BHBA, and urea (**Fig. 2**),[38] indices of energy and protein balance; nevertheless, the recent articles of Chapinal and colleagues[35] and Lomander and colleagues[36] have concluded that, despite their usefulness, the suggested indices (NEFA, BHBA, and Ca) need further research to understand how the thresholds can be applied or which is the best protocol for blood sampling (see also the article of Opsina and colleagues elsewhere in this issue for a discussion of use and interpretation of serum NEFA and BHBA concentrations in transition cows). A potential confounding factor in the interpretation of serum NEFA, BHBA, and other metabolite concentrations is the presence of inflammation and inflammatory mediator substances. Whereas metabolic events can influence inflammation (see the article by Sordillo and colleagues elsewhere in this issue), inflammatory variables are only partly associated with metabolism. Inflammatory variables are, however, strongly associated with health during the transition

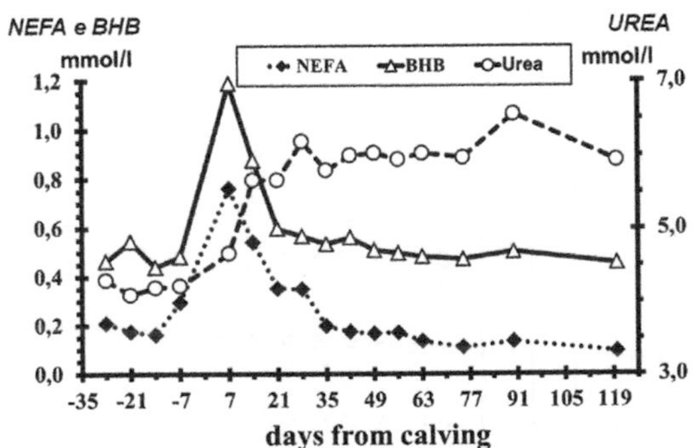

Fig. 2. Pattern of changes of plasma nonesterified fatty acids (NEFA), β-hydroxybutyric acid (BHB), and urea during the last month of pregnancy and the first 4 months of lactation in healthy multiparous dairy cows. (*From* Bertoni G, Lombardelli R, Piccioli-Cappelli F, et al. Main endocrine-metabolic differences between 1st and 2nd lactation of the dairy cows around calving. J Anim Sci 2010;88:E-Suppl 2/J Dairy Sci 2010;93:E-Suppl 1/Poult Sci 2010; 89:E-Suppl 1, 116.)

period.[5,39,40] Recent observations of Van Knegsel and colleagues[41] concerning the concentrations of natural antibodies in blood further support the association of metabolic and inflammatory conditions in transition dairy cows. This aspect is of great interest for several reasons. Inflammatory conditions, not only clinical but also subclinical, occur very often in the transition period and can result in lower milk yield and fertility.[5] Furthermore, inflammation may contribute to reduced feed intake (dry matter intake [DMI]) and efficiency of energy use,[42,43] all of which could contribute to challenges to metabolic adaptation and health.

For all these reasons, blood variables associated with inflammation may be valuable additions to metabolites in the assessment of metabolic disease risk in transition dairy cows. It is important to remember, however, that the interpretation of such analyses requires appropriate reference ranges and an understanding of the underlying physiology associated with each analyte.

Inflammation, liver activity, and cow response

Inflammation is not important in clinical disease only; it can in fact occur in and cause subclinical health problems.[5] Furthermore, the subclinical effects of inflammation may become particularly important in the transition period because they adversely affect other physiologic and metabolic events occurring at this time, including low DMI, increased lipomobilization, impairment of liver function, increase of energy expenditures, and so forth.[44] Therefore any cause of inflammation immediately before and after calving, such as infections, metabolic diseases, trauma, digestive disorders, heat and oxidative stress, dystocia,[45–49] should be avoided. Furthermore, subclinical inflammation may have adverse effects on metabolism, resulting in a higher risk for ketosis[50] and fatty liver.[51] Hence attention to blood variables associated with inflammation may aid in the diagnosis of primary causes of health problems and poor performance, not only in early lactation but later when cows are to be bred.

In the last 30 years, the authors' institution has performed experiments aimed at determining the association between inflammation and measurable blood composition variables (see **Fig. 3**), and also with cow performance.[29,52–57] In general, the indices of inflammation are mainly the acute-phase proteins (APP) of liver origin (see **Fig. 3**). These proteins are designated as positive APP, including haptoglobin, C-reactive protein, serum amyloid A, ceruloplasmin, among others; or negative APP, including albumin, lipoproteins, retinol-binding protein (RBP), cortisol-binding globulin, and some enzymes and other proteins usually synthesized by the liver. The serum concentrations of the positive APP are increased, for a short period, when the liver is activated by proinflammatory cytokines, whereas the serum concentrations of the negative APP are contemporaneously decreased. In the case of the negative APP the change in serum concentration is usually of longer duration than the corresponding change in positive APP concentrations.[58] Cappa and colleagues[59] observed that changes in serum APP concentrations occur quite often around calving and for several different reasons, many of them subclinical.[5]

It is therefore worthwhile to determine the pattern of changes in serum APP, as well as in metabolite concentrations, in the dry period and early lactation of normal cows (**Figs. 2,4,5**). Of the variables in **Fig. 4**, haptoglobin and ceruloplasmin are positive APP, whereas serum zinc is reduced, reflecting its sequestration in liver tissue in response to inflammation. In **Fig. 4** a difference in the temporal pattern of changes is observed. Haptoglobin concentration responds quickly and dramatically within a few hours of the inflammatory event (in this case linked to parturition); its serum concentrations then return to baseline relatively quickly. Serum zinc concentrations follow a temporally similar pattern of change, although opposite in direction of change.

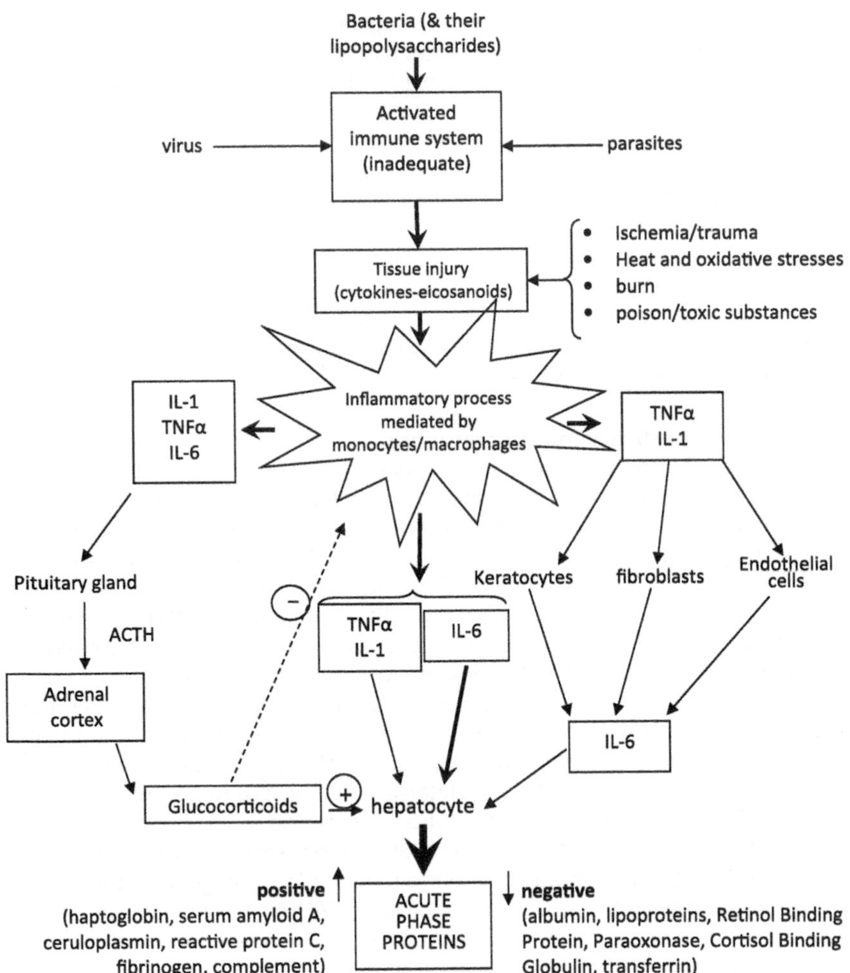

Fig. 3. Causes of the tissue damage and of the inflammatory response, with or without infectious events. Systemic consequences of the inflammation are deviation of the liver synthesis of the acute-phase proteins: increase of the positive ones and reduction of the negative ones. ACTH, corticotropin; IL, interleukin; TNF, tumor necrosis factor.

In healthy cows there are normally low concentrations of haptoglobin, 0.1 to 0.15 g/L except during the peripartum period. After calving a peak occurs around 7 days in milk (DIM), at which time serum haptoglobin concentrations can reach 0.4 to 0.5 g/L; this is followed by a reduction to precalving values in 3 to 5 weeks (see **Fig. 4**). After calving, serum zinc concentrations typically decline quickly from normal values of 13 to 14 μmol/L (0.85–0.92 μg/mL) to 10 to 11 μmol/L (0.65–0.72 μg/mL). These concentrations return to precalving values quickly. Ceruloplasmin (and consequently serum copper) concentrations change more slowly in response to inflammatory events, such as around calving, and also return more slowly (months) to pre-event values. These small changes in serum concentrations of positive APP, as well as the reciprocal changes in negative APP, can be attributed to the small and short-lived inflammatory stimulus associated with calving. The degree of change illustrated in **Fig. 4** can

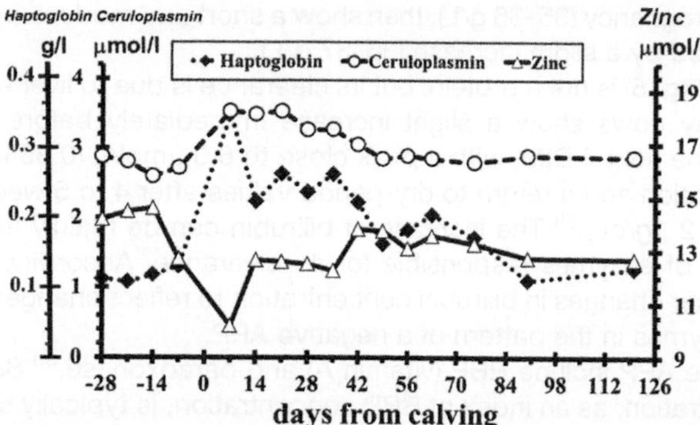

Fig. 4. Pattern of changes of plasma haptoglobin, ceruloplasmin, and zinc during the last month of pregnancy and the first 4 months of lactation in healthy multiparous dairy cows. (*From* Bertoni G, Lombardelli R, Piccioli-Cappelli F, et al. Main endocrine-metabolic differences between 1st and 2nd lactation of the dairy cows around calving. J Anim Sci 2010;88:E-Suppl 2/J Dairy Sci 2010;93:E-Suppl 1/Poult Sci 2010;89:E-Suppl 1, 116.)

be considered physiologic, in healthy cows. Nevertheless, some cows do not show any significant change of positive APP (not more than 15–20% of cow population in our experience).

Serum concentrations of selected negative APP (albumin, cholesterol, and bilirubin) are shown in **Fig. 5**. Serum cholesterol concentration is an index of the serum concentrations of lipoproteins of intestinal and hepatic origin.[60] Hence their values are gradually reduced during the dry period when total feed intake and lipid content of the diet are relatively low. The average values for serum cholesterol of healthy cows at calving time are 2.2 to 2.5 mmol/L (85–96 mg/dL); afterward values remain relatively constant for the first few days, after which a fairly quick increase occurs. Values at the end of the first month to 6 weeks of lactation are typically greater than 4.5 to 5.0 mmol/L (174–193 mg/dL), and may be even higher depending on the lipid concentration of the diet. In normal cows, serum albumin concentrations remain relatively constant in

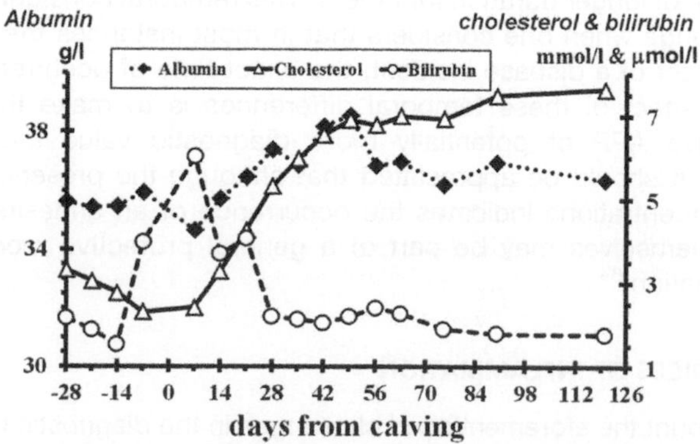

Fig. 5. Pattern of changes of plasma albumin, cholesterol, and total bilirubin during the last month of pregnancy and the first 4 months of lactation in healthy multiparous dairy cows. (*From* Bertoni G, Lombardelli R, Piccioli-Cappelli F, et al. Main endocrine-metabolic differences between 1st and 2nd lactation of the dairy cows around calving. J Anim Sci 2010;88:E-Suppl 2/J Dairy Sci 2010;93:E-Suppl 1/Poult Sci 2010;89:E-Suppl 1, 116.)

the last part of pregnancy (35–36 g/L), then show a short and modest reduction in early lactation, followed by a slight increase (36–37 g/L).

Bilirubin (see **Fig. 5**) is not a protein, but its clearance is due to liver enzymes.[61] The values in healthy cows show a slight increase immediately before calving and a marked one in the next 7 DIM, with a peak close to 6.0 μmol/L (0.35 μg/dL) followed by a quick reduction and a return to dry-period values after 4 to 5 weeks of lactation (~2 μmol/L, 0.12 μg/dL).[38] The increase of bilirubin can be mainly attributed to the lower synthesis of enzymes responsible for its clearance. Accordingly, the authors therefore consider changes in bilirubin concentration to reflect changes in the synthesis of these enzymes in the pattern of a negative APP.

Other negative APP include RBP (vitamin A) and paraoxonase.[30] Serum vitamin A (retinol) concentration, as an index of RBP concentration, is typically slightly reduced in the last days of pregnancy, but remains higher than 40 μg/100 mL. In the first 7 to 10 days of lactation serum vitamin A concentrations continue to decline (30–35 μg/100 mL), with values quickly increasing to 60 to 65 μg/100 mL at the end of the first month of lactation.[5] A small effect in these variations can be attributed to lipoproteins, but are largely the consequence of serum RBP concentration changes attributable to changes in hepatic synthesis rate,[62] which may be modified by inflammation. Paraoxonase is an enzyme, mainly synthesized in the liver, which functions to counteract oxidative metabolites. It is bound to lipoproteins and appears to protect them from oxidative damage. The pattern of changes in its serum concentration relative to calving is close to that shown by vitamin A (RBP), and is probably influenced by similar factors regulating hepatic protein synthesis. Serum paraoxonase values are close to 80 U/mL at calving; a small reduction occurs after parturition (70–75 U/mL), followed by a rapid increase to 90 to 100 U/mL in the first 3 to 4 weeks of lactation.[30]

From the foregoing discussion it can be appreciated that there may be diagnostic utility in the measurement of APP, either positive or negative, in the evaluation of health in transition dairy cows. However, it should be just as obvious that great care would need to be applied in the interpretation of such data because there are clear puerpueral effects on these variables, making the interval between calving and sample collection critical for interpretation. Furthermore, interpretative evaluation must consider the temporal differences in the rate and duration of response of the various APP, as the response is rapid and of short duration for some APP while being slower but of longer duration for others. This temporal consideration creates a particular challenge when one considers that in most instances the objective is to evaluate the effect of a disease incident, the exact time of occurrence of which is unknown. The effect of these temporal differences is to make the more slowly reacting negative APP of potentially more diagnostic value than the positive APP.[5,63] Lastly, it should be appreciated that although the presence of increased serum APP concentrations indicates the occurrence of an undesirable event, the positive APP themselves may be part of a general protective mechanism in the face of inflammation.[64]

COMPOSITE INDICES OF INFLAMMATION

Taking into account the aforementioned challenges in the diagnostic interpretation of serum APP concentrations, the authors have been working on composite indices of transition-cow health using multiple APP concentration values taken over time. The first complex index evaluated includes 3 negative APP, the most useful according to preliminary observations. This index, designated the Liver Activity Index (LAI), has been previously described by Trevisi and colleagues[65] and is outlined in **Box 2**.

Box 2
The Liver Activity Index (LAI)

The LAI includes the average blood level at 7, 14, and 28 days in milk (DIM) of albumin, lipoproteins (indirectly measured as total cholesterol), and retinol binding protein (RBP, measured as retinol whose level in blood is strictly related to RBP synthesized by the liver). Data from these blood parameters are transformed into units of standard deviation for each cow as follows:

- The mean values of the herd population of each plasma parameter (albumin, total cholesterol, and RBP) is subtracted from each cow value at 7, 14, and 28 DIM and divided by the corresponding standard deviation.
- The final LAI score for each cow is the arithmetical mean of the 3 partial values obtained from the 3 selected blood indices from 3 bleedings.
- The LAI values represent an estimation of the consequence of an inflammation that occurs at or around calving time in each cow checked within a defined herd.
- Thus, evaluating the LAI within a herd allows the retrospective ranking of the successful transitioning of cows through calving.

Example of the calculation of LAI

Herd	DIM	Albumin (g/L)	Unit of SD	Cholesterol (mmol/L)	Unit of SD	Vitamin A (μg/100 mL)	Unit of SD
Average of herd		34.05		2.92		27.36	
SD of herd		2.67		1.02		11.36	
Cow XXX	7	33.00	−0.39[a]	1.16	−1.73	11.82	−1.41
	14	34.50	0.17	2.21	−0.69	21.77	−0.51
	21	34.10	0.02	3.23	0.31	24.51	−0.26
Partial value			−0.07		−0.70		−0.72
LAI	Average of the 3 partlal values (albumin, cholesterol, vitamin A) = [(−0.07) + (−0.70) + (0.72)]/3 = −0.49						

Abbreviation: SD, standard deviation.

[a] Example of calculation of the partial index at each day: [(level of the albumin in at 7th DIM) – (average of the albumin in the herd)]/(SD of the albumin in the herd); that is: (33.0 – 34.05)/2.67.

From Trevisi E, Calamari L, Bertoni G. Definition of a liver activity index in the transition dairy cow and its relationship with the reproductive performance. In: Proceedings of X International Symposium of Veterinary Laboratory Diagnosticians. Salsomaggiore (Italy): 2001. p. 118–9.

To validate this index as an indicator of inflammation in transition cows, Bertoni and colleagues[5] retrospectively ranked the cows of 3 farms into quartiles according to their LAI. In the lower quartile 48% of the cows were identified with a clinical problem, whereas in the upper quartile only 5% of the animals had clinical problems. Moreover, the lower vs. upper quartile cows showed:

- Lower milk yield and lower fertility
- Higher haptoglobin at 7 DIM
- Higher serum NEFA and BHBA concentrations. These indices of negative energy balance confirm the higher losses of BCS, but might contradict the lower milk yield. Nevertheless, despite not being directly measured, a lower DMI has also been suggested for low LAI cows. Lower DMI was in fact demonstrated by Trevisi and colleagues[43] in cows with low LAI. Furthermore, Trevisi and colleagues[43,44]

showed that lower LAI is associated with a lower energy efficiency in the first weeks of lactation.

In general, it can be concluded that subclinical inflammation causes several negative consequences in transition cows and that LAI calculation provides an index of the

Box 3
The Liver Functionality Index (LFI)

The LFI includes concentrations of albumin, lipoproteins (indirectly measured as total cholesterol), and bilirubin (as indirect measure of the enzymes synthesized by the liver, which also coordinate bilirubin clearance). LFI measures the relevant changes in concentrations between 3 and 28 DIM, standardized with the optimal pattern of change for the 3 parameters obtained from healthy cows at the same stage of lactation.[5] As with LAI, the LFI allows the evaluation of the consequences of an inflammation occurring at or around calving time. In addition, because it represents an absolute value, the LFI can be used to compare cows from different herds.

Example of the calculation of LFI

Step 1 Albumin (Alb-I) subindex = 50% V3 + 50%(V28 − V3)
Cholesterol (Cho-I) subindex = 50% V3 + 50%(V28 − V3)
Bilirubin (Bil-I) subindex = 67% + 333%(V3 − V28)

Step 2 LFI = (Alb-I − 17.71)/1.08 + (Chol-I − 2.57)/0.43 − (Bil-I − 6.08)/2.17

COW 1 (low LFI)

		V3	V28			Partial LFI Indices
Albumin	g/L	30.00	33.00	Step 1	Alb-I = 0.5 × 30 + 0.5 × (33 − 30) =	16.50
Cholesterol	mmol/L	1.50	3.75		Chol-I = 0.5 × 1.5 + 0.5 × (3.75 − 1.50) =	1.88
Bilirubin	μmol/L	15.50	3.50		Bil-I = 0.67 × 15.5 + 0.33 × (15.5 − 3.5) =	14.35
						LFI
				Step 2	LFI = [(16.5 − 17.71)/1.08] + [(1.88 − 2.57)/0.43] − [(14.35 − 6.08)/2.17]	−6.52

COW 2 (high LFI)

		V3	V28			Partial LFI Indices
Albumin	g/L	35.00	38.00	Step 1	Alb-I = 0.5 × 35 + 0.5 × (38 − 35) =	19.00
Cholesterol	mmol/L	1.80	5.50		Chol-I = 0.5 × 1.8 + 0.5 × (5.5 − 1.80) =	2.75
Bilirubin	μmol/L	6.00	1.50		Bil-I = 0.67 × 6.0 + 0.33 × (8.0 − 1.5) =	6.17
						LFI
				Step 2	LFI = [(19.0 − 17.71)/1.08] + [(2.75 − 2.57)/0.43] − [(6.17 − 6.08)/2.17]	1.57

From Trevisi E, Amadori M, Archetti I, et al. Inflammatory response and acute phase proteins in the transition period of high-yielding dairy cows. In: Veas F, editor. Acute phase protein/book 2. InTech; 2011. p. 355–80.

severity of inflammation. This index - that varies between -1.5 and +1.5 points - can provide a good evaluation of inflammatory phenomena and their consequences, as demonstrated by Trevisi and colleagues.[66,67] Unfortunately, LAI is costly, both in terms of the number of samples required per animal (3) and the price of analytical testing. Furthermore, the index is only comparative within the herd and cannot be applied to general populations.

A new index (**Box 3**),[49] the Liver Functionality Index (LFI), has therefore been proposed as being less costly (2 samplings and 3 more economically determined variables: albumin, cholesterol, and total bilirubin). Moreover, this index is generally applicable across farms and is not dependent on comparison data within the herd. The LFI varies between −12 and +5 points. Values above zero are considered favorable. This new index has been validated relative to the LAI and also in relations to cow performance, inflammatory conditions, and metabolic abnormalities.[44] In a retrospective comparison,[44] cows with lower LFI showed:

- Lower milk yield, slightly higher BCS losses, and lower DMI
- Higher Serum haptoglobin and ceruloplasmin concentrations which latter values and remained elevated longer
- Higher serum concentrations of NEFA and BHBA

The authors conclude that composite indices based on a small number of readily determined negative APP values can be useful in judging the inflammatory state of transition cows. However, as currently developed, these indices are time consuming and costly to determine, and provide information too far after the fact to allow therapeutic or prophylactic intervention (i.e. to improve liver and reproductive functionality). New indices are under development that are expected to provide similar information earlier in lactation and at a lower analytical cost.

SUMMARY

Metabolic profiling as a tool in diagnosing the nutritional-management causes of health problems in dairy farms is of limited use except as part of an IDS (first-step evaluation of the whole farm and animal conditions followed, if needed, by a second step, metabolic profiling). In the 2nd step, great care must be taken in the selection of animals for sampling, timing of sampling relative to feeding, animal handling during the sampling process, sample handling after collection, the analytical procedures used and proper interpretation.

Rather than general profiling of animals across several lactation stages, targeting animals in the transition period appears to hold more promise as a valuable tool in the management of dairy cow health. Information gained from such an approach may be valuable for direct diagnosis of sub-clinical diseases (metabolic and infectious), as well as for enhancing production and fertility, thus efficiency, in herds. The development of metabolic indices for application during the transition period is challenging because of the tremendous physiologic changes taking place during this time. Reference ranges need to be developed that take into careful account the interval between calving and blood sampling. Composite indices based on multiple variables, including variables associated with inflammation, have promise for use as an aid in the diagnosis and correction of management and nutritional problems on dairy farms.

ACKNOWLEDGMENTS

The authors wish to thank Prof. T.H. Herdt (Michigan State University) for the careful and valuable contribution in the revision of the paper.

REFERENCES

1. Goff JP, Horst RL. Physiological changes at parturition and their relationship to metabolic disorders. J Dairy Sci 1997;80:1260–8.
2. Nocek JE. Bovine acidosis: implications on laminitis. J Dairy Sci 1997;80:1005–28.
3. Lacetera N, Scalia D, Bernabucci U, et al. Lymphocyte functions in overconditioned cows around parturition. J Dairy Sci 2005;88:2010–6.
4. Overton TR, Waldron MR. Nutritional management of transition dairy cows: strategies to optimize metabolic health. J Dairy Sci 2004;87(Suppl E):E105–19.
5. Bertoni G, Trevisi E, Han X, et al. Effects of inflammatory conditions on liver activity in the puerperium and consequences for performance in dairy cows. J Dairy Sci 2008;91:3300–10.
6. Bertoni G, Trevisi E, Lombardelli R. Some new aspects of nutrition, health conditions and fertility of intensively reared dairy cows. Ital J Anim Sci 2009;8:491–518.
7. Mulligan FJ, Doherty ML. Production diseases of the transition cows. Vet J 2008. http://dx.doi.org/10.1016/j.tvjl.2007.12.018.
8. Bello NM, Stevenson JS, Tempelman RJ. Invited review: milk production and reproductive performance: modern interdisciplinary insights into an enduring axiom. J Dairy Sci 2012;95:5461–75.
9. Drackley JK. Biology of dairy cows during the transition period: the final frontier? J Dairy Sci 1999;82:2259–73.
10. Varga GA. Feeding strategies for transitioning cows into lactation. In: Penn State Dairy Cattle Nutrition Workshop. Grantville (PA): 2004. p. 57–63.
11. Drackley JK. Advances in transition cow biology: new frontiers in production diseases. In: Joshi N, Herdt TH, editors. Production disease in farms animals. Wageningen (The Netherlands): Wageningen Academic Publ; 2006. p. 24–34.
12. Drackley JK, Dann HM, Douglas GN, et al. Physiological and pathological adaptations in dairy cows that may increase susceptibility to periparturient diseases and disorders. Ital J Anim Sci 2005;4:323–44.
13. NRC. Nutrient requirements of dairy cattle. 7th revised edition. Washington, DC: Natl Acad Sci; 2001.
14. INRA (Institut National de la Recherche Agronomique). Alimentation des bovins ovins et caprins. Paris: INRA; 1988.
15. Payne JM, Dew SM, Manston R, et al. The use of a metabolic profile test in dairy herds. Vet Rec 1970;87:150–7.
16. Bertoni G, Trevisi E. Metabolic profiles in the dairy cows management: a new approach. In: Ubaldi A, editor. Proceedings of 5th Congress of the International Society of Animal Clinical Biochemistry. Parma (Italy): 1992. p. 167–77.
17. Tylutki TP, Fox DG, Durbal VM, et al. Cornell net carbohydrate and protein system: a model for precision feeding of dairy cattle. Anim Feed Sci Technol 2008; 143:174–202.
18. Bertoni G, Calamari L, Trevisi E. Valutazione del benessere delle lattifere: sistema diagnostico integrato per la valutazione delle lattifere. Informatore Agrario 1999; 55(Suppl 35):3–66.
19. Lombardelli R, Bertoni G, Piccioli-Cappelli F. Endocrine and metabolic effects of different feeding frequency in dairy cows. In: Blum J, Gaillard C, editors. Proceeding of VIIIth International Conference of Production disease in farm animals. Berne (Switzerland): 1992. p. 201.
20. Lombardelli R, Bertoni G, Piccioli-Cappelli F. Frequenza dei pasti nelle bovine da latte: effetti a livello metabolico, endocrino e produttivo. Zootecnica e Nutrizione Animale 1993;19:123–30.

21. Trevisi E, Lombardelli R, Cogrossi S, et al. Daily changes of blood insulin and plasma energy indices in early lactating cows fed with Total Mixed Ration. In: 7th International Congress on Farm Animal Endocrinology. Bern (CH), 24–26 August, 2011. p. 54.
22. Calamari L, Bertoni G, Lombardelli R, et al. Variazioni nei parametri del profilo metabolico misurati nel sangue prelevato da vene diverse: giugulare, mammaria e coccigea. Proceedings Società Italiana Scienze Veterinarie 1983;37:439–41.
23. Calamari L, Bertoni G, Maianti MG, et al. Sull'utilità di nuovi parametri ematochimici nella valutazione del profilo metabolico delle lattifere. Zoot Nutr Anim 1989; 15:191–210.
24. Visek WJ. Ammonia: its effects on biological systems, metabolic hormones and reproduction. J Dairy Sci 1984;67:481–98.
25. Ferguson JD, Chalupa W. Impact of protein nutrition on reproduction in dairy cows. J Dairy Sci 1989;72:746–66.
26. Bertoni G, Bani P, Cappa V. Rumen ammonia and blood urea as possible indices of protein degradability. In: Proceedings 4th International Green Crop Drying Congress. Cambridge (United Kingdom): The British Association of Green Crop Driers 1989. p. 122–8.
27. Bani P, Bertoni G, Calamari L, et al. Relationships among dietary proteins, rumen ammonia and blood ammonia and urea. In: Eggum BO, Boise S, Børsting C, et al, editors. 6th International Symposium on Protein Metabolism and Nutrition. Herning (Denmark) EAAP Publication No 59: 1991. p. 167–9.
28. Bertoni G, Calamari L, Cappa V. The diagnostic meaning of blood variation of ceruloplasmin and zinc in the ruminants. In: Borst GHA, Mul AJ, van Knapen F, et al, editors. Proceedings of IVth International Symposium Veterinary Laboratory Diagnosticians, Amsterdam Koninkllijke Nederlandse Maatschappij voor Diergeneeskunde, Utrecht: 1986. p.136–9.
29. Bertoni G, Piccioli-Cappelli F, Calamari L, et al. Digestive upsets of ruminants: possible role of endotoxins and/or histamine. In: Kallfelz FA, editor. Proceedings of VIIth International Conference on Production disease in farm animals. New York: 1989. p. 370–3.
30. Bionaz M, Trevisi E, Calamari L, et al. Plasma paraoxonase, inflammatory conditions, liver functionality and health problems in transition dairy cows. J Dairy Sci 2007;90:1740–50.
31. Cappa V, Bertoni G, Galimberti A. Studio alimentari della ipofertilità bovina mediante l'impiego metabolico. I) Valori normali del profilo metabolico. 1980;6: 199–208.
32. Bertoni G, Calamari L, Trevisi E. Nuovi criteri per l'individuazione dei valori di riferimento di taluni parametri ematici in bovine da latte. La Selezione Veterinaria 2000;(Suppl):S261–8.
33. Collard BL, Boettcher PJ, Dekkers JC, et al. Relationship between energy balance and health traits of dairy cattle in early lactation. J Dairy Sci 2000;83: 2683–90.
34. Grummer RR. Etiology of lipid-related metabolic disorders in periparturient dairy cows. J Dairy Sci 1993;76:3882–96.
35. Chapinal N, LeBlanc SJ, Carson ME, et al. Herd-level association of serum metabolites in the transition period with disease, milk production, and early lactation reproductive performance. J Dairy Sci 2012;95:5676–82.
36. Lomander H, Gustafsson H, Svensson C, et al. Test accuracy of metabolic indicators in predicting decreased fertility in dairy cows. J Dairy Sci 2012. http://dx.doi.org/10.3168/jds.2012-5534.

37. Bauman DE, Currie B. Partitioning of nutrients during pregnancy and lactation: a review of mechanisms involving homeostasis and homeorhesis. J Dairy Sci 1980;63:1514–29.
38. Bertoni G, Lombardelli R, Piccioli-Cappelli F, et al. Main endocrine-metabolic differences between 1st and 2nd lactation of the dairy cows around calving. J Anim Sci 2010;88:E-Suppl 2/J Dairy Sci 2010;93:E-Suppl 1/Poult Sci 2010;89:E-Suppl 1, 116.
39. Loor JJ, Everts RE, Bionaz M, et al. Nutrition-induced ketosis alters metabolic and signaling gene networks in liver of periparturient dairy cows. Physiol Genomics 2007;32:105–16.
40. Trevisi E, Amadori M, Bakudila AM, et al. Metabolic changes in dairy cows induced by oral, low-dose interferon-alpha treatment. J Anim Sci 2009;87: 3020–9.
41. van Knegsel AT, Hostens M, Reilingh GD, et al. Natural antibodies related to metabolic and mammary health in dairy cows. Prev Vet Med 2012;103(4): 287–97.
42. Trevisi E, Han XT, Piccioli-Cappelli F, et al. Intake reduction before calving affects milk yield and metabolism in dairy cows. In: van Honing Y, editor. Proceedings of the 53rd Annual Meeting EAAP. Cairo (Egypt), Wageningen Academic (The Netherlands): 2002. p. 54.
43. Trevisi E, Gubbiotti A, Bertoni G. Effects of inflammation in peripartum dairy cows on milk yield, energy balance and efficiency. EAAP publication No. 124. In: Ortigues-Marty I, editor. Energy and protein metabolism and nutrition. The Netherland: Wageningen Academic Publishers; 2007. p. 395–6.
44. Trevisi E, Ferrari A, Piccioli-Cappelli F, et al. An additional study on the relationship between the inflammatory condition at calving time and net energy efficiency in dairy cows. EAAP publication No. 127. In: Crovetto M, editor. Energy and protein metabolism and nutrition. The Netherlands: Wageningen Academic Publishers; 2010. p. 489–90.
45. Ingvartsen KL. Feeding- and management-related diseases in the transition cow: physiological adaptations around calving and strategies to reduce feeding-related diseases. Anim Feed Sci Technol 2006;126:175–213.
46. Goff JP. Major advances in our understanding of nutritional influences on bovine health. J Dairy Sci 2006;89:1292–301.
47. Trevisi E, Bertoni G. Attenuation with acetylsalicylate treatments of inflammatory conditions in periparturient dairy cows. In: Quinn PI, editor. Aspirin and health research progress. Hauppauge (NY): Nova Science Publishers; 2008. p. 23–37.
48. Bradford BJ. The role of inflammation in metabolic disorders. In: Proceedings of Mid-South Ruminant Nutrition Conference. Texas Animal Nutrition Council. Grapevine (TX): 2011. p. 35–41.
49. Trevisi E, Amadori M, Archetti I, et al. Inflammatory response and acute phase proteins in the transition period of high-yielding dairy cows. In: Veas F, editor. Acute phase protein/book 2. InTech, Rijeka (Croazia); 2011. p. 355–80.
50. D'Angelo A, Trevisi E, Gaviraghi A, et al. Blood inflammatory indices and liver functionality in dairy goats around parturition. In: 13st International Congress of Mediterranean Federation of Health and Production of Ruminants (Fe.Me.S.P.Rum.). Bari, 2005. p. 76–7.
51. Bertoni G, Trevisi E, Calamari L, et al. The inflammation could have a role in the liver lipidosis occurrence in dairy cows. In: Proceedings 12th International Conference of Production Diseases in Farm Animals, East Lansing, Michigan, 2004. Wageningen (The Netherlands): Wageningen Academic Publ; 2006. p. 157–8.

52. Calamari L, Maianti MG, Bertoni G. L'influenza della totale e repentina sostituzione del fieno con mais-silo su alcuni parametri ematochimici. In: Proceeding of Italian Society of Veterinary Science Sorrento (Italy): 1980;34. p. 254.
53. Bertoni G, Maianti MG, Cappa V. Ricerche sui rapporti fra metabolismo lipidico e variazioni dei tassi ematici di vitamina A, caroteni e colesterolo. In: Proceedings of 5th Nat. Congr. of A.S.P.A. (Animal Science and Production Association). Gargnano del Garda (BS), Fondazione Iniziative Zooprofilattiche e Zootecniche, Brescia: 1983. p. 537–43.
54. Bertoni G, Trevisi E, Bani P. Metabolic effects of two different lapses without concentrate in early lactating dairy cows. Livestock Prod Sci 1994;39:139–40.
55. Bertoni G, Calamari L, Maianti MG, et al. Factors others then milk yield that affect the reproductive traits of dairy cows. Livestock Prod Sci 1997;50:99–100.
56. Calamari L, Maianti MG, Bertoni G. Relazioni fra potenzialità produttiva, problemi nel puerperio e fertilità nella vacca da latte. In: 9th National Meeting on "Studio dell'efficienza riproduttiva degli animali di interesse zootecnico". Bergamo, 1997. p. 99–103.
57. Trevisi E, Calamari L, Iamartino N, et al. Sintesi epatiche nel post-parto della bovina: possibili cause di variazione e relazione con la fertilità. In: 10th National Meeting on "Studio della efficienza riproduttiva degli animali di interesse zootecnico". Bergamo, 1998. p. 37–41.
58. Fleck A. Clinical and nutritional aspects of changes in acute phase proteins during inflammation. Proc Nutr Soc 1989;48:347–54.
59. Cappa V, Trevisi E, Bertoni G. Variazioni ematiche e produttive nel 1° mese di lattazione in bovine di allevamenti con o senza problemi "post-partum". Zootecnica e Nutrizione Animale 1989;15:645–60.
60. Bertoni G, Maianti MG, Cappa V. Variazioni nel metabolismo lipidico e glucidico nelle fasi terminali della gravidanza ed iniziali della lattazione nelle bovine. In: Proceedings of Soc. Ital. Buiatria. Modena (Italy), Società Italiana di Buiatria: 1984. 16, 223–36.
61. Tennant BC. Hepatic function. In: Kaneko JJ, Harvey JW, Bruss ML, editors. Clinical biochemistry of domestic animals. San Diego (CA): Academic Press; 1997. p. 327–52.
62. Wolf G. Multiple functions of vitamin A. Physiol Rev 1984;64:873–938.
63. Trevisi E, Amadori M, Cogrossi S, et al. Metabolic stress and inflammatory response in high-yielding, periparturient dairy cows. Res Vet Sci 2012;93: 695–704.
64. Sorci G, Faivre B. Inflammation and oxidative stress in vertebrate host-parasite systems. Philos Trans R Soc Lond B Biol Sci 2009;364:71–83.
65. Trevisi E, Calamari L, Bertoni G. Definition of a liver activity index in the transition dairy cow and its relationship with the reproductive performance. In: Proceedings X International Symposium of Veterinary Laboratory Diagnosticians. Società Italiana di Diagnostica e di Laboratorio Veterinaria, Salsomaggiore (Italy): 2001. p. 118–9.
66. Trevisi E, Bionaz M, Librandi F, et al. Periparturient health conditions of dairy cows: metabolic effects and performances. Livestock Prod Sci 2005;98:193.
67. Trevisi E, Zecconi A, Bertoni G, et al. Blood and milk immune and inflammatory responses in periparturient dairy cows showing a different liver activity index. J Dairy Res 2010;77:310–7.

Ketosis Treatment in Lactating Dairy Cattle

Jessica L. Gordon, BS, DVM*, Stephen J. LeBlanc, BSc, DVM, DVSc,
Todd F. Duffield, DVM, DVSc

KEYWORDS

• Ketosis • Treatment • Systematic review • Propylene glycol

KEY POINTS

- Ketosis is a common disease in dairy cattle in early lactation.
- Multiple treatments have been used in dairy cattle, with varying levels of support of efficacy and varying results.
- There is a lack of well-designed ketosis treatment clinical trials.
- The best recommendation for treatment is 300 mL of 100% propylene glycol orally once daily for 5 days.
- Further research is required to determine the most effective ketosis treatment regimen for economically important outcomes.

INTRODUCTION

Subclinical ketosis is a common disease of the transition period in dairy cattle, affecting approximately 40% of lactations in North America.[1,2] The incidence on individual farms varies widely and may be as high as 80%.[2] The costs associated with ketosis include treatment of the disease, increased risk and treatment of other diseases, decreased milk production, worse reproductive performance, and higher risk of culling in the first 30 days of lactation.[3,4]

CLASSIFICATION

Historically, ketosis was classified as primary or secondary based on when signs commenced and what concurrent diseases were facing the animal.[5] Recently, this nomenclature has fallen out of favor, because most ketosis is seen in the first

Funding Sources: OMAFRA, Bayer Animal Health, AABP Research Assistantship.
Conflict of Interest: None.
Department of Population Medicine, Ontario Veterinary College, University of Guelph, 2509 Stewart Building (#45), Guelph, Ontario N1G2W1, Canada
* Corresponding author.
E-mail address: jgordo04@uoguelph.ca

Vet Clin Food Anim 29 (2013) 433–445
http://dx.doi.org/10.1016/j.cvfa.2013.03.001 **vetfood.theclinics.com**

10 days after calving in North America and may or may not be accompanied by other disease.[1] The terms subclinical and clinical are favored for ketosis definition. Clinical ketosis is characterized by an increase in blood, urine, or milk ketone bodies in conjunction with other visible signs, such as inappetence, obvious rapid weight loss, and dry manure. Subclinical ketosis is defined as an increase in blood, urine, or milk ketone bodies, above a threshold shown to be associated with undesirable outcomes, in the absence of obvious clinical signs.

Because of the housing system used in many North American dairies (large groups of loose-housed cattle), it has become difficult or impossible to determine if a specific animal is showing clinical signs of ketosis. Attempts have been made to classify ketosis as clinical or subclinical based on blood β-hydroxybutyrate (BHB) concentrations.[3] However, our experience is that when examined, animals with high levels of ketonemia may show no clinical signs and animals with low levels may be obviously ill. The severity of clinical effect seems to depend on the individual animal's ability to process and tolerate ketone bodies.[5] The disease may therefore be best described as hyperketonemia rather than trying to distinguish clinical from subclinical.

Classification of ketosis is most relevant for clarity and consistency in comparing incidence risk rates. Depending on the methods and frequency of screening, incidence rates of clinical ketosis are expected to be 2% to 15% in the first month of lactation, whereas 40% cumulative incidence of subclinical ketosis is typical if cows are screened weekly during the same period.[2] There is some evidence that greater ketonemia is associated with higher risk of negative outcomes, such as subsequent disease and culling.[1] However, the importance of the distinction between clinical and subclinical ketosis with regard to treatment is unclear. To our knowledge, there are no well-designed studies that have shown a difference in efficacy of treatments based on the initial level of ketonemia.

PHYSIOLOGY OF EARLY LACTATION AND KETOSIS

When considering effective treatment of ketosis, it is critical to consider the physiology of the animal during this period. At the beginning of lactation, animals are faced with a sudden and drastic increase in energy demand.[5] This demand is coupled with a decrease in feed intake, which generally starts in the dry period. The rate of increase of feed intake post partum lags behind the demands of lactation, leading to a period of negative energy balance. Fat is mobilized from body stores in the form of nonesterified fatty acids (NEFA) to meet energy requirements. NEFA travel to the liver destined for 1 of 3 pathways, complete oxidation for energy, incomplete oxidation to ketone bodies, or re-esterification to fatty acids. All of these pathways are stimulated in the transition animal, but the magnitude of fat breakdown and tolerance of the individual determine the relative distribution of the paths.[5]

In early lactation, homeorhesis is the driving physiologic force.[6] Homeorhesis was defined by Bauman and Currie as "the orchestrated or coordinated changes in metabolism of body tissues necessary to support a physiologic state."[7] These processes facilitate breakdown of body stores of fat and protein in excess of what would be allowed based on homeostatic regulation. This situation leads to a period of insulin resistance, which is nearly universal in early lactation animals.[6] Milk production requires large amounts of glucose. Because ruminants absorb only minimal amounts of glucose from their diet, gluconeogenesis is required to meet this need. This process is generally diminished in animals affected by ketosis, leading to hypoglycemia. Providing glucose, stimulating gluconeogenesis, and decreasing fat breakdown form the foundation for rational ketosis treatment.[8]

SYSTEMATIC REVIEW OF KETOSIS TREATMENT

Background

Reviews have long been used to summarize the body of literature on a given topic. This material can be especially helpful for practitioners who have limited time to read primary scientific articles or require the information in a short period while working on a clinical case.[9] Historically, these reviews were narrative reviews conducted by an expert on the subject.[10,11] Even high-quality reviews are inherently biased, because selection of papers and interpretation of the information are consciously or unconsciously influenced by the author's opinions at the outset.

Systematic reviews help remove the bias of the reviewers by following a rigorous method in selection of materials to be included.[9,11] Investigators provide a detailed framework for conducting the review that can be repeated and examined for accuracy. A specific question is formulated and an exhaustive search of the literature is performed. Methods for inclusion of materials are clearly defined and laid out before initiation of the review. The quality of all materials included is determined through specified criteria. Inclusion of all high-quality relevant material is the framework for a systematic review, so small studies that are well designed are not excluded because of lack of power.

Materials and Methods

A systematic review of ketosis treatment was performed in February 2011 to determine the most effective treatment(s) for ketosis in lactating dairy cattle. The search phrases "ketosis treatment cattle" and "acetonemia treatment cattle" were entered into 4 databases: CAB, PubMed, Agricola, and Google Scholar. These databases included references from 1900 to present in all languages. A complete list of references from the search was obtained from each database and abstracts were obtained for all references. Titles and abstracts were used to determine the relevance of each reference to the question. If abstracts were unavailable and the title was suggestive that the reference was relevant, the full reference was obtained and analyzed. Materials that seemed relevant based on the title or abstract were obtained in full and analyzed. In addition, a manual search of relevant conference proceedings (American Dairy Science Association, American Association of Bovine Practitioners) was conducted, and studies known to us that were not yet published in the peer-reviewed domain were solicited for evaluation.[3,4,12]

The following criteria were used to determine the appropriateness of materials for the review:

1. Study animals were lactating dairy cattle
2. Animals experienced naturally occurring ketosis
3. Animals were diagnosed before initiation of treatment and method of diagnosis was clearly defined
4. A control group was included that was positive for ketosis
5. Control group was untreated or treated with a baseline treatment common to both groups (eg, dextrose vs dextrose and insulin)
6. Any intervention was considered: oral, injectable, or feed additive
7. Any outcome was considered, but must be clearly defined: ketosis cure, health data, milk production, reproductive performance

Results of the Review

A total of 1395 references were obtained from the search (**Fig. 1**). These references included journal articles, theses, conference proceedings, abstracts, and book

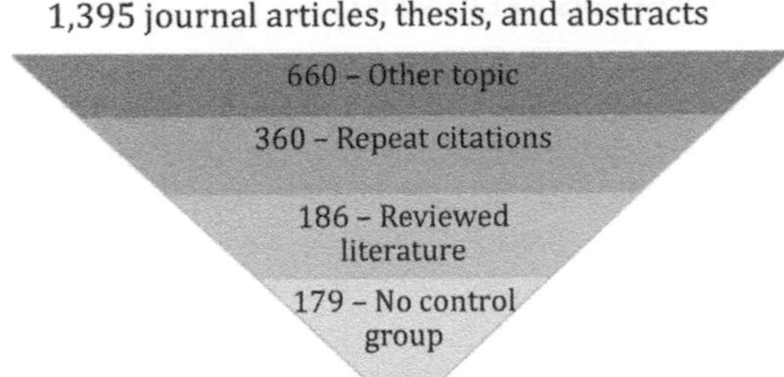

Fig. 1. Total number of articles and articles excluded by reason for exclusion.

articles. Of these references, 660 were excluded because they covered another topic, such as ketosis prevention, and 360 were excluded as duplicate citations. A further 186 were excluded because they reviewed the literature without presenting novel data. Of the 189 that remained, 179 did not include a control group, leaving just 10 articles considered appropriate for the review (**Table 1**).

One of the most striking aspects of this venture was the lack of well-designed ketosis treatment literature. During the past 15 years, the extent of ketosis observed in North America has been clearly defined and the prevalence of ketosis initially surprised many veterinarians and producers. Because of the relative frequency of clinical and subclinical ketosis, it is surprising that there has been so little advancement in the body of evidence for treatment of a ketotic cow. Much treatment of ketosis is based on disease principles or past experience. Although both of these factors are critical

Table 1
Studies remaining after exclusion criteria were applied

Study	Treatment	Control Group	Random
McArt et al,[3,4] 2011, 2012	Propylene glycol	Untreated	Yes
Carrier et al,[12] personal communication	Dextrose + dexamethasone + B_{12} + propylene glycol	Untreated	Yes
Sahoo et al,[40] 2009	Dextrose + dexamethasone, Dextrose + dexamethasone + E/Se	Untreated	No
Seifi et al,[23] 2007	Isoflupredone, isoflupredone + insulin (Ultralente, Eli Lily)	Untreated	Yes
Lohr et al,[29] 2006	Catosal	Untreated	Yes
Fetrow et al,[41] 1999	rBST	Untreated	Yes
Shpigel et al,[42] 1996	Dextrose + dexamethasone, dextrose + flumethasone	Dexamethasone or flumethasone	No
Sakai et al,[25] 1993	Dextrose + insulin (lente)	Dextrose	No
Ruegsegger & Shultz,[35] 1986	Propylene glycol, niacin	Untreated	Yes
Robertson,[22] 1966	Dexamethasone/flumethasone + insulin (protamine zinc), dexamethasone/flumethasone alone	Untreated	Yes

Abbreviations: E/Se,Vitamin E/Selenium; rBST, recombinant bovine somatotropin.

components for development of treatment strategies, stronger evidence is required to ensure rational and effective treatment.[13] Because of the small number of studies that met the inclusion criteria and the large number of treatments represented by these studies, it is difficult to provide concrete information on many common treatments. However, some of the common treatments are discussed in relation to the findings of the review.

DEXTROSE

Background

The presence of hypoglycemia in ketosis was well established by the 1930s.[14] Since that time, dextrose has been considered a staple in ketosis treatment. This treatment seems physiologically sound, because the requirement for glucose for milk production drives fat metabolism and hypoglycemia.[8]

There are concerns that the amount of glucose in a standard 500-mL bottle of 50% dextrose is excessive. A bolus of 500 mL 50% dextrose increases the blood glucose concentrations to about 8 times normal immediately after administration and returns to pretreatment concentrations by about 2 hours after administration.[15] This increase is paired with an immediate 5-fold increase in circulating insulin concentration and a 12-fold increase after 15 minutes.[15] Any glucose not used by the animal during this period is excreted via the kidneys, increasing the excretion of electrolytes and potentially increasing the risk of electrolyte imbalances.[16] The decrease in blood BHB levels caused by dextrose treatment is short lived (<24 hours) and must be repeated or followed with another treatment for lasting effect.[16]

Some have expressed concern with the high level of glucose leading to abomasal dysfunction. There is evidence that high levels of glucose can lead to decreased abomasal motility, and displaced abomasum has been correlated with hyperglycemia.[17–20] However, such effects of 1 treatment with dextrose have not been established.

Systematic Review

Dextrose was studied extensively early on (in the 1940s and 1950s) in case series or small studies without controls in which all affected animals were treated and the number that improved with treatment was determined. Since then, dextrose has been studied only in combination with other treatments or as the baseline for a positive control group. It has never been studied in a randomized clinical trial to determine efficacy as a standard treatment of all cases. None of the articles successfully passing the review process examined the efficacy of dextrose without the addition of other treatments.

Recommendations

Use of dextrose should be considered a second-line treatment of cases of ketosis. Animals with severe ketonemia with concurrent hypoglycemia may benefit from treatment with dextrose. Animals with ketosis suffering from nervous signs (such as abnormal licking, chewing on pipes or concrete, gait abnormalities, and aggression) should also be treated promptly with dextrose to alleviate hypoglycemia and nervous signs. These animals should then be followed up with other treatments for longer-term effectiveness.[8,16]

GLUCOCORTICOIDS

Background

Glucocorticoids have been used in ketosis treatment because of their ability to produce hyperglycemia as a result of changes in glucose use.[8] Steroids also block the effects of insulin, allowing for increased catabolism of fat and protein stores. Plasma concentrations of both glucose and insulin increase significantly about 48 hours after injection with dexamethasone.[21]

Systematic Review

Two studies in the review used a glucocorticoid alone. One of these studies was the oldest study of the group and was well designed.[22] In this study, enrolled animals were randomly assigned to receive dexamethasone or flumethasone, dexamethasone or flumethasone plus protamine zinc insulin, or no treatment. Animals were then followed for 5 days after treatment to determine milk production, presence of clinical signs of ketosis, and appetite. There was no difference between dexamethasone and flumethasone, so these treatments were grouped together as glucocorticoids. Treated animals were more than twice as likely to improve clinically compared with untreated controls based on appetite, behavior, and digestive examination coded subjectively (68% for glucocorticoid + insulin and 55% for glucocorticoid alone vs 23% for untreated animals). Treated animals also had increased milk yields in the first week after treatment (6.07 $\pm$ 0.79 kg/d for glucocorticoid + insulin and 3.73 $\pm$ 1.04 kg/d for glucocorticoid alone vs 1.11 $\pm$ 0.91 kg/d for untreated animals). This study was revolutionary in its time because of the use of an untreated control group, something not previously used in ketosis treatment studies. The major downfalls of this study are the short follow-up time and the lack of proper statistical methods available at the time to examine the influence of potential confounders such as parity.

The second study points to concerns for use of glucocorticoids.[23] Animals enrolled in this study were randomly assigned to treatment with 20 mg of isoflupredone (Predef 2x, Pfizer, Zoetis, Madison, NJ), 20 mg of isoflupredone plus 100 IU insulin, or a placebo, each treatment given once between calving and 8 days in milk [DIM]. This study was not designed as a ketosis treatment study, because all fresh animals were enrolled. However, blood was collected before enrollment and animals were later classified as subclinically ketotic or not based on serum BHB 1.4 mmol/L or greater. Animals that were ketotic at enrollment and were treated with isoflupredone and insulin were more likely than controls to remain ketotic in the 2 weeks after treatment. Animals that were not ketotic at the start and were treated with isoflupredone alone or isoflupredone and insulin were respectively 1.6 and 1.7 times more likely to become ketotic 1 week after treatment. There was no effect of treatment on reproduction or test-day milk production. This study suggests that there is no benefit of routine use of corticosteroids at the time of calving, and metabolic state may be impaired with their use. Furthermore, care should be exercised when using these products for ketosis treatment, because they may impair the animal's ability to overcome the disease.

Recommendations

Evidence for corticosteroids as therapy for ketosis is at best equivocal and indicates that steroids with insulin decreases cure. The lack of efficacy, combined with the risk of adverse side effects, does not support inclusion of corticosteroids in treatment of ketosis.

INSULIN

Background

Dairy cattle in early lactation are inherently insulin resistant.[6] This characteristic is part of the complex mechanism of homeorhesis that allows dairy cattle to produce a large amount of milk during a period of negative energy balance. Animals with ketosis show increased insulin resistance compared with their healthy herdmates.[15] Insulin is used in the treatment of ketosis because of the anabolic effects of the hormone.[24] Insulin decreases fat breakdown, increases fat synthesis, and increases use of ketone bodies as energy sources, which should decrease the level and consequences of ketonemia.

Systematic Review

Insulin is never given as the sole treatment of ketosis, because of the risk of hypoglycemia. There were 3 studies from the review of the literature that used insulin as an adjunct therapy in which the added benefits of insulin could be examined. Two of these studies are discussed in the glucocorticoid section.[22,23] Results from the Robertson study[22] indicated that the addition of insulin increased cure rate and milk production compared with treatment with glucocorticoids alone. Beyond the concerns that were mentioned earlier regarding this study, the insulin used was an animal-source protamine zinc formulation that is no longer available. It is difficult to say if recombinant human forms of insulin would yield the same results. In a study from 2007 by Seifi and colleagues,[23] treatment with a recombinant insulin (Humulin Ultralente, Eli Lily, Indianapolis, IN) increased the risk of animals developing and remaining ketotic compared with animals treated with isoflupredone alone.

The third study was performed by Sakai and colleagues[25] to examine the effects of insulin when added to dextrose therapy. Animals were diagnosed with ketosis using a combination of urine ketone body concentrations and clinical signs. All animals received 500 mL 50% dextrose intravenously (IV) once a day for 5 days after diagnosis. Half of the cows were assigned to receive 200 IU of lente insulin subcutaneously for 3 days from day 2 to 4 after enrollment. On day 6 after enrollment, urine ketone body concentrations were measured to determine the effectiveness of treatment. Blood was collected on enrollment and at day 6 and later analyzed for BHB concentrations. In this study, animals treated with insulin had significantly lower blood BHB concentrations and significantly higher glucose and insulin concentrations at day 6 after enrollment than cows treated with dextrose alone. However, this study had a short follow-up period and did not look at any economically important outcomes, such as milk production and culling.

We conducted a ketosis treatment study in the summer of 2011, in which we used insulin glargine (Lantus, Sanofi Aventis, Lavla, Quebec, Canada) or a placebo in addition to propylene glycol in animals diagnosed with ketosis using 1.2 mmol/L or greater blood BHB with a validated hand-held meter (Precision Xtra, Abbott, Abbott Park, IL). Based on preliminary results, insulin had no effect on blood ketone body concentrations 1 or 2 weeks after treatment or on the likelihood of cure of ketosis based on blood BHB concentrations.[26]

Recommendations

There is limited evidence in support of insulin therapy as part of a ketosis treatment regimen. This finding, coupled with the high cost of most insulin preparations, precludes wide-scale use of insulin in ketosis treatment. It is possible that there may be some benefit in refractory cases, especially those involving hepatic lipidosis,[24] but more research is needed in this area.

VITAMIN B_{12}/PHOSPHORUS COMBINATION PRODUCT

Background

Cyanocobalamin (a form of vitamin B_{12}) has been used as an adjunct therapy in ketosis treatment because of its role in gluconeogenesis. It has been hypothesized that administration of vitamin B_{12} may increase gluconeogenesis by increasing the activity of methylmalonyl-coenzyme A (CoA) mutase, a vitamin B_{12}-dependent enzyme and important component of the Krebs or tricarboxylic acid (TCA) cycle.[27] With an increase in the activity of this enzyme, energy may be produced more efficiently and TCA cycle activity and gluconeogenesis may be increased.

Butaphosphan, an organic phosphorus source, has been also been used because of its presumed role in gluconeogenesis.[28] Phosphorus is required at many stages in the gluconeogenic pathway, because all intermediate compounds must be phosphorylated to continue the cycle. However, it is unclear if this form of phosphorus is available to the animal.

Systematic Review

One study from the review used a vitamin B_{12} product.[29] One hundred and twenty lactating cows were enrolled in the study when they were presented to veterinary clinics in Germany for left displaced abomasum (LDA) and were determined to have ketosis based on a urine test. After correction of the LDA, animals were randomly assigned to receive 3 days of a commercial combination butaphosphan and cyanocobalamin (Catosal, Bayer, Shawnee Mission, KS) product or a placebo. Blood samples were collected during treatment and animals were monitored for feed intake, milk production, and rumination. Animals were considered to have healthy rumination if there were at least 3 ruminations/min. Individuals evaluating the animals were blind to treatment. Treatment with this product resulted in a significant increase in proportion of animals with healthy rumination at days 2 (65 vs 48%) and 3 (82 vs 63%) after treatment. Treated animals also tended to have a larger decrease in plasma BHB concentrations compared with values on the day of enrollment.

It is challenging to determine the usefulness of a butaphosphan cyanocobalamin combination product for ketosis treatment based on this study. The outcomes found to be different between treatments are subjective (ruminations) and have questionable economic significance. It is also difficult to determine if animals with ketosis, but without an LDA, would respond in the same manner. A large study using this product at calving showed a decreased risk of ketosis in treated cows that were in their third or higher lactation,[28] but this does not prove efficacy in ketosis treatment.

In a recent study,[26] we treated animals with 3 days of butaphosphan and cyanocobalamin or a placebo; all cows received propylene glycol. Based on preliminary results, this product tends to increase the likelihood of cure of ketosis (blood BHB <1.2 mmol/L in the week after treatment), decrease blood BHB concentrations 1 week after treatment, and increase milk production in the first 30 days.[26]

Recommendations

This butaphophan-cyanocobalamin combination product may prove useful in ketosis treatment in the future, if effects on milk production, culling, and disease risk can be confirmed. There is insufficient evidence to suggest routine use of this product for ketosis treatment.

PROPYLENE GLYCOL

Background

Propylene glycol was first described as a treatment of ketosis in 1954.[30,31] It is generally given as an oral drench once a day. When propylene glycol enters the rumen, it is either absorbed directly or converted to propionate.[32] Propylene glycol that is absorbed directly enters the TCA cycle to increase oxidation of acetyl CoA and stimulate gluconeogenesis. Propionate from propylene glycol can also be used for gluconeogenesis and helps stimulate insulin release.[33] There is a significant increase in insulin by 15 minutes after administration, and insulin remains increased for 2 hours or more after drenching.[33] This spike in insulin helps decrease fat breakdown and hepatic ketone body production.

Because of the physical labor required to administer propylene glycol, many producers and veterinarians have expressed interest in propylene glycol feed additives.[32] The concern with this method of delivery is that there is no resultant insulin spike caused by the small, relatively steady amount of propylene glycol that is supplied to the rumen throughout the day.[32] This chronic delivery of propylene glycol also alters the environment in the rumen to favor more propionate production.[32] According to the hepatic oxidation theory, this situation would likely decrease feed intake, increasing fat mobilization and perpetuating the problem of ketosis, although the clinical relevance of this has not been determined.[34]

Systematic Review

Previously, much of the work carried out with propylene glycol and ketosis involved prevention of ketosis.[32] Two of the studies that remained at the end of the systematic review selection process used propylene glycol without other treatments.[3,4,35] In the study conducted in 1986 by Ruegsegger and Shultz,[35] cows from study herds were tested once a week for milk ketone bodies and enrolled if they had ketosis without other complicating diseases. Enrolled animals were randomly assigned to receive no treatment, 125 mL propylene glycol, or 125 mL propylene glycol with 12 g of niacin daily for 7 days. There were no differences in blood BHB, milk production, or milk composition between any of the groups. The small sample size may have resulted in a lack of power to detect these differences, and the low amount of propylene glycol used in this trial is insufficient for lactating cattle.[32]

One of the best-designed and highest-impact trials on ketosis treatment was conducted in 2010 by researchers at Cornell University.[3,4] For this trial, all animals 3 to 16 DIM were tested for ketosis on Mondays, Wednesdays, and Fridays using a hand-held meter (Precision Xtra). All animals with 1.2 to 2.9 mmol/L blood BHB that had not been previously treated for ketosis by farm personnel were enrolled. Cows were randomly assigned to receive 300 mL (310 g) propylene glycol or 300 mL water daily until their blood BHB levels were less than 1.2 mmol/L or greater than 3.0 mmol/L or they reached 16 DIM. Blood BHB was measured 3 times a week until 16 DIM and daily milk weights, culling, and reproductive records were collected.

Animals that were treated with propylene glycol were 1.5 times more likely to be cured of subclinical ketosis (blood BHB <1.2 mmol/L) and half as likely to progress to blood BHB greater than 3.0 than control cows. Treated animals were also 40% less likely to develop a displaced abomasum and half as likely to die or be sold in the first 30 days of lactation. Milk production was increased by 1.3 and 1.6 kg/d in treated cows in the first 30 days of lactation in 2 of the herds, whereas the third herd showed no difference in milk production between groups.

This study clearly showed the potential benefits of oral propylene glycol in treatment of subclinical ketosis. The identification of significant differences in economically important outcomes was a first for the ketosis treatment literature and is a trait that future studies should strive to emulate. A limitation of this study was the failure to treat animals with blood BHB levels 3.0 mmol/L or greater. It can be expected that propylene glycol would be efficacious in animals with higher blood BHB levels, but higher initial BHB levels might decrease the cure rate and milk response. The variable amount of time that animals were treated in this study can also prove challenging for interpretation. Although the median time for treatment was 5 days, it varied from 2 to 13 days. Many producers would like a specific protocol for treatment and few would likely be willing to drench animals for 13 days.

Recommendations

Treatment of ketotic animals with 300 g of propylene glycol daily should be considered the base of ketosis treatment. The length of time that animals should be treated still needs to be determined, but based on results of the McArt study[3] and other studies in propylene glycol use,[32] 5 days of treatment seems to be sufficient without being overly taxing on farm labor. When choosing a product, it is critical to examine the concentration of propylene glycol in the product and ensure that animals are being treated with sufficient volume to provide 300 g of propylene glycol. Propylene glycol should be considered for treatment of all ketotic animals, although more research is needed to determine the efficacy for animals with BHB higher than 3.0 mmol/L.

COMBINATION THERAPIES

Background

Many studies of ketosis treatment have used combinations of therapies. Many of these studies have shown that animals treated with more than 1 product have better outcomes than animals treated with only 1 treatment. However, many of these studies have used short follow-up periods and outcomes that were not economically important.

Systematic Review

An excellent example of a trial involving multiple treatment modalities was conducted at the University of Minnesota.[12] Urine was collected daily from all animals in the first 15 days of lactation for ketone body testing using Ketostix (Bayer, Pittsburgh, PA). Animals that were classified with a small level of ketosis or higher were enrolled in the study and randomly assigned to the treatment or control groups. Treated cows (n = 279) were given 20 mg dexamethasone, 500 mL 50% dextrose, 5 mg vitamin B_{12} (all IV), and 500 mL propylene glycol orally on the day of enrollment and for 2 days after enrollment. Control animals (n = 282) were left untreated. In this study, treatment tended ($P = .1$) to lower milk production (1 kg/d over the lactation) and significantly increased the risk of culling (by 40%) in the first 60 days. Although outcomes were not different or poorer for treated animals, treatment did decrease BHB and NEFA values in treated animals in the first week after treatment compared with controls. This study is a critical addition to the ketosis treatment literature for 2 reasons: it shows the importance of long-term follow-up and use of economically important outcomes, and it requires us to reconsider common ketosis treatment regimens.

Recommendations

No combination therapy can be recommended. It is essential that future work tests individual treatments alone or in factorial study designs, so the efficacy of each product can be determined. Any combination that is studied should be based on treatments previously proved efficacious (ie, propylene glycol) and with the addition of 1 other treatment. By taking this stepwise approach, the efficacy of treatment combinations can be established.

Summary of Treatment Recommendations

The only treatment of ketosis that has been shown to improve resolution of ketosis, cow health, and productivity is oral propylene glycol.[3,4] The concentration of propylene glycol in the product should ensure that animals are receiving 300 g once a day for 5 days. Dosing once a day is sufficient and decreases the labor requirement for treatment. Use of a drenching gun increases the ease with which animals can be treated, increasing producer compliance. Subclinically ketotic animals should not receive other treatments, because the risk of detriment likely outweighs the benefit. Animals experiencing nervous signs of clinical ketosis may also benefit from a single treatment with 500 mL 50% dextrose IV.

SUMMARY

There is a scarcity of well-designed ketosis treatment trials and information on effective ketosis treatment. In the past, the focus was on treating ketonemia, rather than improving productivity. Research has shown that blood BHB concentrations 1.2 mmol/L or greater in the first 2 weeks post partum increase the risk of disease and culling and decrease milk production.[36–39] Increased emphasis on economically important outcomes (disease risk, milk production, culling, and reproductive performance) is required in subsequent research to increase understanding of effective ketosis treatment.

REFERENCES

1. McArt JA, Nydam DV, Oetzel GR. Epidemiology of subclinical ketosis in early lactation dairy cattle. J Dairy Sci 2012;95(9):5056–66.
2. Duffield TF. Subclinical ketosis in lactating dairy cattle. Vet Clin North Am Food Anim Pract 2000;16(2):231–53.
3. McArt JA, Nydam DV, Ospina PA, et al. A field trial on the effect of propylene glycol on milk yield and resolution of ketosis in fresh cows diagnosed with subclinical ketosis. J Dairy Sci 2011;94(12):6011–20.
4. McArt JA, Nydam DV, Oetzel GR. A field trial on the effect of propylene glycol on displaced abomasum, removal from herd, and reproduction in fresh cows diagnosed with subclinical ketosis. J Dairy Sci 2012;95(5):2505–12.
5. Herdt TH. Ruminant adaptation to negative energy balance. Vet Clin North Am Food Anim Pract 2000;16(2):215–30.
6. Bauman DE. Regulation of nutrient partitioning during lactation: homeostasis and homeorhesis revisited. In: Cronje PB, editor. Ruminant physiology: digestion, metabolism, growth and reproduction. Wallingford, Oxfordshire, UK: Publisher CABI; 2000. p. 311–28.
7. Bauman DE, Currie WB. Partitioning of nutrients during pregnancy and lactation: a review of mechanisms involving homeostasis and homeorhesis. J Dairy Sci 1980;63(9):1514–29.
8. Herdt TH, Emery RS. Therapy of diseases of ruminant intermediary metabolism. Vet Clin North Am Food Anim Pract 1992;8(1):91–106.
9. Vandeweerd JM, Clegg P, Hougardy V, et al. Using systematic reviews to critically appraise the scientific information for the bovine veterinarian. Vet Clin North Am Food Anim Pract 2012;28(1):13–21.
10. Cook DJ, Mulrow CD, Haynes RB. Systematic reviews: synthesis of best evidence for clinical decisions. Ann Intern Med 1997;126(5):376–80.
11. Sargeant JM, Rajic A, Read S, et al. The process of systematic review and its application in agri-food public-health. Prev Vet Med 2006;75(3–4):141–51.
12. Carrier J, Godden S, Fetrow JP, et al. Clinical trial of early ketosis detection and therapy in fresh cows. Paper presented at: American Association of Bovine Practitioners. St Louis, Sept 22–24, 2011.

13. Vandeweerd JM, Gustin P, Buczinski S. Evidence-based practice? An evolution is necessary for bovine practitioners, teachers, and researchers. Vet Clin North Am Food Anim Pract 2012;28(1):133–9.
14. McSherry BJ, Maplesden DC, Branion HD. Ketosis in cattle–a review. Can Vet J 1960;1(5):208–13.
15. Sakai T, Hamakawa M, Kubo S. Glucose and xylitol tolerance tests for ketotic and healthy dairy cows. J Dairy Sci 1996;79(3):372–7.
16. Wagner SA, Schimek DE. Evaluation of the effect of bolus administration of 50% dextrose solution on measures of electrolyte and energy balance in postpartum dairy cows. Am J Vet Res 2010;71(9):1074–80.
17. Holtenius K, Sternbauer K, Holtenius P. The effect of the plasma glucose level on the abomasal function in dairy cows. J Anim Sci 2000;78(7):1930–5.
18. Samanac H, Stojic V, Kirovski D, et al. Glucose tolerance test in the assessment of endocrine pancreatic function in cows before and after surgical correction of left displaced abomasum. Acta Vet 2009;59(5/6):513–23.
19. Sahinduran S, Albay MK. Haematological and biochemical profiles in right displacement of abomasum in cattle. Rev Med Vet 2006;157(7):352–6.
20. Zadnik T. A comparative study of the hemato-biochemical parameters between clinically healthy cows and cows with displacement of the abomasum. Acta Vet 2003;53(5–6):297–309.
21. Jorritsma R, Thanasak J, Houweling M, et al. Effects of a single dose of dexamethasone-21-isonicotinate on the metabolism of heifers in early lactation. Vet Rec 2004;155(17):521–3.
22. Robertson JM. The evaluation of a therapeutic trial on bovine ketosis. J Am Vet Med Assoc 1966;149:1620–3.
23. Seifi HA, LeBlanc SJ, Vernooy E, et al. Effect of isoflupredone acetate with or without insulin on energy metabolism, reproduction, milk production, and health in dairy cows in early lactation. J Dairy Sci 2007;90(9):4181–91.
24. Hayirli A. The role of exogenous insulin in the complex of hepatic lipidosis and ketosis associated with insulin resistance phenomenon in postpartum dairy cattle. Vet Res Commun 2006;30(7):749–74.
25. Sakai T, Hayakawa T, Hamakawa M, et al. Therapeutic effects of simultaneous use of dextrose and insulin in ketotic dairy cows. J Dairy Sci 1993;76(1):109–14.
26. Gordon JL, LeBlanc SJ, Neuder L, et al. Efficacy of a combination butaphosphan and cyanocobalamin product and insulin for ketosis treatment. J Dairy Sci 2012; 95(Suppl 2):177.
27. Kennedy DG, Cannavan A, Molloy A, et al. Methylmalonyl-CoA mutase (EC 5.4.99.2) and methionine synthetase (EC 2.1.1.13) in the tissues of cobalt-vitamin 12 deficient sheep. Br J Nutr 1990;64:721–32.
28. Rollin E, Berghaus RD, Rapnicki P, et al. The effect of injectable butaphosphan and cyanocobalamin on postpartum serum beta-hydroxybutyrate, calcium, and phosphorus concentrations in dairy cattle. J Dairy Sci 2010;93(3):978–87.
29. Lohr B, Brunner B, Janowitz H, et al. Clinical efficacy of Catosal in the treatment of ketosis in cows with left abomasal displacement. Tierarztl Umsch 2006;61: 187–90.
30. Johnson RB. The treatment of ketosis with glycerol and propylene glycol. Cornell Vet 1954;44:6–21.
31. Maplesden DC. Propylene glycol in the treatment of ketosis. Can J Comp Med 1954;18(8):287–93.
32. Nielsen NI, Ingvartsen KL. Propylene glycol for dairy cows. Anim Feed Sci Technol 2004;115(3–4):191–213.

33. Studer VA, Grummer RR, Bertics SJ. Effect of prepartum propylene glycol administration on periparturient fatty liver in dairy cows. J Dairy Sci 1993; 76(10):2931–9.
34. Allen MS, Bradford BJ, Oba M. Board invited review: the hepatic oxidation theory of the control of feed intake and its application to ruminants. J Anim Sci 2009; 87(10):3317–34.
35. Ruegsegger GJ, Shultz LH. Use of a combination of propylene glycol and niacin for subclinical ketosis. J Dairy Sci 1986;69(5):1411–5.
36. Chapinal N, Carson ME, LeBlanc SJ, et al. The association of serum metabolites in the transition period with milk production and early-lactation reproductive performance. J Dairy Sci 2012;95(3):1301–9.
37. Chapinal N, Carson M, Duffield TF, et al. The association of serum metabolites with clinical disease during the transition period. J Dairy Sci 2011;94(10): 4897–903.
38. Ospina PA, Nydam DV, Stokol T, et al. Association between the proportion of sampled transition cows with increased nonesterified fatty acids and beta-hydroxybutyrate and disease incidence, pregnancy rate, and milk production at the herd level. J Dairy Sci 2010;93(8):3595–601.
39. Ospina PA, Nydam DV, Stokol T, et al. Evaluation of nonesterified fatty acids and beta-hydroxybutyrate in transition dairy cattle in the northeastern United States: critical thresholds for prediction of clinical diseases. J Dairy Sci 2010;93(2): 546–54.
40. Sahoo SS, Patra RC, Behera PC, et al. Oxidative stress indices in the erythrocytes from lactating cows after treatment for subclinical ketosis with antioxidant incorporated in the therapeutic regime. Veterinary research communications 2009; 33(3):281–90.
41. Fetrow JP, Pankowski JW, Vicini JL, et al. Use of bovine somatotropin at the time of surgery for left displacement of the abomasum in dairy cows. J Am Vet Med Assoc 1999;214:529–31.
42. Shpigel NY, Chen R, Avidar Y, et al. Use of corticosteroids alone or combined with glucose to treat ketosis in dairy cows. J Am Vet Med Assoc 1996;208:1702–4.

Oral Calcium Supplementation in Peripartum Dairy Cows

Garrett R. Oetzel, DVM, MS

KEYWORDS

- Milk fever • Subclinical hypocalcemia • Hypocalcemia treatments
- Sources of calcium for oral supplementation
- Oral calcium supplementation strategies

KEY POINTS

- Most second and greater lactation cows have a transient hypocalcemia around calving.
- Subclinical hypocalcemia has greater associated costs for dairy producers than clinical cases of milk fever.
- Oral calcium supplements vary in their ability to support blood calcium concentrations; not all forms are appropriate supplements for dairy cows.
- Supplementation with oral calcium is the preferred approach for supporting cows that are exhibiting early signs of milk fever but are still standing.
- Prophylactic treatment with oral calcium around calving can reduce the risk for postpartum problems and increase milk yield in targeted populations of dairy cows.

INTRODUCTION

The initiation of lactation challenges a dairy cow's ability to maintain normal blood calcium concentrations. Milk (including colostrum) is rich in calcium, and cows must quickly shift their priorities to adjust for this sudden calcium outflow. Average blood calcium concentrations noticeably decline in second or greater lactation cows around calving, with the lowest concentrations occurring approximately 12 to 24 hours after calving (**Fig. 1**).[1,2] The extent to which hypocalcemia occurs around calving is an important determinant of fresh cow health and milk production.

CLINICAL MILK FEVER VERSUS SUBCLINICAL HYPOCALCEMIA

Clinical milk fever is one of the most recognized diseases of dairy cattle. The clinical signs of milk fever may, for convenience, be divided into 3 stages. Stage I clinical milk

Funding Sources: Boehringer Ingelheim Vetmedica.
Conflict of Interest: Consultant and speaker for Boehringer Ingelheim Vetmedica.
Food Animal Production Medicine, Department of Medical Sciences, School of Veterinary Medicine, University of Wisconsin–Madison, 2015 Linden Drive, Madison, WI 53706, USA
E-mail address: groetzel@wisc.edu

Vet Clin Food Anim 29 (2013) 447–455
http://dx.doi.org/10.1016/j.cvfa.2013.03.006 vetfood.theclinics.com
0749-0720/13/$ – see front matter

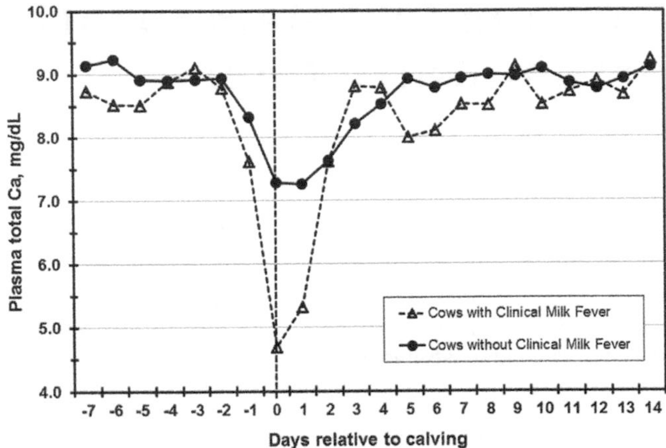

Fig. 1. Plasma concentrations of total calcium before and after calving. Data are from mature Jersey cows with clinical milk fever (n = 8) or without clinical milk fever (n = 19). (*Data from* Kimura K, Reinhardt TA, Goff JP. Parturition and hypocalcemia blunts calcium signals in immune cells of dairy cattle. J Dairy Sci 2006;89:2588–95.)

fever is early signs without recumbency. It may go unnoticed because its signs are subtle and transient. Affected cattle may appear excitable, nervous, or weak. Some may shift their weight frequently and shuffle their hind feet.[3] Cows in stage II milk fever are in sternal recumbency. They exhibit moderate to severe depression and partial paralysis and typically lie with their head turned into their flank.[3] Cows in stage III clinical milk fever are in lateral recumbency, completely paralyzed, typically bloated, and severely depressed (to the point of coma). They die within a few hours without treatment.[3]

Subclinical hypocalcemia is defined as low blood calcium concentrations without clinical signs of milk fever. Subclinical hypocalcemia affects approximately 50% of second and greater lactation dairy cattle fed typical prefresh diets. If anions are supplemented to reduce the risk for milk fever, the percentage of hypocalcemic cows is reduced to approximately 15% to 25%.[4]

A cow does not necessarily have to become recumbent (down) to be negatively affected by hypocalcemia. With or without obvious clinical signs, hypocalcemia has been linked to a variety of secondary problems in postfresh cows.[1,3] This happens because blood calcium is essential for muscle and nerve function—in particular, functions that support skeletal muscle strength and gastrointestinal motility. Problems in either of these areas can trigger a cascade of negative events that ultimately reduce dry matter intake, increase metabolic diseases, and decrease milk yield.[1] The pathways by which hypocalcemia may negatively affect cow health and milk production are illustrated in **Fig. 2**.

Subclinical hypocalcemia is more costly than clinical milk fever because it affects a much higher percentage of cows in the herd.[3] For example, if a 2000-cow herd has a 2% annual incidence of clinical milk fever and each case of clinical milk fever costs $300,[5] the loss to the dairy from clinical cases is approximately $12,000 per year. If the same herd has a 30% annual incidence of subclinical hypocalcemia in second and greater lactation cows (assume 65% of cows in the herd) and each case costs $125 (an estimate that accounts for milk yield reduction and direct costs due to increased ketosis and displaced abomasum), then the total herd loss from subclinical hypocalcemia is approximately $48,750 per year. This is approximately 4 times greater than the cost of the clinical cases.

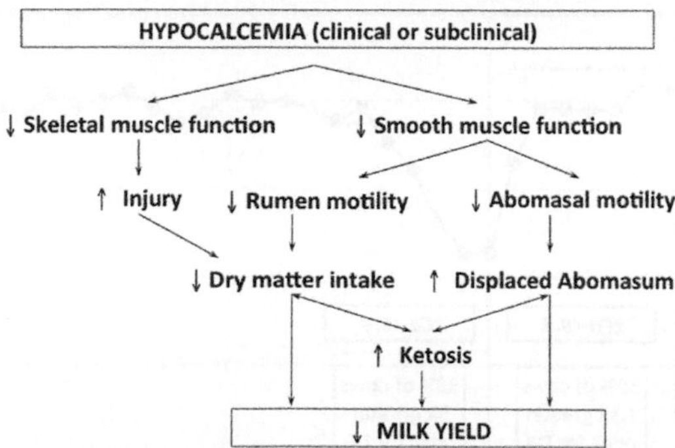

Fig. 2. Proposed mechanisms for reduction in milk yield in early lactation cows due to hypocalcemia.

A recently published, large multisite study shows that hypocalcemia around calving was associated with reduced milk yield[6] and increased risk for displaced abomasum.[7] These studies also demonstrated that the cutpoint for serum total calcium is approximately 8.5 mg/dL, which is a higher concentration than had been previously assumed (**Figs. 3** and **4**).

TYPES OF ORAL CALCIUM SUPPLEMENTATION

The source of calcium in an oral supplement and its physical form greatly influence calcium absorption and blood calcium responses. Calcium chloride has the greatest ability to support blood calcium concentrations.[8,9] This is explained by its high calcium

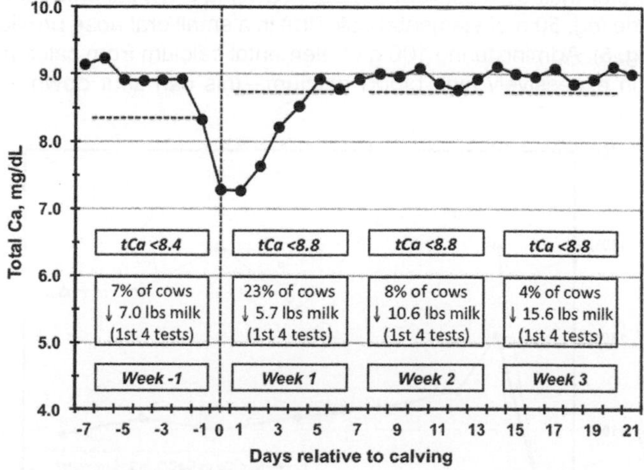

Fig. 3. Effect of serum total calcium on milk yield for the first 4 dairy herd improvement tests after calving. Different cutpoints were derived for serum samples collected on weeks −1, 1, 2, and 3 after calving. Data are from 2365 cows in 55 Holstein herds in Canada and the United States. Reference levels for blood calcium are from mature Jersey cows without clinical milk fever (n = 19). (*Data from* Chapinal N, Carson ME, LeBlanc SJ, et al. The association of serum metabolites in the transition period with milk production and early-lactation reproductive performance. J Dairy Sci 2012;95:1301–9; and Kimura K, Reinhardt TA, Goff JP. Parturition and hypocalcemia blunts calcium signals in immune cells of dairy cattle. J Dairy Sci 2006;89:2588–95.)

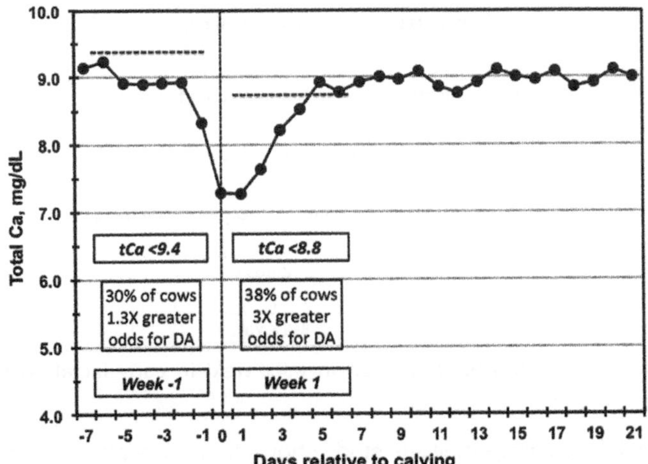

Fig. 4. Effect of serum total calcium on the odds for displaced abomasum after calving. Different cutpoints were derived for serum samples collected on weeks −1, 1, 2, and 3 after calving. Data are from 2365 cows in 55 Holstein herds in Canada and the United States. Reference levels for blood calcium are from mature Jersey cows without clinical milk fever (n = 19). (*Data from* Chapinal N, Carson M, Duffield TF, et al. The association of serum metabolites with clinical disease during the transition period. J Dairy Sci 2011;94:4897–903; and Kimura K, Reinhardt TA, Goff JP. Parturition and hypocalcemia blunts calcium signals in immune cells of dairy cattle. J Dairy Sci 2006;89:2588–95.)

bioavailability and its ability to invoke an acidic response in cows, which causes mobilizing more of their own calcium stores. Providing a typical amount of elemental calcium chloride (eg, 50 g of elemental calcium) in a small oral dose provides the best absorption (**Fig. 5**). Administering 100 g of elemental calcium from calcium chloride in water results in excessively high blood calcium—this can shut down a cow's own

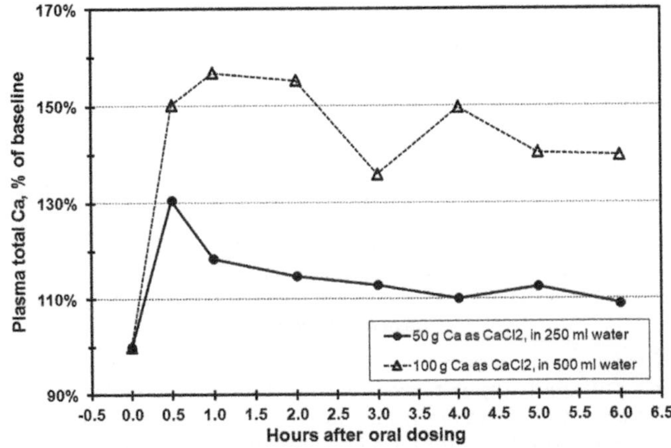

Fig. 5. Effect of 2 different doses of oral calcium chloride on plasma total calcium concentrations, expressed as percent of baseline values. Data are from nonpregnant, nonlactating Jersey cows (n = 8 for the 50-g dose and n = 4 for the 100-g dose). (*Data from* Goff JP, Horst RL. Oral administration of calcium salts for treatment of hypocalcemia in cattle. J Dairy Sci 1993;76:101–8.)

calcium homeostatic mechanisms and invoke a calcitonin response to protect from hypercalcemia.

The risk of aspiration is great when thin liquids are given orally, and calcium chloride is caustic to upper respiratory tissues. Calcium propionate is absorbed more slowly and must be given at higher doses of elemental calcium (usually 75–125 g).

Calcium carbonate in water as an oral calcium supplement does not increase blood calcium concentrations (**Fig. 6**).[8] This may be explained by its poorer bioavailability and by its potential to evoke an alkalogenic response, which would blunt the cow's own ability to mobilize calcium from bone.[3] Calcium carbonate is used as a feed source of calcium for dairy cows to meet longer-term calcium needs. It not an appropriate choice, however, for oral supplement of postpartum cows that need rapid access to additional blood calcium.

A combination of calcium chloride and calcium sulfate delivered in a fat-coated bolus (Bovikalc, Boehringer Ingelheim Vetmedica, St. Joseph, MO) resulted in more sustained improvements in blood calcium concentrations (**Fig. 7**) than observed in previous studies with oral calcium chloride or calcium propionate in water.[10]

SUBCUTANEOUS CALCIUM TREATMENT

Subcutaneous calcium is used to support blood calcium concentrations around calving but has substantial limitations.[11] Absorption of calcium from subcutaneous administration requires adequate peripheral perfusion. It may be ineffective in cows that are severely hypocalcemic or dehydrated. Subcutaneous calcium injections are irritating and may cause tissue necrosis; administration should be limited to no more than 75 mL of a 23% calcium gluconate solution (approximately 1.5 g elemental calcium) per site. Calcium solutions that also contain glucose should not be given subcutaneously. Glucose is poorly absorbed when given by this route. Abscessation and tissue sloughing may result when glucose is given subcutaneously.

The kinetics of subcutaneously administered calcium indicate that it is well absorbed initially but that blood concentrations fall back to baseline values in

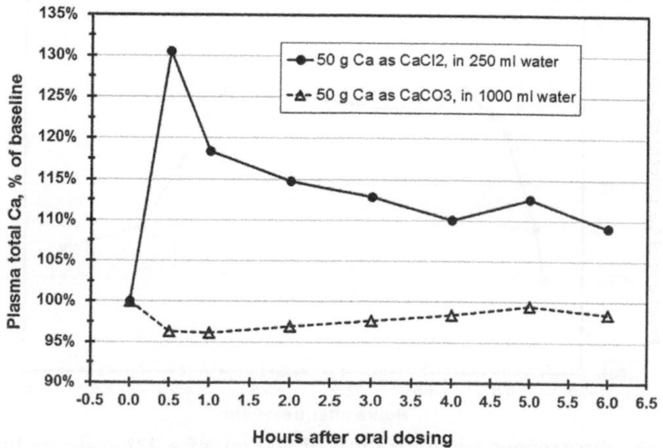

Fig. 6. Effect of oral calcium chloride and oral calcium carbonate on plasma calcium, expressed as percent of baseline values. Data are from 8 nonpregnant, nonlactating Jersey cows. (*Data from* Goff JP, Horst RL. Oral administration of calcium salts for treatment of hypocalcemia in cattle. J Dairy Sci 1993;76:101–8.)

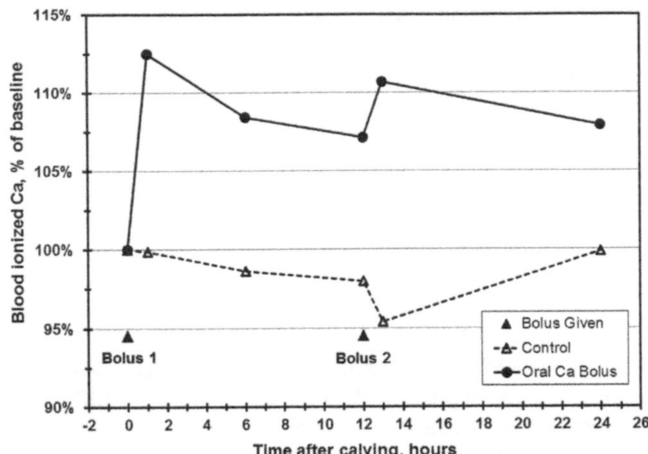

Fig. 7. Effect of administration of 2 oral calcium boluses (Bovikalc, Boehringer Ingelheim Vetmedica) on blood ionized calcium concentrations (expressed as percent of baseline). Data are from Holstein cows (n = 20) with hypocalcemia at calving. (*Data from* Sampson JD, Spain JN, Jones C, et al. Effects of calcium chloride and calcium sulfate in an oral bolus given as a supplement to postpartum dairy cows. Vet Ther 2009;10:131–9.)

approximately 6 hours (**Fig. 8**).[11] Thus, repeat doses are necessary to equal the sustained blood calcium support that is possible with oral calcium boluses.

TREATMENTS OF SUBCLINICAL HYPOCALCEMIA AND CLINICAL MILK FEVER

Oral calcium supplementation is the best approach for hypocalcemic cows that are still standing, such as cows in stage 1 hypocalcemia or who have undetected subclinical hypocalcemia.[3] Cows absorb an effective amount of calcium into the bloodstream within approximately 30 minutes of supplementation. Blood calcium concentrations

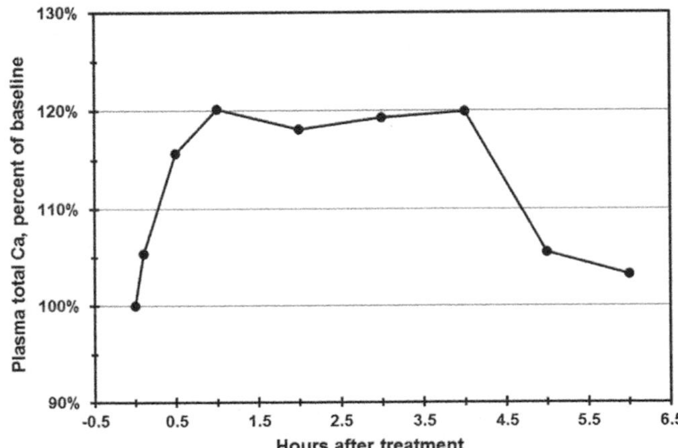

Fig. 8. Effect of subcutaneous administration of 500 mL of a 23% calcium borogluconate solution (10.5 g of calcium) on plasma total calcium, expressed as percent of baseline concentration. The 500-mL solution was divided into 10 different sites. Data are from 6 Jersey cows. (*Data from* Goff JP. Treatment of calcium, phosphorus, and magnesium balance disorders. Vet Clin North Am Food Anim Pract 1999;15:619–39.)

are supported for only approximately 4 to 6 hours afterward[8,9] for most forms of oral calcium supplementation.

Intravenous (IV) calcium is not recommended for treating cows that are still standing.[3] Treatment with IV calcium rapidly increases blood calcium concentrations to extremely high and potentially dangerous levels.[11] Extremely high blood calcium concentrations may cause fatal cardiac complications and (perhaps most importantly) shut down a cow's own ability to mobilize the calcium needed at this critical time.[3] Cows treated with IV calcium often suffer a hypocalcemic relapse 12 to 18 hours later.[12,13] The kinetics of blood calcium concentrations after IV treatment is illustrated in **Fig. 9**.

Stage II and stage III cases of milk fever should be treated immediately with slow IV administration of 500 mL of a 23% calcium gluconate solution. This provides 10.8 g of elemental calcium, which is more than sufficient to correct a cow's entire deficit of extracellular calcium (approximately 4–6 g). Administering larger doses of calcium in the IV treatment has no benefit.[14] Treatment with IV calcium should be given as soon as possible, because recumbency can quickly cause severe musculoskeletal damage.

To reduce the risk for relapse, recumbent cows that respond favorably to IV treatment need additional oral calcium supplementation once they are alert and able to swallow, followed by a second oral supplement approximately 12 hours later.[3,13]

Transient hypocalcemia occurs in cows whenever they go off feed or have periods of decreased intestinal motility.[15] It can be difficult to tell which comes first—the hypocalcemia or the gastrointestinal stasis. Whatever the case, the 2 problems positively reinforce each other. During the experimental induction of hypocalcemia, researchers[16] noted that ruminal contractions ceased well before the onset of clinical signs of milk fever. Off-feed cows, particularly in early lactation, are likely to benefit from prompt oral calcium supplementation.

Oral calcium supplements can be beneficial in most dairy herds - even herds with successful acidogenic prepartum diets and minimal cases of clinical milk fever. Producers should start by giving oral calcium to all standing cows with clinical signs of

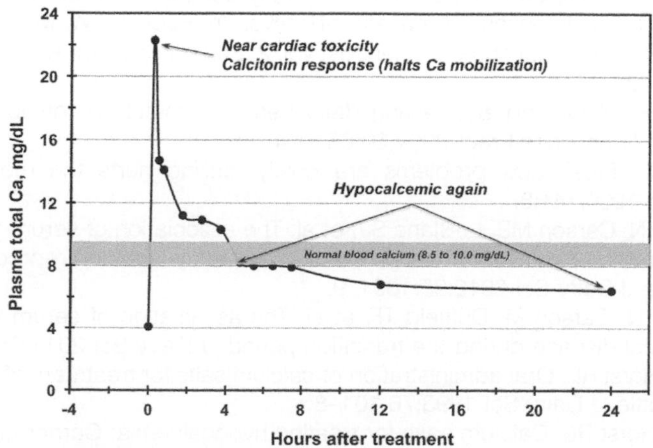

Fig. 9. Effect of IV calcium treatment with 10.8 g of elemental calcium on serum total calcium concentrations. Data are from a mature Jersey cow with clinical milk fever. (*Data from* Goff JP. Treatment of calcium, phosphorus, and magnesium balance disorders. Vet Clin North Am Food Anim Pract 1999;15:619–39.)

hypocalcemia and to all down cows following successful IV treatment. For herds with a high incidence of hypocalcemia, it may also be economically beneficial to strategically supplement all fresh cows with oral calcium. Finally, cows with high milk yield in the previous lactation (>105% of herd average mature equivalent milk production) and lame cows have the best response to oral calcium supplementation. Cows with high previous lactation milk yield and lame cows that were supplemented with oral calcium produced 3.1 kg more daily milk at their first monthly test after calving compared with control cows that had the same previous previous lactation milk yield and lameness status.[17]

TIMING OF ORAL CALCIUM SUPPLEMENTATION RELATIVE TO CALVING

Strategies for giving oral calcium supplements around calving should include at least 2 doses—1 at calving and a second dose the next day. The expected nadir in blood calcium concentrations occurs between 12 and 24 hours after calving.[1,10] Giving a single dose of oral calcium supplement at approximately calving time leaves cows without support when their blood calcium concentrations are naturally the lowest. The original protocols for oral calcium supplementation called for 4 doses—1 approximately 12 hours before calving, 1 at calving, 1 at 12 hours postcalving, and 1 at 24 hours postcalving. It was difficult to predict when at cow was approximately 12 hours from expected calving, and many cows calved without receiving this dose.[18] The dose at calving is not practically challenging to administer, and providing a dose sometime the day after calving provides critical support at approximately the time of nadir and is practical in large dairies where the postfresh pen is locked up only once daily.

REFERENCES

1. Goff JP. The monitoring, prevention, and treatment of milk fever and subclinical hypocalcemia in dairy cows. Vet J 2008;176:50–7.
2. Kimura K, Reinhardt TA, Goff JP. Parturition and hypocalcemia blunts calcium signals in immune cells of dairy cattle. J Dairy Sci 2006;89:2588–95.
3. Oetzel GR. Non-infectious diseases: milk fever. In: Fuquay JW, McSweeney PL, editors. Encyclopedia of dairy sciences, vol. 2. San Diego (CA): Academic Press; 2011. p. 239–45.
4. Oetzel GR. Monitoring and testing dairy herds for metabolic disease. Vet Clin North Am Food Anim Pract 2004;20:651–74.
5. Guard CL. Fresh cow problems are costly; culling hurts the most. Hoard's Dairyman 1996;141:8.
6. Chapinal N, Carson ME, LeBlanc SJ, et al. The association of serum metabolites in the transition period with milk production and early-lactation reproductive performance. J Dairy Sci 2012;95:1301–9.
7. Chapinal N, Carson M, Duffield TF, et al. The association of serum metabolites with clinical disease during the transition period. J Dairy Sci 2011;94:4897–903.
8. Goff JP, Horst RL. Oral administration of calcium salts for treatment of hypocalcemia in cattle. J Dairy Sci 1993;76:101–8.
9. Goff JP, Horst RL. Calcium salts for treating hypocalcemia: Carrier effects, acid-base balance, and oral versus rectal administration. J Dairy Sci 1994;77:1451–6.
10. Sampson JD, Spain JN, Jones C, et al. Effects of calcium chloride and calcium sulfate in an oral bolus given as a supplement to postpartum dairy cows. Vet Ther 2009;10:131–9.

11. Goff JP. Treatment of calcium, phosphorus, and magnesium balance disorders. Vet Clin North Am Food Anim Pract 1999;15:619–39.
12. Curtis RA, Cote JF, McLennan MC, et al. Relationship of methods of treatment to relapse rate and serum levels of calcium and phosphorous in parturient hypocalcaemia. Can Vet J 1978;19:155–8.
13. Thilsing-Hansen T, Jørgensen RJ, Østergaard S. Milk fever control principles: a review. Acta Vet Scand 2002;43:1–19.
14. Doze JG, Donders R, van der Kolk JH. Effects of intravenous administration of two volumes of calcium solution on plasma ionized calcium concentration and recovery from naturally occurring hypocalcemia in lactating dairy cows. Am J Vet Res 2008;69:1346–50.
15. DeGaris PJ, Lean IJ. Milk fever in dairy cows: a review of pathophysiology and control principles. Vet J 2008;176:58–69.
16. Huber TL, Wilson RC, Stattleman AJ, et al. Effect of hypocalcemia on motility of the ruminant stomach. Am J Vet Res 1981;42:1488–90.
17. Oetzel GR, Miller BE. Effect of oral calcium bolus supplementation on early lactation health and milk yield in commercial dairy herds. J Dairy Sci 2012;95:7051–65.
18. Oetzel GR. Effect of calcium chloride gel treatment in dairy cows on incidence of periparturient diseases. J Am Vet Med Assoc 1996;209:958–61.

Index

Note: Page numbers of article titles are in **boldface** type.

Vet Clin Food Anim 29 (2013) 457–467
http://dx.doi.org/10.1016/S0749-0720(13)00046-7
0749-0720/13/$ – see front matter

N

O

P

V

Z

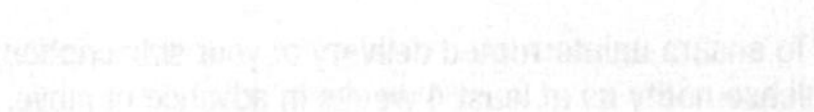